Practical Soft Tissue Management

for Dental Implants
and Natural Teeth

Arun K. Garg, D.M.D.

Lilibeth Ayangco, D.M.D., M.S.

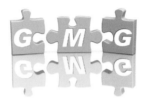

GARG MULTIMEDIA GROUP

MIAMI

Garg Multimedia Group, inc.

1840 NE 153rd Street

North Miami Beach, FL 33162

ISBN: 978-0-9820953-5-5

Cover and interior design by

Robert Mott for Robert Mott & Associates

www.RobertMottDesigns.com

Printed in the United States of America.

13 14 15 16 17 10 9 8 7 6 5 4 3 2 1

First Edition

Contents

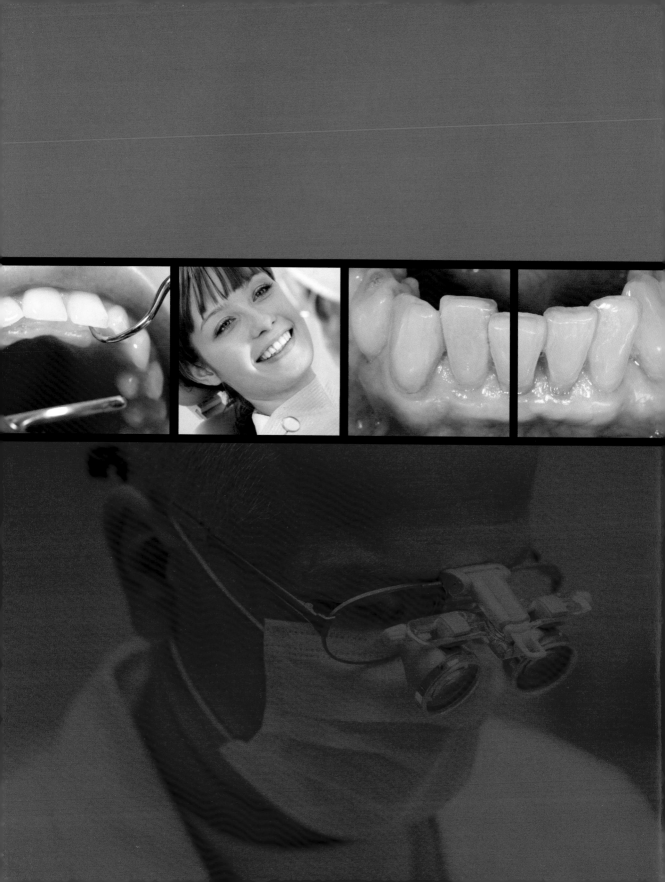

Biology and Rationale for Soft Tissue Management for Esthetics and Function

Gingival tissues, the soft tissue frame of dentition, play a major role in dental esthetics. Variations in the form and regularity of gingival tissue can significantly alter the appearance of the natural dentition or prosthetic tooth replacement. Soft tissue appearance can be affected by developmental, pathologic, or iatrogenic factors.[1-4] The clinician who ignores any of these causative factors does so at his or her peril, and that of the patient. Esthetics, in particular, is increasingly becoming a primary goal of dental treatment. Current treatment philosophy holds that the healthy appearance of soft tissues is indispensable for achieving an optimal esthetic outcome for many kinds of dental surgery. Therefore, a successful soft tissue management program should aim for a complete and predictable recession-free healing of gingival tissue, with equal considerations for both esthetics and function.

Both the appearance of the smile and tooth function are critical elements of soft tissue management. While, appearance is an essential element of nearly all social interaction, dental function can never be a second-tier concern for the clinician. In implant-supported restorations in particular, the long-term clinical and esthetic success of procedures are measured by the extent of osseointegration and optimum level of remodeling of peri-implant soft tissues. Knowledge of the proliferative processes in wound healing is necessary to attain superior soft tissue conditions.[5-8] Lack of knowledge of these processes can result in patient dissatisfaction with the esthetic as well as with the functional outcome of the procedures. The clinician, therefore, must aim for a complete and comprehensive outcome of both form and function.

Non-invasive Approach to Soft Tissue Management

Soft tissue management (STM) involves: (a) identification of host risk factors, such as systemic diseases, smoking habits, medications, and genetic predisposition; (b) detailed patient education about disease and treatment; (c) active therapy, including (but not 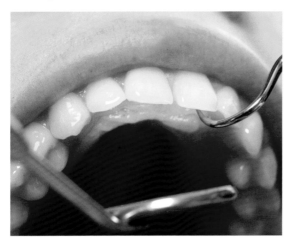 limited to) nonsurgical therapy and surgical therapy with or without antibiotic therapy; (d) oral home care instruction to promote daily periodontal health; (e) and regular dental and periodontal maintenance visits and checkups.[9-13] Prevention often plays a significant role in soft tissue management as well as in a host of other dental and medical conditions. Obviously, single modalities must be avoided when not indicated, and an assortment of therapies and procedures, both surgical and non-surgical, must be considered, working in harmony to satisfy both patient and professional concerns.

In addition to the non-surgical methods of soft tissue management, surgical techniques have been employed to achieve periodontal health. These procedures, referred to as mucogingival surgery, include surgeries performed to enhance function and provide esthetic integrity of the soft tissue. This balance of function and esthetics must never be forgotten. The new term "periodontal plastic surgery" was suggested by the American Academy of Periodontology in 1989 to replace "mucogingival surgery."[14-17] Pasquinelli rightly notes that "periodontal plastic surgery has been part of the effort" to meet the increased demand by the public for esthetic dentistry techniques.[14] In addition, the new term obviously captures the complexity of balancing both the functional and esthetic concerns of patients. The "plastic surgery" element of the definition reminds the clinician of the social and esthetic elements of the equation while "periodontal" clearly refers to satisfying the demanding functional aspects of each case.

Mucogingival Surgery (Periodontal Plastic Surgery)

The aim of mucogingival surgery is to maintain adequate mucogingival complex with a primary focus on the importance of a healthy and adequate gingiva. It is no coincidence that a healthy and adequate gingiva is an essential element of an esthetically pleasing outcome. The concept was based on long-term observations that periodontal health is directly associated with the amount of gingival tissue present. The term "mucogingival surgery" was coined by Freidman to refer to any surgery "designed to preserve attached gingiva, to remove aberrant frenum or muscle attachment, and to increase the depth of the vestibule." [18,19] The focus of surgery thus defined is on the functional aspects of cases almost exclusively, and herein lies a possible shortcoming in the definition. If the patient is satisfied with functional outcomes but not esthetic results, then the surgery, no matter how technically successful, cannot be considered a complete success. These considerations are especially relevant in the esthetic, or smile zone of the patient. This

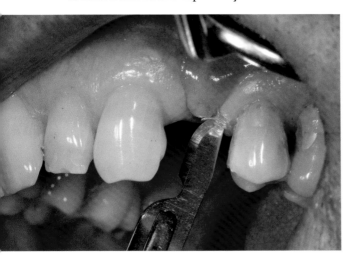

zone is concerned not exclusively with what the patient sees, but how the patient perceives himself or herself to be seen by others.

The term "periodontal plastic surgery" has a much broader application, including recent developments in surgical techniques that help improve the function and esthetics of the periodontal tissues. Inherent in the definition is the double concern of both function and esthetics, the "what" as well as the "how" of surgery. These procedures aim to prevent or treat defects of the gingiva, alveolar bone, and mucosa usually caused by anatomical, developmental, traumatic, or plaque-induced factors.[20-23] However, of equal importance is that these procedures should also address the esthetic concerns of the patients. Periodontal plastic surgeries are usually performed in conjunction with restorative and/or orthodontic therapy to achieve and enhance soft tissue functions and esthetics.

The following procedures[24,25] fall under the category of periodontal plastic surgery:

- **VESTIBULAR DEEPENING** for the treatment of shallow vestibule, to increase optimal levels of oral hygiene

- **FRENECTOMY** for the treatment of aberrant frenum, both lingually and labially

- **SOFT TISSUE GRAFTING** for the treatment of marginal tissue recession resulting from any number of etiologies

- **CROWN LENGTHENING** for the reduction of excessive gingival display

- **RIDGE AUGMENTATION** for the treatment of deficient ridges, including a number of different surgical techniques and procedures

- **GRAFTING EXTRACTION SITES** to prevent ridge collapse following extraction of periodontally involved teeth

- **PAPILLA RECONSTRUCTION** for the treatment of loss interdental papillae "Black Triangle," one of the most challenging of periodontal procedures

- **SURGICAL EXPOSURE OF UNERUPTED TEETH** prior to orthodontic treatment, to optimize orthodontic correction

- **BONE AND/OR SOFT TISSUE AUGMENTATION** for the treatment of esthetic defects around dental implants, including both one-stage and two-stage procedures

Noteworthy in this list of procedures is the fact that both function and esthetics play integral and complementary roles in producing both patient and clinical satisfaction.

A Brief History of Periodontal Plastic Surgery

The history of periodontal plastic surgery begins in the early 1930s, when frenectomies, as well as procedures to deepen the mucobuccal fold, were performed. The first gingivoplasty was performed by Dr. Henry M. Goldman in 1948.[26] Dr. Goldman

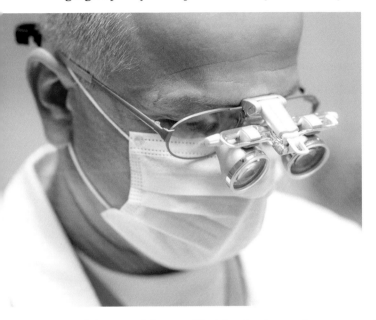

emphasized the importance of soft tissue development and its physiologic contours for the success of any periodontal treatment, noting that "while the elimination of periodontal pockets with resolution of gingival inflammation and the establishment of physiologic function to the tooth are essential requisites for successful periodontal therapy, the achievement of a self-cleansing ability by a physiologic gingival architectural form will aid ... in the maintenance of health." He further notes that this cleansing ability "must...in no way discourage the patient's participation in a home care routine to aid in the cleansing."[26]

Periodontal plastic surgery underwent a major reform when HE Warren and RF Grupe showcased the Laterally Positioned Flap in 1956.[27] This technique is indicated when keratinized tissue lying next to the gingival recession is wide enough, and sufficiently long and thick enough, to cover a relatively narrow exposure of tooth root. Warren and Grupe's technique was followed by the introduction of Apically Positioned Flap and the internal beveled incision by Dr. Nathan Friedman in 1962. Friedman's other notable work in dentistry was the development of precise terms for his innovations in periodontics, along with his pioneering efforts in addressing dental patient fears. In 1963, Dr. Hilding Bjorn was the first to perform the Free Gingival Graft (FGG) for soft tissue management,[28] using tissue directly from the roof of the mouth and attaching the tissue to the recession. This technique was then built upon by Dr. P. D. Miller (1982), who used it for root coverage.[29] Dr. Pini Prato (1992) performed the first Guided Tissue Regeneration (GTR) procedure to enrich the field of periodontal plastic surgery.[30] This description was the first such description in the literature indicating that "a guided tissue regeneration procedure can be used to successfully treat recession....compar[ing] favorably with the mucogingival surgery in the treatment of deep recession."[30]

Though brief, this history shows the important synergistic developments of periodontal plastic surgery, with a clear emphasis on satisfying both form and function in patient outcomes.

Factors Affecting Periodontal Plastic Surgery Outcomes

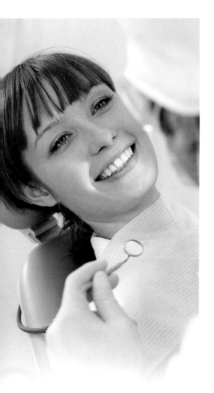

The proposed surgical site must be free of plaque, calculus, and inflammation prior to surgery to decrease the risk of post-operative complications and to ensure good healing. Knowledge of anatomy is important, including the location of the mental foramen to prevent unnecessary nerve damage resulting in paresthesia. Adherence to good surgical techniques includes:

- Good incision design to ensure adequate blood supply,
- Tension free flap reflection and closure, and
- Primary stability of the grafted site.

All of these factors determine the successful outcome of any periodontal plastic surgery. The factors complement each other and deficiencies or weaknesses in any could easily compromise the effectiveness of the others.

Indications for Periodontal Plastic Surgery

The following procedures have become routinely associated with periodontal plastic surgery.

Gingival Augmentation

Gingival augmentation and regeneration are performed to increase the thickness of the gingiva, to increase the width of the keratinized tissue, to establish a proper vestibular depth, and to prevent and/or correct soft tissue recession to facilitate plaque control and for root coverage.[31,32] Improving the appearance of the esthetic, or smile zone is often the genesis for gingival augmentation, even when functional considerations, such as supporting bone damage due to recession, are not otherwise a medical concern. Tissue grafts are often the treatment of choice for gingival augmentation, including subepithelial connective tissue and free gingival grafts — both of which are harvested from the patient's palate — and pedicle grafts, which use tissue near the targeted area needing coverage when the patient's natural tissue amount is sufficient to cover the recessed gingiva. These autologous grafts are often preferred to tissue regeneration or the use of grafts from a tissue bank.

Elimination of the Aberrant Frenum Pull

The condition of an aberrant frenum pull is determined by the presence of marginal gingival tissue mobility when the frenum is depressed. Tension, poor location, or other impairments of the frenum necessitate its removal or modification, as in the case of short frenum beneath the tongue (ankyloglossia). Anterior lower labial frenum tension could cause gingival recession near the incisors. A frenectomy is most often performed in conjunction with a soft tissue graft to increase keratinized gingiva and to eliminate the aberrant frenum pull at the same time.[33-35]

Coverage of Exposed Roots

Lack of attached gingiva, trauma, inflammatory periodontal disease, and tooth location outside the alveolar housing often result in recession of gingival tissue, accompanied by root exposure. Periodontal soft tissue procedures are employed to achieve root coverage, to increase keratinized gingiva, and to decrease root sensitivity. The height of the adjacent interdental gingiva determines the amount of root coverage that can be achieved.[36,37] Ideally, both root coverage and restorative techniques are needed to

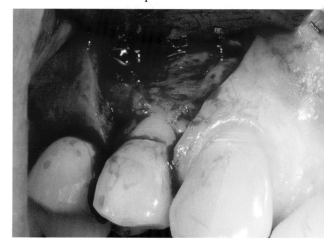

reestablish a proper tooth length and to repair the cervical defect. The clinician should note that periodontal procedures to achieve root coverage should be performed prior to restorative procedures. The following are periodontal soft tissue procedures employed for root coverage: Coronally Positioned Flap, Semilunar Flap, Laterally Positioned Flap, Double Papilla Flap, Free Gingival Graft, Connective Tissue Graft, and Guided Tissue Regeneration.

Alveolar Socket/Ridge Preservation and Augmentation

Alveolar ridge defects occur most commonly when the loss of teeth results in a dimensional loss of bone and soft tissue surrounding the alveolus. Ridge defects can lead to esthetic compromise and may create functional problems as well. Evidence suggests that rapid and severe resorption of the ridge will occur immediately following tooth extraction unless therapeutic measures are taken by the clinician to preserve the ridge and thus to minimize or avoid resorption.[38-40]

If a tooth is treatment-planned for extraction in addition to dental implant restoration, the clinician must plan to provide hard tissue as well as soft tissue preservation and regeneration at the time of tooth removal to prevent an esthetic or functional defect. It is much easier to preserve the ridge and prevent a cosmetic or functional defect than to try to regenerate a deficient ridge. Historically, tooth

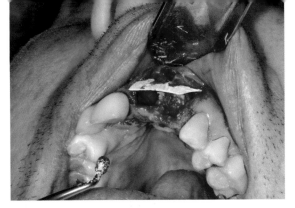

Socket preservation/ridge augmentation of Maxillary central incisors.

extractions rank as perhaps the most often performed dental procedures, so alveolar ridge preservation around the extraction site has long been a concern of general dentists, periodontists, and implantologists. Implantologists in particular wish to preserve as much dimensional bone structure as possible to optimize implant stability and osseointegration over time. Ridge preservation and augmentation, along with preservation of the keratinized tissue, can have significant effects on not only function and phonetics but the esthetics of the site, especially in the smile zone.

Esthetic Crown Lengthening

When anterior teeth are shorter than normal or when excessive gingival tissue is displayed, esthetic crown lengthening may help the patient to regain a more perfect set of dentition.[41-45] A gummy smile can result from gingival enlargement, altered or delayed passive eruption, short clinical crowns, vertical maxillary excess, a short upper lip, or orthodontic deformities. This panoply of anti-esthetic conditions can be a nightmare for patients desiring to have optimal appearance. The clinician, then, is faced with the esthetic and moral challenges of satisfying the patient's needs.

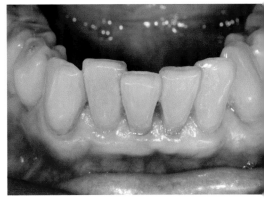

Esthetic crown lengthening involves the shaping of the gingival and alveolar bone to achieve improved esthetics. When restorations are anticipated, crown lengthening will allow the clinician to fabricate restorations of proper length and shape, producing an esthetically pleasing smile. The product of such a smile cannot be underestimated by the clinician, as the literature and practical clinical experience have shown. A recent study concludes, in fact, that "excessive gingival display did positively affect how attractive a person's smile is judged to be."[46] Furthermore, the report notes that "how friendly, trustworthy, intelligent, and self-confident a person was perceived to be was inversely related to the amount of gingival display." Remarkably, according to the study, "Untrained laypeople were just as sensitive to these differences as senior dental students."

Summary

An optimally-functioning and esthetically-appealing dentition requires the gingival contours to be regular and in harmony with the upper lip. In addition, the anterior and posterior segments should be in proportion to each other, and the length and width of the teeth should be normal. The long-term success of any prosthetic treatment is assessed by the strategies adopted to identify and eliminate etiologic factors. Fundamental prosthetic and surgical principles, the clinician's experience, and current scientific literature should be the basis for planning treatment to ensure a predictable and successful long-term outcome.

References

1. Chen ST. Periodontics and its influence on aesthetics. Ann R Australas Coll Dent Surg. 1998 Oct; 14:81-5.

2. Reddy MS. Achieving gingival esthetics. J Am Dent Assoc. 2003 Mar;134(3):295-304; quiz 337-8.

3. McNeely TE. Coronally repositioning the cemento-enamel junction to address gingival margin discrepancies. J Periodontol. 2005 Jan;76(1):138-42.

4. Oh SL. Biologic width and crown lengthening: case reports and review. Gen Dent. 2010 Sep-Oct;58(5):e200-5. Review.

5. Schultze-Mosgau S, Blatz MB, Wehrhan F, Schlegel KA, Thorwart M, Holst S. Principles and mechanisms of peri-implant soft tissue healing. Quintessence Int. 2005 Nov-Dec; 36(10):759-69.

6. Schultze-Mosgau S, Wehrhan F, Wichmann M, Schlegel KA, Holst S, Thorwarth M. Expression of interleukin 1-beta, transforming growth factor beta-1, and vascular endothelial growth factor in soft tissue over the implant before uncovering. Oral Surg Oral Med Oral Pathol Oral Radiol Endod. 2006 May;101(5):565-71. Epub 2006 Feb 21.

7. Galli F, Capelli M, Zuffetti F, Testori T, Esposito M. Immediate non-occlusal vs. early loading of dental implants in partially edentulous patients: a multicentre randomized clinical trial. Peri-implant bone and soft-tissue levels. Clin Oral Implants Res. 2008 Jun;19(6):546-52.

8. Geurs NC, Vassilopoulos PJ, Reddy MS. Soft tissue considerations in implant site development. Oral Maxillofac Surg Clin North Am. 2010 Aug;22(3):387-405, vi-vii.

9. Bhaskar SN. Four steps to soft tissue management: non-surgical periodontal therapy. Dent Today. 1995 Oct; 14(10):30, 32, 34-9.

10. Drisko CH. Nonsurgical periodontal therapy. Periodontol 2000. 2001;25:77-88. Review.

11. Bonito AJ, Lohr KN, Lux L, Sutton S, Jackman A, Whitener L, Evensen C. Effectiveness of antimicrobial adjuncts to scaling and root-planing therapy for periodontitis. Evid Rep Technol Assess (Summ). 2004 Jan;(88):1-4.

12. American Academy of Periodontology— Research, Science, and Therapy Committee; American Academy of Pediatric Dentistry. Treatment of plaque-induced gingivitis, chronic periodontitis, and other clinical conditions. Pediatr Dent. 2005-2006; 27(7 Suppl):202-11. Review.

13. Madden TE, Herriges B, Boyd LD, Laughlin G, Chiodo G, Rosenstein D. Alterations in HbA1c following minimal or enhanced non-surgical, non-antibiotic treatment of gingivitis or mild periodontitis in type 2 diabetic patients: a pilot trial. J Contemp Dent Pract. 2008 Jul 1 ;9(5):9-16.

14. Pasquinelli KL. Periodontal plastic surgery. J Calif Dent Assoc. 1999 Aug;27(8):597-610. Review.

15. Blue AH. Periodontal plastic procedures in esthetic dentistry. Tex Dent J. 2001 Oct; 118(10):972-6. Review.

16. Townsend C. Prerestorative periodontal plastic surgery. Creating the gingival framework for the ideal smile. Dent Today. 2004 Feb;23(2):130-3.

17. Pasquinelli LK. Periodontal plastic surgery as an adjunctive therapeutic modality for esthetic restorative dentistry. J Calif Dent Assoc. 2005 Mar;33(3):217-21. Review.

18. Friedman, N. Mucogingival surgery. Texas Dental Journal. 1957, 75, 358-362.

19. Bains VK, Gupta V, Singh GP, Bains R. Mucogingival surgery: where we stand today. J Calif Dent Assoc. 2011 Aug;39(8):573-83. Review.

20. Oringer RJ, Iacono VJ. Current periodontal plastic procedures around teeth and dental implants. N Y State Dent J. 1999 Jun-Jul; 65(6):26-31.

21. Prato GP. Advances in mucogingival surgery. J Int Acad Periodontol. 2000 Jan; 2(1):24-7.

22. Pini Prato GP, De Sanctis M. Soft-tissue plastic surgery. Curr Opin Dent. 1991 Feb; 1(1): 98-103.

23. Allen AL. Use of the gingival unit transfer in soft tissue grafting: report of three cases. Int J Periodontics Restorative Dent. 2004 Apr;24(2):165-75.

24. Miller PD Jr. A classification of marginal tissue recession. Int J Periodontics Restorative Dent. 1985; 5(2):8-13.

25. Miller PD Jr, Allen EP. The development of periodontal plastic surgery. Periodontol 2000. 1996 Jun;11:7-17. Review.

26. Goldman HM. The development of physiologic gingival contours by gingivoplasty. Oral Surg Oral Med Oral Pathol. 1950 Jul; 3(7):879-88.

27. Grupe HE, Warren RF Jr. Repair of gingival defects by a sliding flap operation. Journal of Periodontology 1956; 27:92-5.

28. Bjorn H. Free transplantation of gingiva propria. Sverges tandlaek tidn. 1963; 22: 648-63.

29. Miller PD Jr. Root coverage using the free soft tissue autograft following citric acid application. III. A successful and predictable procedure in areas of deep-wide recession. Int J Periodontics Restorative Dent. 1985; 5(2):14-37.

30. Pini Prato G, Tinti C, Vincenzi G, Magnani C, Cortellini P, Clauser C. Guided tissue regeneration versus mucogingival surgery in the treatment of human buccal recession. J Periodontol 1992; 63:919–28.

31. Hirsch A. Root coverage techniques—a literature review and a case report. Refuat Hapeh Vehashinayim. 2006 Jul;24(3):59-69, 95. Review. Hebrew.

32. Greenwell H, Fiorellini J, Giannobile W, Offenbacher S, Salkin L, Townsend C, Sheridan P, Genco R; Research, Science and Therapy Committee. Oral reconstructive and corrective considerations in periodontal therapy. J Periodontol. 2005 Sep;76(9):1588-600. Review.

33. Devishree, Gujjari SK, Shubhashini PV. Frenectomy: a review with the reports of surgical techniques. J Clin Diagn Res. 2012 Nov;6(9):1587-92.

34. Zadeh HH. Minimally invasive treatment of maxillary anterior gingival recession defects by vestibular incision subperiosteal tunnel access and platelet-derived growth factor BB. Int J Periodontics Restorative Dent. 2011 Nov-Dec;31(6):653-60.

35. Park JB. Correcting the frenal pull and increasing the width of keratinized mucosa around endosseous implants using denudation procedure. Indian J Dent Res. 2008 Oct-Dec;19(4):362-5.

36. Hofmänner P, Alessandri R, Laugisch O, Aroca S, Salvi GE, Stavropoulos A, Sculean A. Predictability of surgical techniques used for coverage of multiple adjacent gingival recessions--A systematic review. Quintessence Int. 2012 Jul-Aug;43(7):545-54. Review.

37. Cortellini P, Pini Prato G. Coronally advanced flap and combination therapy for root coverage. Clinical strategies based on scientific evidence and clinical experience. Periodontol 2000. 2012 Jun;59(1):158-84. Review.

38. Horváth A, Mardas N, Mezzomo LA, Needleman IG, Donos N. Alveolar ridge preservation. A systematic review. Clin Oral Investig. 2012 Jul 20.

39. Sanz I, Garcia-Gargallo M, Herrera D, Martin C, Figuero E, Sanz M. Surgical protocols for early implant placement in post-extraction sockets: a systematic review. Clin Oral Implants Res. 2012 Feb;23 Suppl 5:67-79.

40. Vignoletti F, Matesanz P, Rodrigo D, Figuero E, Martin C, Sanz M. Surgical protocols for ridge preservation after tooth extraction. A systematic review. Clin Oral Implants Res. 2012 Feb;23 Suppl 5:22-38.

41. Ittipuriphat I, Leevailoj C. Anterior space management: interdisciplinary concepts. J Esthet Restor Dent. 2013 Feb;25(1):16-30.

42. Malkinson S, Waldrop TC, Gunsolley JC, Lanning SK, Sabatini R. The Effect of Esthetic Crown Lengthening on Perceptions of a Patient's Attractiveness, Friendliness, Trustworthiness, Intelligence, and Self-Confidence. J Periodontol. 2012 Nov 9.

43. Afshar A. A systematic approach to recreate a patient's former smile. Compend Contin Educ Dent. 2012 Sep;33(8):606, 608, 610 passim.

44. Fletcher P. Biologic rationale of esthetic crown lengthening using innovative proportion gauges. Int J Periodontics Restorative Dent. 2011 Sep-Oct;31(5):523-32.

45. Borges I Jr, Ribas TR, Duarte PM. Guided esthetic crown lengthening: case reports. Gen Dent. 2009 Nov-Dec;57(6):666-71.

46. Malkinson S, Waldrop TC, Gunsolley JC, Lanning SK, Sabatini R. The Effect of Esthetic Crown Lengthening on Perceptions of a Patient's Attractiveness, Friendliness, Trustworthiness, Intelligence, and Self-Confidence. J Periodontol. 2012 Nov 9. [Epub ahead of print].

Notes

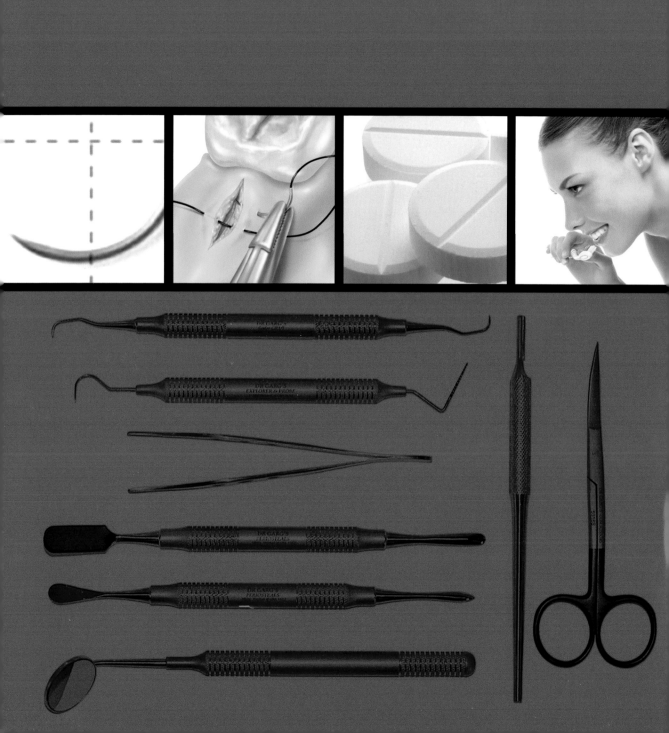

Surgical Armamentarium, Sutures and Suturing Techniques, Anesthesia, and Post-Operative Care

Tension-free primary wound closure of various soft tissue flaps is essential to uneventful and predictable wound healing after periodontal plastic surgery. Procedures that necessitate clinical flap manipulation require professional execution and a detailed knowledge of the various perioperative techniques of surgery, suturing, anesthesia, and the materials currently available for the desired clinical results.

The first half of this chapter describes the various instruments used in periodontal procedures in general, types of suture material used, and the various suturing techniques being practiced. The second half deals with the anesthetic considerations and the post-operative management of the patient after periodontal procedures.

This chapter excludes details about microsurgery, which are covered in Chapter 3.

Surgical Armamentarium for Periodontal Plastic Surgery

Since periodontal surgery can range from the simplest of procedures for preserving healthy gingiva to extensive periodontal plastic surgery, the clinician's reliance on surgical experience must be complemented by advancements in both surgical techniques and armamentarium, including, for example, the latest advances in periodontal tissue engineering and regeneration, whose three most promising areas include "a range of regenerative surgical procedures, the development of a variety of grafting materials, and the use of recombinant growth factors."[1] Generally, studies have found that "sound understanding of first [surgical] principles will simplify periodontal surgical management," and "careful surgical preparation will render surgical procedures more predictable and reduce post-operative discomfort."[2] Surgical armamentarium in many ways is significantly different and more available than its predecessors of only a decade ago. Minimizing trauma in periodontal surgery requires the handling of soft tissues in a way that reflects predictable, standard surgical management, which in turn leads to the improved quality of surgical outcomes.[3]

General surgical armamentarium for periodontal plastic surgery (Fig. 2-1) includes the mouth mirror, periodontal probe, tissue forceps, round scalpel handle, Allen periosteal elevator, Orban periodontal knife, bone condenser, small defect bone condenser, 15 and 15C scalpel blades, ZAP Laser Pro, and Styla Laser. Several of these items and other armamentariums are discussed below.

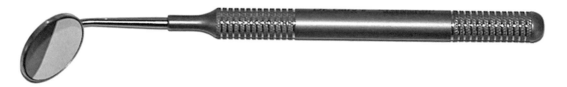

MOUTH MIRROR

A mouth mirror is the most widely used instrument in dental practice. By using a mouth mirror, a dentist can view all sides of the teeth and all areas of the mouth, including areas that may not be seen on direct manual inspection. While the mouth mirror can also be used to retract tissue such as the cheek or tongue, its primary use is to reflect light onto dental surfaces for better viewing, or to view dental surfaces otherwise out of the clinician's field of vision. The most popular mouth mirror in dentistry is the front-surface reflecting mirror, whose glass surface of reflection is relatively undistorted, as opposed to the concave (magnified) model and flat surface model (where the reflective surface is on the back of the mirror), whose surfaces distort the image.

COTTON PLIERS

A cotton plier is an important instrument in any dental procedure because it helps to pick up and remove small items from the mouth, including cotton items used for absorption as well as larger pieces of debris in the oral cavity. The structure of cotton pliers resembles tweezers, having two long arms, with tapering and sometimes bent edges, to enhance grip over the items to be removed. The edges of the gripping surfaces can be smooth or serrated for gripping. Sometimes the handles of the pliers can be self-locking. Made of stainless steel, the pliers can be sterilized. Use of cotton pliers also helps avoid contamination of the surgical wound when the clinician or assistant is transporting items to and from the oral cavity during surgery.

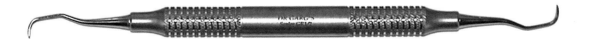

PERIODONTAL CURETTE

A periodontal curette should be sharp and spoon-shaped for removing calculus, cleaning infected cavities in bone, and removing debris from the tooth sockets. Curettes are used in both surgical and non-surgical procedures. The curette cutting surfaces must be sharpened regularly to maintain their efficiency. Periodontal curettes are available in various sizes and are straight or angled. The choice of curette depends on its intended use and the anatomy of the tissue on which it will be used. Curettes are usually round-tipped to minimize the trauma to gingival tissue during any procedure. Classically, there are two recognized groups of curettes, Universal and Gracey.

Universal curettes get their name from the varied purposes they serve. The blade of the curette is perpendicular to the terminal shanks, enabling both sides of the blade to be used. This kind of curette can reach all areas of dentition in the oral cavity. The cutting action of this kind of curette occurs either on the outer or inner edges. Types of universal curettes are the Barhart curette and the Columbia curette.

Gracey curettes, by contrast, are types of periodontal curettes with flexible shanks. Unlike universal curettes, the blade of the Gracey curette is offset by 70 degrees; therefore, it has two edges: a lower, cutting edge and an upper, non-cutting edge. This dual property makes it a site-specific instrument. Some curettes, such as Molt curettes, are single-ended and have large handles. Other curettes may be double-ended and have slender handles.

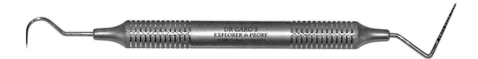

PERIODONTAL PROBE

Also known as a dental probe, this instrument is long and thin, with a blunt end. The probe has three parts: a handle, a distal portion, and a measuring needle. Usually, a periodontal probe is used to determine pocket depths around a tooth; the markings on the instrument make the measurement more accurate and reliable. The flexible end of the instrument enables it to move around corners in tortuous blind pockets. The instrument gives a high reading in patients with gingivitis because the gingival tissue is swollen from inflammation. There might be some gingival bleeding upon probing the inflamed tissues. The readings are even higher in patients with periodontal disease due to the surrounding bone loss in addition to the inflammation of the gingival tissue.

A periodontal probe may give inaccurate readings if not used properly. The clinician should apply light pressure when keeping the tip of the instrument on the gingival sulcus, keeping the periodontal probe parallel to the form of the root of the tooth, and then introduce the probe down to the base of the pocket. As a result, a part of the tip of the instrument gets covered by the tissue, and the first visible reading above it is the measurement of the pocket depth. Normal, healthy probing measures 0 mm to 3 mm. A probing depth measurement higher than 3 mm may indicate periodontal disease.

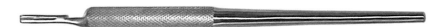

SCALPEL

Scalpel blades are sharp knives made of hardened and tempered steel and come in various sizes. They find their uses in every periodontal procedure ranging from free gingival grafts to soft tissue and hard tissue regeneration. The blade sizes used in periodontal procedures are 12, 12B, 15, and 15C. Blades 12 and 15 are single-edged whereas blade 12B is double-edged. The tip of the scalpel handle is designed to have a number of different blades inserted for various types of incisions. A holder must be used to place the blade on the handle to avoid injury. After surgery, the cutting blade is discarded. No sterilization and re-use is permitted. Because the blade could become dulled after contact with the dentition or bone, several blades may be used during a single surgery.

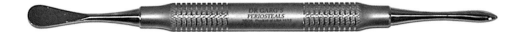

PERIOSTEAL ELEVATOR

A periosteal elevator has a sharp, pointed end and a broader, flat end. It is used to elevate gingival tissue to expose the surgical site without causing trauma. Usually the pointed end is used to start lifting the soft tissue flap, directing it towards the bone; the broader end is then used to continue elevating the soft tissue from the underlying bone. The standard instrument for flap reflection after an incision is the Molt #9 periosteal elevator. Its most common use is to reflect mucosa and periosteum away from the underlying bone. This kind of elevator has a broad, flat end and also a pointed end, which is very sharp. The two ends work in concert to lift the soft tissue flap (the pointed end) and then to continue to dissect the tissue from the bone (the broad end). Periosteal elevators can also be used for retraction.

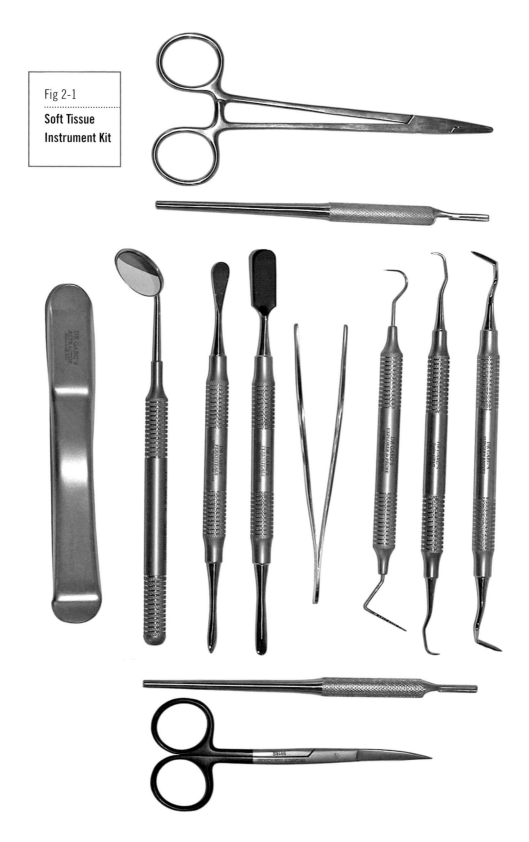

The suturing needle has three parts: the point, the body, and the swaged end. Needles are classified based on their curvature, radius, and shape. Usually, three-eighths (3/8) and one-half (1/2) circle needles are most commonly used for intraoral procedures. The three-eighths (3/8) needle is used to close tissue in the oral cavity whereas a one-half (1/2) circle needle is traditionally used in more restricted areas. The one-half (1/2) circle needle is most commonly used in periodontal and mucogingival surgery. Suturing needles are also classified based on the cutting edges they have. In a conventional suturing needle, the inner concave curvature is sharp, which increases the possibility of tearing when the needle is pulled through the tissue.

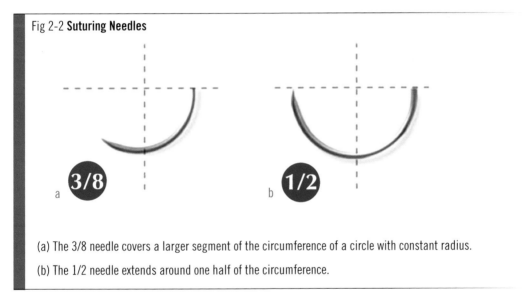

Fig 2-2 **Suturing Needles**

(a) The 3/8 needle covers a larger segment of the circumference of a circle with constant radius.

(b) The 1/2 needle extends around one half of the circumference.

Therefore, a conventional needle may not be appropriate for periodontal plastic surgery. A reverse cutting needle, unlike the conventional needle, has a smooth inner curvature with a third cutting edge located on the outside. This feature prevents tearing of the tissue during suturing.

Types of Sutures and Suturing Techniques

Suture materials and suturing techniques play an important role in the successful outcome of periodontal plastic surgery. The clinician should be well-informed about the nature of the suture material, the physiology of wound healing, the biologic and mechanical forces exerted on the healing wound, and the chemical and physiologic interaction between the suture and the soft tissue.[4-6] If the suture material and the suturing techniques are not appropriate to the procedure being performed, the suture material may break or the knots may untie, resulting in dehiscence of the wound.[7-10]

An ideal suture should have adequate strength to prevent breakage during suturing. A proper knot that is compatible with the material being used will prevent untying or knot slippage. In addition, to keep the wound edges together, the clinician must choose a suture that is able to retain its strength until the tissues of the flaps regain sufficient stability: selecting the suture material and diameter based on the thickness of the tissue to be sutured and whether there is a need for flap tension.

TYPES OF SUTURES

Suture material can be resorbable or non-resorbable based on its ability to break down and to be resorbed by the body.

Resorbable Sutures

As the name suggests, resorbable sutures tend to lose tensile strength over a period of time, from several days to several weeks. Therefore, the suture selected should be such that the breakdown of the resorbable material should equal the healing rate of the tissue being held together by the material. A tissue that heals rapidly should be sutured with a material which resorbs at about the same rate as the tissue regains strength. As a result, when the wound heals, there will not be any foreign material left. The surgical gut or the rapidly resorbable polyglycolic acid sutures (PGA) are the most commonly used resorbable sutures.

A 2012 study consisting of 50 random patients requiring minor surgery compared nonabsorbable black silk suture and absorbable polyglycolic acid sutures clinically and histologically on an assortment of criteria.[11] The aim was to determine, among other findings, the inflammatory reaction within tissue based on the kind of suture used in the oral cavity. The results revealed that all the polyglycolic acid sutures were retained, but four patients did not retain the black silk suture. All but seven of the polyglycolic acid sutures had mild to moderate inflammatory reaction, half of them mild. The black silk

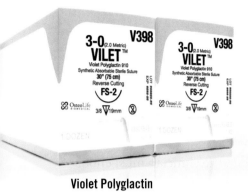

**Violet Polyglactin
Synthetic Absorbale Suture**

revealed forty-one mild to moderate cases, split nearly evenly with only six severe cases. Histologically, the results for both types of sutures were predominantly mild, including forty-one for the black silk. The study concluded that the polyglycolic acid suture was superior to the black silk since all 50 patients given the former retained them. The polyglycolic acid suture also led to less tissue reaction while exhibiting superior handling and knotting characteristics.

There are two mechanisms through which the resorbable sutures resorb. Sutures such as plain and chromic gut are of biological origin and therefore undergo gradual digestion by the enzymes in the patient's blood. On the other hand, sutures that are fabricated from synthetic materials, such as polyglycolic acid, are resorbed through hydrolysis. Gut is an animal protein and has been shown to cause tissue irritation due to its antigenic properties. Plain gut sutures lose tensile strength in 24 to 48 hours, while chromic gut resorbs in five days.

A clinician needs to carefully consider the selection of suture material when used on a patient with low intraoral pH. A low intraoral pH may cause rapid breakage of the material during the resorption process, thus preventing healing and apposition of the wound. Conditions that may lead to low intraoral pH are epigastric reflux, hiatal hernia, bulimia, certain medications, and certain therapeutic modalities such as chemotherapy and radiation therapy. In these patients, a fast-absorbing PGA suture is appropriate since it is not affected by intraoral pH. The suture is hydrolyzed in five days at the same time as the intraoral wound healing process.

Nonresorbable Sutures

Nonresorbable sutures do not lose their tensile strength during the resorption process and must be removed after a period of time. Silk is an example of natural nonresorbable suture. Suture materials like nylon, polyester, polyethylene, polypropylene, or expanded polytetrafluoroethylene (e-PTFE) are synthetic sutures.

Silk is the most widely used suture material. The advantage of this material is that it has high tensile strength, easy handling characteristics, low tendency for knot slippage, and low expense.[12,13] However, because silk is a multifilament thread, it has a tendency to pull microorganisms and fluids into the wound, creating a "wick effect."[14-16] Therefore, silk cannot be used in surgeries that involve placing foreign materials such as dental implants or bone grafts under a mucoperiosteal flap, or when active infection is present at the time of surgery. Silk sutures must be removed within 7 to 10 days after surgery to prevent suture abscess.

Synthetic nonresorbable suture material is used in conditions where silk is contraindicated. A polyester suture is made of multiple filaments braided into a single strand, and, therefore, possesses high tensile strength and does not weaken when

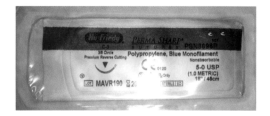

moistened. These materials must be coated with a biologically inert material to be able to pass through the tissues easier. The coating, however, makes the material slippery and the knots to untie easily. These coated suture materials should be secured with a surgeon's knot. Nonresorbable e-PTFE suture material is a monofilament with high tensile strength, good handling properties, and good knot security; however, it is expensive compared to other nonresorbable suture materials.

Suture materials are available in varying thicknesses, identified by the numbers 1 through 10. The higher the number is, the thinner and more delicate the thread. In most of the periodontal plastic surgeries, a 5-0 thread diameter is often used to secure soft tissue grafts and pedicle flaps while a 4-0 thread diameter is most often used in securing mucoperiosteal flaps.

SUTURING TECHNIQUES

Correct suturing techniques help in accurate apposition of surgical flaps, which is essential to patient comfort, hemostasis, reduction of wound size, and prevention of unnecessary bone resorption. Surgical wound edges may not be held in close proximity if inappropriate suturing techniques are used, thereby compromising hemostasis. Accumulation of blood or serum under the flap may result in a space between the underlying soft tissue and bone, thus delaying the healing process. In such cases, because the healing occurs by secondary intention, the soft tissue may be scarred or have irregular contours.

Surgical knots are essential to keep the flaps apposed to each other. The choice of surgical knots depends on the type of suture material used. When an appropriate surgical knot is used based on the type of material used, the knot should ideally be secure and should not untie. A slip surgical knot could be used for e-PTFE, chromic gut, or plain gut suture material whereas a surgeon's knot must be used with synthetic resorbable and nonresorbable suture materials.

The following are types of suturing techniques used in periodontal procedures:

- **INTERRUPTED SUTURES:** used for tension-free mobile flaps[17,18] (Fig. 2-3)

- **SIMPLE LOOP INTERRUPTED SUTURE:** used to coapt tension-free, mobile surgical flaps in surgery of edentulous ridge areas, to coapt vertical releasing incisions, for periosteal suturing, and to coapt flaps as part of certain periodontal surgical procedures

- **FIGURE-8 SUTURE:** used when suturing on the lingual aspect of the mandibular molars, especially in a patient with an active gag reflex or a large tongue and for suturing extraction sockets (Fig. 2-6)

- **INTERRUPTED SUSPENSORY SUTURE OR SLING SUTURE:** used when performing coronally repositioned sliding flaps

- **CONTINUOUS SUTURE:** used to attach two surgical flap edges with more stability[17]

- **MATTRESS SUTURE:** resists pulls caused by muscle attachments. Horizontal mattress (Fig. 2-4) and the apically or coronally repositioned vertical mattress (Fig. 2-5) are variations of the mattress sutures.

Fig 2-3 **Interrupted Suturing Technique**

a

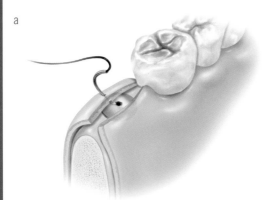

(a) The first step consists of passing the needle through the first flap from the outside inwards. Where there is one movable flap and one immovable flap, the needle should pass through the movable flap first.

a

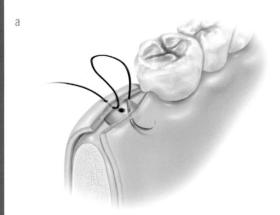

(b) The needle pierces the second flap from the inside out. Approximately the same penetration distance of the flap must be maintained so as to avoid asymmetry between the two flaps, which might compromise the esthetic results.

c

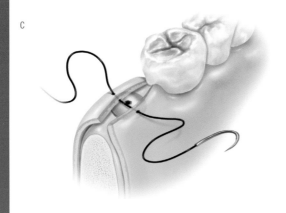

(c) The depth of penetration and the distance from the margin must be evaluated for each case. For healthy tissues, the depth and distance should be between 1.5 mm-2 mm from the free margin. For more fragile tissues, the distance may be increased.

▼

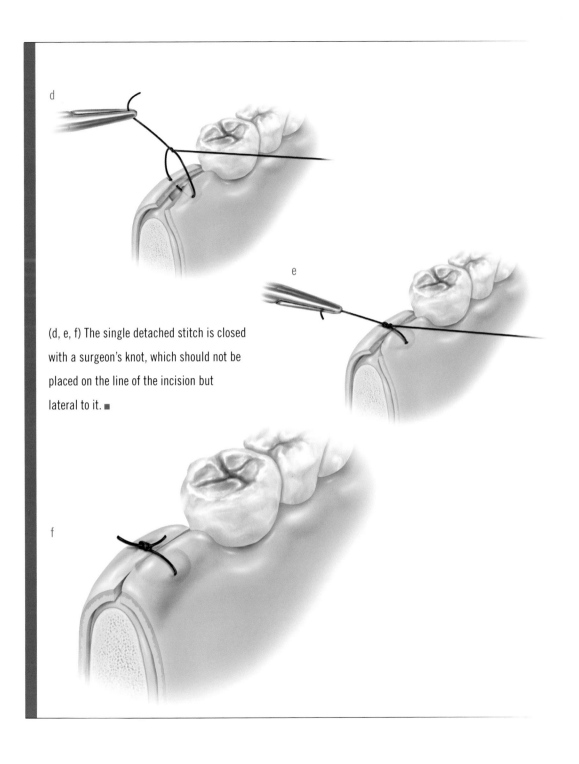

(d, e, f) The single detached stitch is closed with a surgeon's knot, which should not be placed on the line of the incision but lateral to it. ■

Fig 2-4 Horizontal Mattress Suturing Technique

a

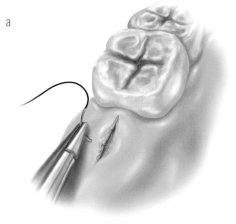

(a) The clinician should pierce the flap on the external mucosal side with the needle approximately 3 mm from the incision line.

b

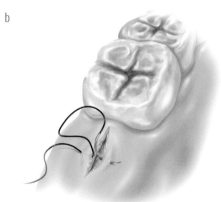

(b) The needle is passed across the free space between the two flaps and pierces the inner mucosal surface of the second flap with the same distance from the incision line (3 mm) to ensure uniform traction.

c

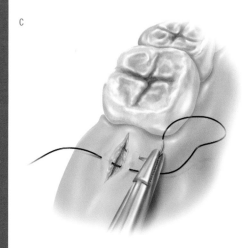

(c) The clinician turns the needle on a plane parallel to the free margin of the flap and pierces the second flap from the external mucosal side inwards, maintaining a distance of 2 mm to 3 mm from the initial exit point.

▼

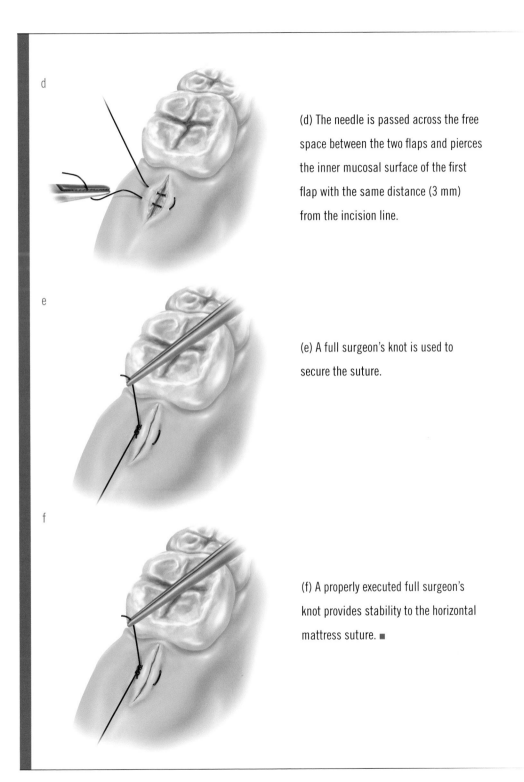

(d) The needle is passed across the free space between the two flaps and pierces the inner mucosal surface of the first flap with the same distance (3 mm) from the incision line.

(e) A full surgeon's knot is used to secure the suture.

(f) A properly executed full surgeon's knot provides stability to the horizontal mattress suture. ■

Vertical Mattress Suturing Technique

This suturing technique applies a method known as "far-far, near-near" suturing.

Fig 2-5 Vertical Mattress Suturing Technique

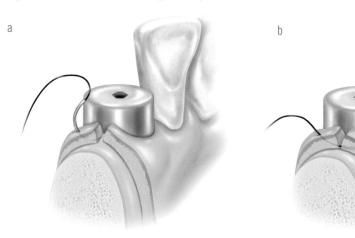

a

b

(a) and (b) The first step in the "far-far, near-near" vertical mattress suture involves the clinician placing the needle in the needle holder in a forward position, then passing the suture ("far-far") through both of the wound edges (at approximately 6 mm from the wound edges).

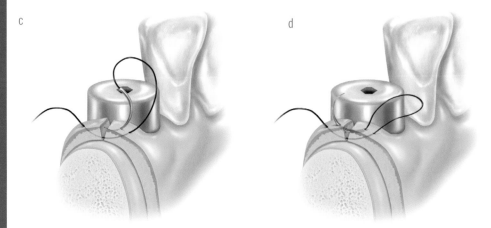

c

d

(c) and (d) Next, the needle is positioned in reverse in the holder so that the "near-near" suture placement can occur, less deeply (1 mm-2 mm), and similarly within 1 mm-2 mm of the edges of the wound. ▼

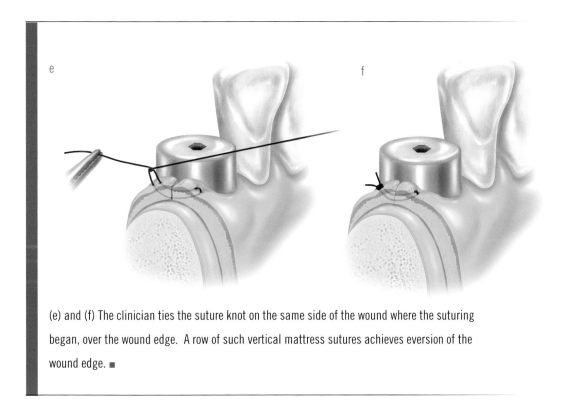

(e) and (f) The clinician ties the suture knot on the same side of the wound where the suturing began, over the wound edge. A row of such vertical mattress sutures achieves eversion of the wound edge. ■

To recap and to clarify, we must note that the clinician places the far-far suture approximately 6 mm (+2 mm or – 2mm) from the edge of the wound. The placement is made relatively deeply below the skin of the wound in order to securely place the sutures. The needle is then placed in the needle holder in the opposite position so that once this far-far placement has occurred on the sides of the wound (and before the suture is tied), the "near-near" suturing can occur at a depth more shallow (approximately 1 mm deep) in the upper skin, and 1 mm to 2 mm from the edge of the wound, followed by tying of the suture on the side of the wound where the suturing began.

Figure-8 Suturing Technique

Fig 2-6 **Figure-8 Suturing Technique**

a

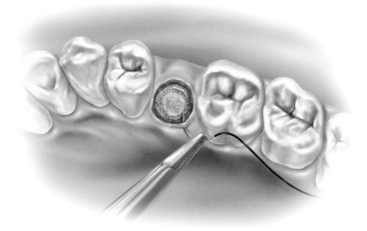

(a) The needle passes through the interdental space without piercing the tissue, mesial to the point where it is intended to place the first stitch.

b

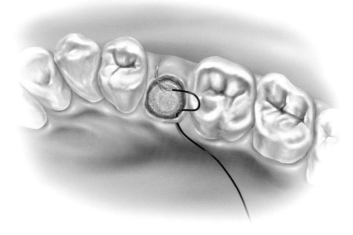

(b) The second step begins exactly as the first, by the clinician's passing the needle and thread through the proximal interdental space of the adjacent tooth mesially without piercing the soft tissues. The direction of the needle is the same as it enters the palatal flap, the clinician taking care to pierce it approximately 2 mm distal to the exit hole of the first thread and emerging some 2 mm mesial of this hole. ▼

c

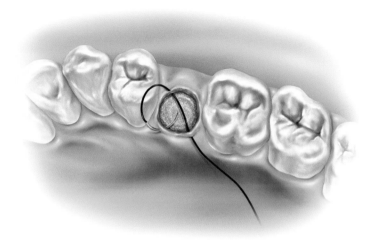

(c) Needle and thread pass external to the palatal flap, and the needle pierces the flap, at least 2 mm to 3 mm apical of the apical edge of the area where the graft was harvested.

d

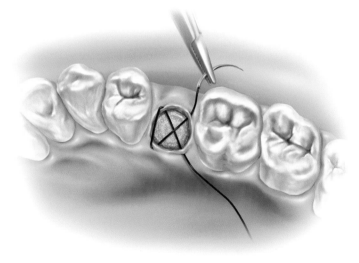

(d) The thread is crossed over and emerges again in the distal interdental space or, in any case, as in this illustration, distal to the tooth to be treated. ▼

Fig 2-6 **Criss-Cross Suturing Technique** (CONT.)

e

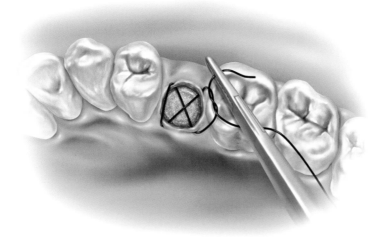

(e) The thread is again crossed over, and the needle passes through the distal interdental space without piercing the soft tissues.

f

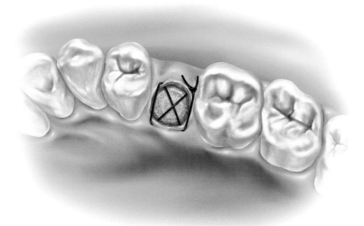

(f) A full surgeon's knot tied on the vestibular face of the tooth provides the second point of anchorage. It is clear that the traction of this suture acting on the two anchorage points, which are almost completely inextensible (periosteum and tooth), enables compression to be exercised on the deeper layers. ■

Sling Suturing has two versions: the single interrupted sling suturing technique, and the continuous, independent sling suturing technique. Both techniques "sling" the suture around one tooth or two or more teeth as part of an attempt to bind gingiva that has been removed from both sides of the tooth/teeth. Sling suturing is used if flap position is not an essential element of surgery due to the location of the sutures. The critical criterion in such cases is often optimal closure. Other critical factors include buccal flap stability and position.

Once the clinician has made the initial lingual and buccal tie, he or she passes the suture around the tooth neck between the adjacent teeth, and then through the lingual flap. The suture is moved between the teeth and through the papilla on the buccal side and then back again between the teeth around the lingual tooth surface to the buccal papilla. The suture is then moved around the lingual papilla and around the buccal tooth surface. This lingual/buccal rotation continues until an end loop at a terminus is secured with a knot.

Anesthesia

Anesthesia is necessary not only to carry out the procedure pain-free but also to achieve tissue rigidity and hemostasis. Both local and block forms of anesthesia are used widely in faciomaxillary and oral surgical procedures. A clinician is professionally obligated to learn which forms and techniques are most suitable to his or her abilities as well as for patient needs. For example, one study notes the "advantages of using the regional blocks over … [local infiltration] anesthesia include reduced dosage and number of needle pricks."[19] Another study points out that while "local anesthesia usually is used in surgical procedures, field or nerve blocks can provide more effective anesthesia in some situations," necessitating the clinician's professional "review of regional anatomy and the location of nerves and other important structures…before administering the injection."[20] Applications of infiltration anesthetic techniques can differ between the mandible and maxilla,[21] and the search for superior anesthetic agents is ongoing.[22]

INSTRUMENTS FOR LOCAL ANESTHESIA

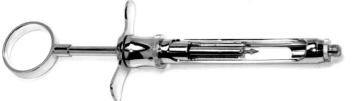

Anesthetic syringes are designed to support and expel anesthetic solution from carpules.

Topical anesthetic in a gel or ointment form is used to numb the area where the actual local anesthetic injection is to be made. A cotton-tip applicator is used to apply the topical anesthetic over the area to be anesthetized. Topical anesthetics are used to reduce the pain and discomfort caused by the local anesthetic injection.

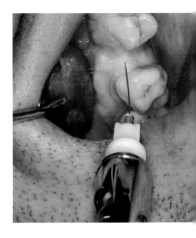

Local anesthetics like lidocaine hydrochloride with epinephrine (1:50,000 to 1:100,000) are used to anesthetize the operative area. The ratio of the epinephrine in the local anesthetic determines the duration of the anesthetic effect. Epinephrine also acts on the capillaries to constrict them and to slow the blood flow. This vasoconstrictor property of epinephrine is useful when hemostasis is required.

Before giving anesthesia, the clinician should instruct the patient to rinse his mouth with chlorhexidine gluconate for one minute. Using a gauze pad, the clinician will dry the area to be anesthetized. The topical anesthetic is applied on the oral tissue for approximately three minutes by a cotton-tip applicator. This application will anesthetize the area superficially. Thereafter, the clinician infiltrates the surgical site with the local anesthetic (lidocaine hydrochloride with epinephrine, 1:100,000).

Vibraject

The clinician gently presses the oral tissues at some distance away from the planned puncture site to distract the patient from pain caused by puncture of the site. The anesthetic is injected into the vestibular fold and then into the interdental papilla of the operative area. Blanching of the soft tissues would indicate that the area to be operated on is anesthetized. The clinician may gently massage the tissues to diffuse the anesthetic and promote rapid anesthesia. If the clinician is expecting hemorrhage during the procedure, lidocaine with epinephrine (1:50,000) can be infiltrated to obtain a blood-free surgical site.

Post-Operative Management

The patient should be given a mild analgesic before he or she leaves the clinic. The patient should also be advised to follow these instructions:

GENERAL CARE

The patient should relax as much as possible and avoid exerting himself or herself. No strenuous activity should be taken for the next few days.

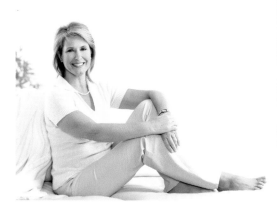

DISCOMFORT

Periodontal surgery may be associated with various degrees of discomfort. The patient should take the prescribed analgesics (Ibuprofen 600 mg or acetaminophen 300 mg and codeine phosphate 30 mg), preferably before the pain starts again.

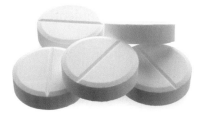

SWELLING

Swelling can be minimized by patient's applying an icepack to the outside of the face approximately 15 minutes on/15 minutes off, immediately following the surgery. The patient can fill a plastic bag with ice, wrap it in a towel, and use it as an ice pack. The patient is also instructed to keep his/her head elevated when lying down.

BLEEDING

There could be minor bleeding from the surgical site. In case of active bleeding, gauze should be placed over the operative site and gentle pressure applied for 15 to 30 minutes.

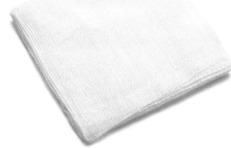

DRESSING

The patient should be instructed not to disturb the periodontal dressing. The patient should be advised to avoid chewing in the operated area side to prevent dislodgement of the dressing. A soft diet will help prevent dislodgement of the dressing.

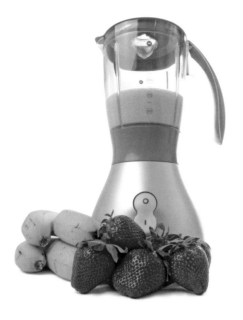

DIET

The patient should be advised to follow a soft diet. Soft foods that do not require chewing are tolerated best. The patient should avoid hot foods and hot liquids. It is also important to drink plenty of fluids.

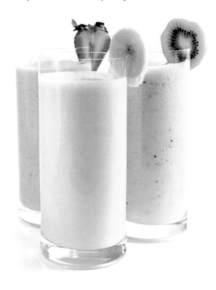

SMOKING AND ALCOHOL

Smoking and alcohol are prohibited postoperatively as they may delay wound healing and complicate recovery.

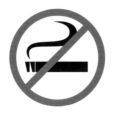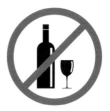

ORAL HYGIENE

The patient should not use a prescribed mouthwash for the first week postoperatively. Thereafter, the mouthwash can be used to rinse the mouth. Teeth in the non-affected area should be brushed and flossed as usual.

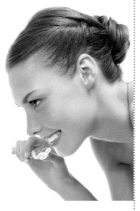

Summary

The clinician must obtain knowledge and practical clinical experience regarding the various instruments used in periodontal procedures in general, the types of suture material used, and the various suturing techniques being practiced. Anesthetic considerations and the post-operative management of the patient after periodontal procedures are also crucial clinical elements to learn and practice. The introduction of new and advanced suture materials and the development of different suturing techniques suited for specific purposes help clinicians to ease some of the difficulties previously encountered during periodontal surgeries. Clinicians need to be well-informed about the various types of suturing materials and their proper use to bring about predictable procedural outcomes. The use of the appropriate suturing material and technique contributes to the success of periodontal surgery and helps to prevent complications like wound dehiscence, bleeding, graft mobility, and infection. There is a need for clinicians to be able to make logical decisions regarding which suture materials to use for each given procedure because the choice of wound closure materials may make all the difference in wound healing and the final functional and aesthetic result obtained. Anesthesia application and post-operative care are also essential elements of professional periodontal plastic surgery.

References

1. Chen FM, Jin Y. Periodontal tissue engineering and regeneration: current approaches and expanding opportunities. Tissue Eng Part B Rev. 2010 Apr;16(2):219-55.

2. Bateman GJ, Saha S, Pearson D. Contemporary periodontal surgery: 1. Surgical principles. Dent Update. 2008 Jul-Aug;35(6):411-3.

3. Bateman GJ, Saha S, Pearson D. Contemporary periodontal surgery: 2. Surgical practice. Dent Update. 2008 Sep;35(7):470-2, 475-6, 478.

4. Levin MP. Periodontal suture materials and surgical dressings. Dent Clin North Am 1980; 24:767-81.

5. Silverstein LH, Kurtzman GM, Kurtzman D. Suturing for optimal soft tissue management. Gen Dent. 2007 Mar- Apr;55(2):95-100.

6. O'Neal RB, Alleyn CD. Suture materials and techniques. Curr Opin Periodontol. 1997; 4:89-95.

7. Silverstein LH. Preserving needle edges during dental suturing. Pract Proced Aesthet Dent. 2005 Sep;17(8):562, 564.

8. Silverstein LH, Kurtzman GM. A review of dental suturing for optimal soft-tissue management. Compend Contin Educ Dent. 2005 Mar;26(3):163-6, 169-70; quiz 171, 209. Review.

9. Silverstein LH. Essential principles of dental suturing for the implant surgeon. Dent Implantol Update. 2005 Jan;16(1):1-7.

10. Minozzi F, Bollero P, Unfer V, Dolci A, Galli M. The sutures in dentistry. Eur Rev Med Pharmacol Sci. 2009 May-Jun;13(3):217-26. Review.

11. Balamurugan R, Mohamed M, Pandey V, Katikaneni HK, Kumar KR. Clinical and histological comparison of polyglycolic acid suture with black silk suture after minor oral surgical procedure. J Contemp Dent Pract. 2012 Jul 1;13(4):521-7.

12. Kulkarni SS, Chava VK. Comparison of cyanoacrylate and silk sutures on healing of oral wounds--an animal model study. Indian J Dent Res. 2003 Oct-Dec;14(4):254-8.

13. Kulkarni S, Dodwad V, Chava V. Healing of periodontal flaps when closed with silk sutures and N-butyl cyanoacrylate: a clinical and histological study. Indian J Dent Res. 2007 Apr-Jun;18(2):72-7.

14. Selvig KA, Biagiotti GR, Leknes KN, Wikesjö UM. Oral tissue reactions to suture materials. Int J Periodontics Restorative Dent. 1998 Oct;18(5):474-87.

15. Leknes KN, Røynstrand IT, Selvig KA. Human gingival tissue reactions to silk and expanded polytetrafluoroethylene sutures. J Periodontol. 2005 Jan;76(1):34-42.

16. Leknes KN, Selvig KA, Bøe OE, Wikesjö UM. Tissue reactions to sutures in the presence and absence of anti-infective therapy. J Clin Periodontol. 2005 Feb;32(2):130-8.

17. Nelson EH, Funakoshi E, O'Leary TJ. A comparison of the continuous and interrupted suturing techniques. J Periodontol. 1977 May; 48(5):273-81.

18. Amarante ES, Leknes KN, Skavland J, Lie T. Coronally positioned flap procedures with or without a bioabsorbable membrane in the treatment of human gingival recession. J Periodontol. 2000 Jun;71(6):989-98.

19. Kanakaraj M, Shanmugasundaram N, Chandramohan M, Kannan R, Perumal SM, Nagendran J. Regional anesthesia in faciomaxillary and oral surgery. J Pharm Bioallied Sci. 2012 Aug;4(Suppl 2):S264-9.

20. Salam GA. Regional anesthesia for office procedures: part I. Head and neck surgeries. Am Fam Physician. 2004 Feb 1;69(3):585-90.

21. Meechan JG. The use of the mandibular infiltration anesthetic technique in adults. J Am Dent Assoc. 2011 Sep;142 Suppl 3: 19S-24S. Review.

22. Katyal V. The efficacy and safety of articaine versus lignocaine in dental treatments: a meta-analysis. J Dent. 2010 Apr;38(4):307-17.

Notes

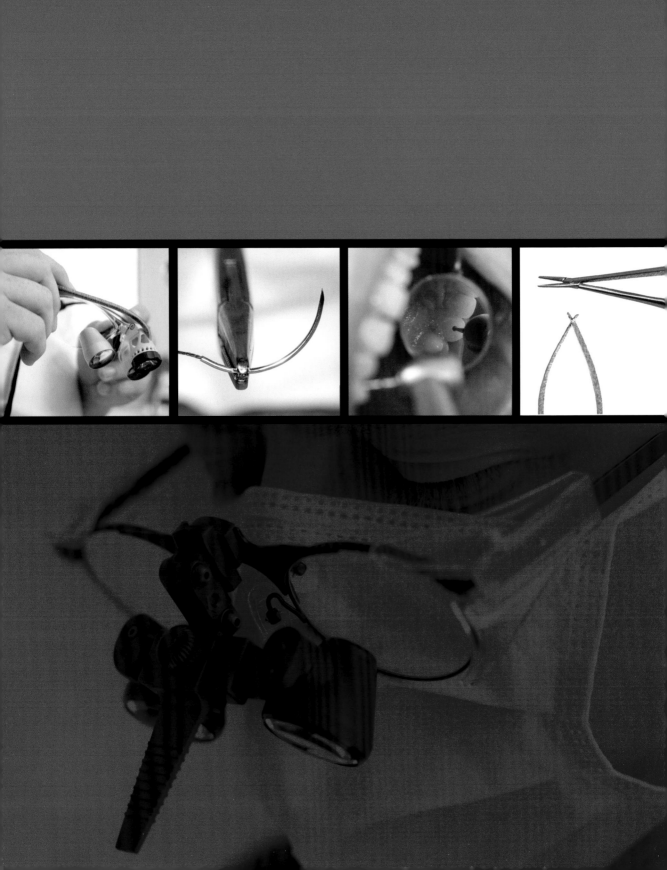

Introduction to Microsurgery

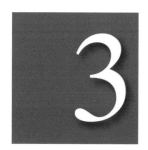

With the increasing patient demand for both mucogingival esthetics and dental function, periodontal clinical procedures and general perioperative practices must be optimized so that patient satisfaction is one of the highest priorities—if not the highest priority. This optimization is especially true for the patients who elect to undergo cosmetic dental procedures. In such cases, the patient's esthetics and the clinician's ethics are intertwined: Elective surgery necessarily requires thoughtful ethical considerations on the part of the clinician. The clinician must recognize that what the patient wants and what the patient needs may be vastly divergent concerns. While the clinician cannot assume a pseudo-parental role with regard to the patient's wishes, he or she must nevertheless provide the mature, balanced, and reasonable counsel the patient may need to make realistic esthetic choices.[1-4]

Use of a surgical microscope in periodontal surgeries is one of the best ways to optimize such esthetic periodontal practices because the microscope enhances complete visualization of the operative field and helps the clinician to perform procedures with maximum precision. As the name suggests, microsurgery involves minimal invasion and is performed with the help of a surgical microscope and specialized instruments as well as suturing materials. Because familiarity with these adapted instruments is necessary to bring about the expected outcomes, it is mandatory for a clinician to undergo an extended period of systematic training to handle the microinstruments.[5] It has even been suggested that "[t]he surgical community should follow the example of other high-risk industries such as aviation, where continuous assessment on simulators is a part of training, but further research is necessary before such methods can be used for summative assessment and revalidation."[6]

Historical Milestones in Microsurgery

Microsurgery was the result of various improvements brought about in vascular surgery techniques. Development of the operating microscope, modified instruments, microsutures, and novel operating techniques equally contributed to the refinement and sophistication of microsurgery. Although the vascular anastomosis was first performed by Dr. J.B. Murphy in 1897, Dr. Alexis Carrel originated the method for triangulation of blood vessels to perform arterial and venous repairs in 1902. By 1908, Carrel had devised methods for the transplantation of whole organs. Thereafter, there were many procedures of reimplantation of amputated body parts performed throughout the world.[7]

The term "microvascular surgery" was coined by Dr. Jules Jacobson, a vascular surgeon, in 1960. Using a microscope, Jacobson was successful at anastomosing extremely small vessels (1.4 millimeters). Jacobson's accomplishment was a turning point in the field of microsurgery. Use of magnification in surgery is not a new concept; in fact, it has been cited in many historical literatures. Zaccharias Janssen was a Dutch spectacle maker and the inventor of the compound microscope. Anthony Leeuwenhoek and Robert Hooke

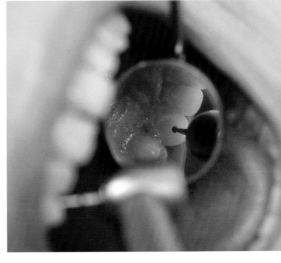

contributed to improving the design and capabilities of the microscope. In 1921, Dr. Carl Nylen was the first to use a microscope to perform ear surgery, thereby opening the way to several microsurgical procedures. However, the use of microscopes in medicine gained popularity only after the vascular anastomosis performed by Jacobson in 1960.[8]

Microsurgery in Dentistry

The microscope in dental practice was introduced in 1982 by Dr. Harvey Apothekar, who created the first dentoscope and coined the terms "microscope dentistry" and "micro dentistry."[9]

In 1992, Dr. Gary B. Carr described the use of microscopic techniques in endodontics, including "applications [such as] removal of fractured instruments, localizing calcified canals, soft tissue management and root-end procedures."[10]

Dr. Dennis Shanelec was the first to perform periodontal microsurgery, in 1993. Tibbetts and Shanelec described in a seminal article how "the quiet trend toward microdentistry" allowed them to "use microsurgical principles to improve visual acuity and the precision of existing surgical techniques to broaden the scope and character of periodontics, with knowledge and technology borrowed from medicine." These clinicians accurately predicted that "effect of periodontal microsurgery may include more predictable therapeutic results, less invasive procedures with reduced patient discomfort, more rapid healing, improved cosmetic results, and greater patient acceptance."[11]

They note in subsequent literature that "[s]ubtle basic microsuturing techniques offer vast improvement in wound closure through magnification and good visual feedback, as opposed to the tactile information traditionally taught in conventional suturing."[12] Subsequently, there were many studies published describing the role of the microscope in dental practice. The overwhelming conclusions of such studies were that for enhanced visibility, reduced trauma, and improved surgical results, periodontal surgeries should be coupled with optical magnification.

The use of a surgical microscope in periodontal surgeries provides the periodontist a better illumination and enhanced visual acuity of the operative area. Microsurgical techniques, when used in gingival transplantation for treating recession, significantly improve the aesthetic outcomes. These techniques also aid in complex procedures like papillary reconstruction, where high level magnification is required. Stretching, distorting, and tearing of gingival tissue that usually occur during flap reflection and suturing may be minimized by use of microsurgical procedures. Periodontal microsurgery has been shown to bring about improved therapeutic results, including minimally-invasive techniques, enhanced patient comfort, reduced recovery time, and, therefore, improved esthetic results.[13]

Root preparation is an important modality in periodontal therapy. Evidence suggests that root planing is enhanced when the procedure is aided by fiber optic illumination.[14,15] Studies also demonstrate that prosthodontic procedures performed with magnification are associated with significantly fewer errors. In fact, one study concluded that "[d]ental students who performed fixed prosthodontic procedures while using magnifiers were found to have committed half as many errors as students who performed the same preparation without the aid of a magnifier."[16]

In periodontics, microscopes have been successfully employed in the treatment of buccal recession by the free rotated papilla autograft technique combined with the coronally advanced flap. A study based on this technique demonstrated excellent gain in root coverage with microsurgery; the patients did not require a second surgical site, consequently reducing patient morbidity.[17]

The tunnel approach is one of the techniques of root coverage. A modification of the approach performed microscopically along with an undermining split flap preparation of the buccal tissues yielded better results, including minimal trauma and enhanced blood supply to the connective tissue graft. The authors of the study noted, "The use of a microsurgical concept, including microsurgical blades and suture material, improves wound healing and establishes a better esthetic result." Additionally, they indicated that "[b]ecause these modifications simplify the tunnel approach, the spectrum of indications for the tunnel technique may be expanded and a broader application achieved."[18] Furthermore, when the macroscopic approach was compared to the microsurgical approach in root surface coverage, the latter was found to significantly improve the vascularization of the grafts and the percentages of root coverage.[19]

Outcomes of regenerative periodontal surgery are directly associated with improvements in flap design and soft tissue manipulation. A study demonstrated that the ability to obtain and maintain primary closure of the interdental tissues was enhanced with microsurgical approach. As a result, there were minimal recessions, and clinically important amounts of clinical attachment gains were reported.[20]

Periodontal regeneration can be achieved through principles of guided tissue regeneration and the use of enamel matrix derivative. A microsurgical approach to flap procedure in both these treatment modalities resulted in high percentage of primary flap closure and maximum tissue preservation.[21]

In a case completed half a decade later, the aims "were to clinically and radio-graphically evaluate the effect of a microsurgical approach for the treatment of intra-bony defects with and without an enamel matrix derivative." These same researchers concluded that "[t]he combination of a microsurgical access flap with [enamel matrix derivative] seems to be superior to open flap debridement in terms of [probing pocket depth] reduction, [clinical attachment level] gain and radiographic bone fill." Additionally, in both the control and test groups, "primary wound closure was successfully achieved."[22]

Microsurgical Armamentarium

Instruments used in microsurgeries are small and, therefore, correspondingly very delicate and expensive. These instruments should be selected and bought carefully, and should be handled with extreme care. Surgical stainless steel and titanium are the most common metals used for microsurgical instruments. Instruments made of titanium are lightweight but expensive and tend to deform easily. Stainless steel instruments, on the other hand, may not be expensive, but they are prone to magnetization. The variety of stainless steel instruments is greater than instruments fashioned from titanium.

Among the many types and designs of microsurgical instruments used in periodontal plastic surgery, some of the most commonly used are knives, retractors, scissors, needle holders, and tying forceps.[23-25]

All instruments for microsurgery are designed based on the pinch mechanism. These instruments are handled and maneuvered with the thumb and index finger. Common characteristics of these instruments include lightness in weight, small precision tips, balanced proportions, pinch closure, and surfaces that do not reflect light. All the instruments are downsized, including knives, retractors, elevators, scissors, needle holders and needles, and tying forceps. Knives used in microsurgery are small in size and extremely sharp. They are designed to allow small, accurate incisions and easy maneuvering in spatially tight areas of the oral cavity.

Microneedle Holder

A microneedle holder is used to hold the needle steadily and prevent it from slipping.[26] The needle, thus secured by a needle holder, can be pulled through the tissue, and a knot can be tied. Needle holders usually have a locking-type variety to ensure that the needle is held firmly. The locks in the needle holder should be closed slowly and released promptly to reduce jerky movements. An ideal microneedle holder should be light in weight and of appropriate length to facilitate maneuvering with minimal force from a hand. Titanium microneedle holders are preferred to the stainless steel ones. The most commonly used needle holders are 14 cm and 18 cm in size. Needle holders with gently curved tips are preferred to the straight models. The type of needle holder a clinician uses depends on the type of sutures that are needed in the procedure. For 5-0 and 6-0 sutures, 1 mm tip needle holders are used, and for 8-0 and 10-0 sutures, 0.3 mm needle holder tips are used.

The clinician should hold the needle between its middle and lower thirds at its distal tip, through a needle holder. A grip too close to the top may prevent apposing two surfaces with a single stitch; a grip that is too distal may make the needle unsteady and change its direction.

Microforceps

Microforceps allow clinicians to work on delicate and minute tissues without causing trauma to them, and they also allow clinicians to perform movements that may not be possible with hands. Microforceps are also used to hold sutures while the clinician ties knots. The choice of forceps depends on the procedure being performed. Microforceps are usually 15 cm long, and have smooth and strong tips of 0.2 mm to 0.3 mm. The rounded handle of microforceps allows easy manipulation and maneuvering required when dissecting and tying knots. Microforceps may also have platforms or teeth to firm the grip.

While the basic design of microforceps has remained essentially unchanged for the last several decades, some important modifications, particularly in conjunction with complementary microsurgery instruments, have been implemented.[27-29]

Microscissors

Microscissors of different sizes are used for the purposes of cutting and dissecting. Microscissors of 14 cm and 18 cm are used for cutting microsutures and tissues as well as for repairing blood vessels and nerves. Microscissors of size 9 cm are used to handle delicate tissues. The scissors, which have straight tip blades, are used to cut sutures and tissues attached to vessels and nerve endings. Curved-tip scissors are used for dissection of nerves and vessels. The sides of the scissor blades are also used for cutting and trimming.

Microscissors have evolved in some medical/surgical disciplines to facilitate the clinician's tasks, for example, in neurosurgery, where bipolar scissors assist "in the management (coagulation and cutting) of cerebral microvessels during the resection of brain tumors rich in vascularity."[30] Another innovation driven by the challenges of

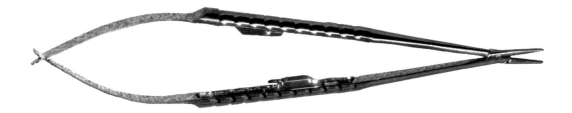

neurosurgery has been the creation of low-profile, coaxial microinstruments, including "microscissors and microforceps, as well as tumor-grasping forceps" to increase visibility and tactile manipulation via ergonomic design.[31]

Needles and Sutures

A three-eighths (3/8) inch (10 mm) curvature needle is the most commonly used needle followed by the one-half (1/2) inch (12.7 mm) needle. Large needles are suitable for procedures that are not associated with esthetic compromise or do not require the clinician to take minute details under consideration. However, for procedures which require precise closure or involve the area that directly influences esthetic outcomes, small needles are by far the best choice. Most of the periodontal microsurgeries use a 6.6 mm long spatula needle, which has a curvature of 140 degrees.

A 2011 technical note contends that "[m]icrosuturing in a narrow and/or a deep operating space is technically challenging, and classical microinstruments such as a bayonet microneedle-holder have their limitation, mainly related to their [built-in] rigidity." The note advocates a "flexible and 360° rotating shaft microneedle-holder made from nitinol" to accommodate such conditions.[32] Interestingly, a study in 2010 points out the "[a]dvantages of virtual-reality simulators [for] surgical skill assessment and training." The benefits include additional "training time, no risk to patient, repeatable difficulty level, reliable feedback, without the resource demands, and ethical issues of animal-based training." The study compared simulator results with those performed in a traditional setting. Suturing performance was compared for four different groups, including "experienced surgeons and naive subjects, on a custom-made virtual-reality simulator." The range of testing revealed that "[i]n all traditional parameters such as time, number of attempts, and motion quantity, the medical surgeons outperformed the other three groups, though differences were not significant." However, the study indicated that for the trained group, "motion smoothness, penetration and exit angles, tear size areas, and orientation change were statistically significant" when contrasted with the untrained group, suggesting strongly that such training on simulators should definitely be considered as part of microsurgery training.[33] Additionally, it has been noted that while traditional surgical approaches stress handling tissues gently to reduce trauma, and to optimize healing as the product of a "predictable operative environment," the plethora of microsurgical instruments generally available now suggests that their principles of use in special cases have extended to general surgery practices, precipitated in great part, no doubt, by the presence of the instrumentation itself.

Bateman has rightly noted that "[c]ontemporary surgical techniques emphasize gentle tissue handling with a minimum of trauma." These techniques, as a result, make the perioperative experience "predictable," most importantly regarding the healing process. Modern surgical armamentarium may be very different from that encountered a decade ago. This is clear from the greater availability of dental microsurgical instruments. So, while the complexity of microsurgery may not be routinely necessary in general dental practice, many of the principles and equipment used may make standard surgical management easier and more predictable. The clinical relevance of the study, therefore, is that "[a] greater understanding of the evidence base behind periodontal surgery will allow [clinicians and researchers] to improve flap design, closure and operative management. Also, the use of microsurgical techniques and equipment will improve the quality and outcomes of periodontal surgery in practice."[34] This "correspondence" of principles and practices from microsurgery to general surgery extends to the use of other armamentarium, such as the surgical microscope, which "offers the periodontist increased illumination and visual acuity to perform procedures with greater precision than with other methods of magnification." Coupled with "smaller instruments and sutures," such magnification offers "enhanced calculus removal."[35]

Sutures used in periodontal microsurgery should be able to hold the tissues together without causing any deformation in the tissues. Therefore, small sutures (6-0, 7-0, and 8-0) are most often used. A large suture tends to damage the tissues and may not close the opening caused by the needle. Sutures can be nonresorbable (silk, nylon, and polyester) or resorbable (plain and chromic gut, polyglactin 910, poliglecaprone 25, and polydioxanone), monofilament or multifilament. Studies demonstrate superiority of poliglecaprone 25 over others in periodontal microsurgeries.[36]

Instruments used in microsurgery are designed in such a way that they are most stable and easy to use when held like a writing instrument. A clinician should be aware of several principles, such as needle gripping and needle penetration into the tissue, when dealing with microsurgical tying of both dominant and non-dominant tying techniques, and with the guiding of sutures through delicate tissues.

A needle should enter the tissue at right angles to the incision line, keeping equal distance on exit. A general rule is that the proper amount of tissue to engage is approximately two times that of the diameter of the needle. Failure to observe this rule may result in improper tissue closure. Similar to the needle, the suture should be pulled through the tissue, keeping it perpendicular to the incision. Square knots are most preferred in microsurgery owing to the security it provides.

Recent literature concerning microsurgical tying involves a number of important innovations, belying the notion that the traditional tying methods in macrosurgery are often most suitable for microsurgical venues. For example, rudimentary elements of knot-tying vary between dry and most fields of operation.[37] A 2010 study rightly points out that "there are no human randomized, controlled clinical trials comparing the efficacy and clinical outcomes of each of the various suture techniques, and therefore one's comfort and familiarity should dictate his or her microsurgical technique."[38] Finally, though its wide application in dental surgery may still be decades away, telemicrosurgery (combining telesurgery and traditional microsurgery) offers a number of compelling benefits, including "three-dimensional high definition vision, abolition of physiological tremor, motion scaling of gestures down to 5 times, use of three instruments at once, and extreme mobility."[39]

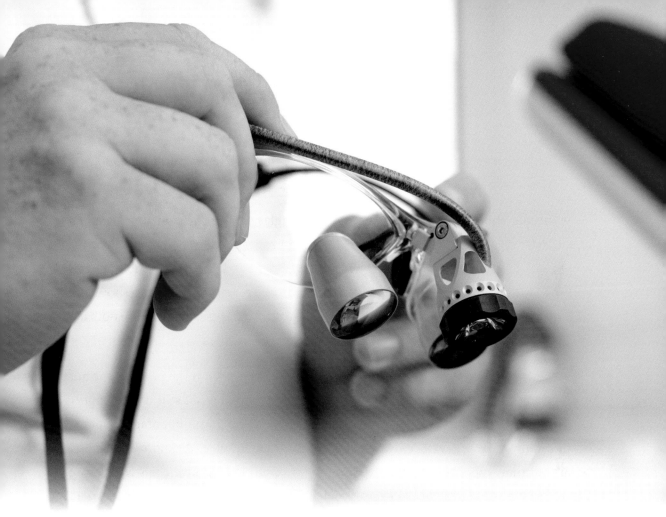

Magnification in Periodontal Plastic Surgery

Various ranges of magnification are used for microsurgeries in periodontics. Commonly, a magnification of up to x20 is sufficient for improving treatment outcomes for procedures that have a limited operating field.[40-42]

Clinicians who perform periodontal plastic surgery should be aware of various health-related problems due to the nature of the work. The poor body mechanics maintained during these procedures may cause musculoskeletal problems, particularly in the neck, shoulders, and back.[43] Maintaining a good posture when operating is very important for the musculoskeletal health of the clinician. The most important factor that influences the posture is the focal distance between the clinician's eyes and the surgical field. Therefore, the focal length of the magnifying device should be matched accordingly. If the focal length is too short or too long, the clinician may strain the muscles of his neck, shoulders, and back, resulting in muscle pain. Another important factor is alignment of binocular loupe optics. The clinician may strain his/her eyes if the loupes are not aligned properly.

When operating under magnification, the clinician must control trembling of the hands. Proper hand control is the first step in the training phase of microsurgery because if the hands are not controlled, the result can adversely affect the procedural outcomes. For example, it has been shown that recent exercising by the surgeon increases tremors.[44]

In a macroscopic procedure, the clinician has to get closer to the operative site to have a clear view; however, this creates poor posture, resulting in back, neck, and shoulder pain. In microsurgery, the clinician has an optically magnified view of the operative area, thereby allowing him to sit in a relatively comfortable posture.[45] Evidence supports the fact that surgical loupes allow the clinician to adopt the best ergonomic position while performing the procedure.

A common myth among clinicians is that use of magnification weakens the eye. However, studies suggest that the eyes are not affected, but the clinician becomes so accustomed to seeing large images that normal image may seem to be less detailed. This phenomenon may give the clinician the sensation that the eyes have become weak.[43] Nevertheless, the literature does contain evidence that "[s]tereoacuity and depth perception decrease when viewing a test target with loupes or with a microscope, with the effect worsening as magnification increases."[46]

Most magnifying loupes have a protective covering over their lenses to protect them from damage by debris produced during the procedure. The debris consists of broken pieces of tooth and metals, which can cause significant damage to the lenses. After the procedure, the lenses should be cleaned carefully. A water lavage is advisable for water-resistant lenses; for other lenses, a moist, lens-cleaning cloth provided by loupe manufacturers can be used. This procedure should be followed by sterilization. Experts recommend sterilizing all areas of the loupe after each procedure.

Surgical Loupes

Optical magnification in microsurgery not only enlarges the operating site but also provides powerful homogenous lighting. Both surgical loupes and surgical microscopes allow the clinician to visualize anatomical details which may not be otherwise observable through the naked eye. It is, therefore, universally accepted that microsurgery improves the quality of care provided to patients as well as widens the treatment options that can be offered.

Among the many advantages of magnification, some worth mentioning are magnified image with brilliant illumination, better posture and improved comfort for the clinician, increased precision, improved care, wide range of treatment options, and improved profitability. Many dental procedures that do not require high-level magnification can be easily performed with surgical loupes. Acceptance of loupes among clinicians is better than that of surgical microscopes because they are more portable and practical, easier to use, and less expensive.

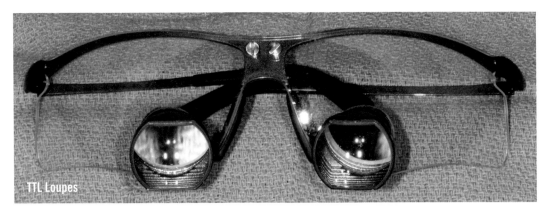

TTL Loupes

Surgical loupes provide marked visibility when compared to that of the naked eye. A surgical loupe is usually available with a magnification range of 2.0X to 6.0X. The level of magnification depends upon the type of procedure being undertaken. A magnification of 2.5X to 3.5X is sufficient for general dental procedures, whereas most of the microsurgery procedures require a magnification in the range of 4.5X and 6.0X. Resolution, the ability to distinguish one small thing from another, is an important feature of any surgical loupe and depends upon the design and quality of the lenses used in manufacturing the loupes.

It is important that the loupes provide good visual acuity of the entire field. Because it is very difficult to determine which loupe has the best resolution, experts recommend that the clinician request a trial period to assess the loupes and compare them with other loupes.[47]

The loupes are available in two designs: Through The Lens loupes (TTL) and Flip-up loupes.

TTL Loupes

The TTL loupes have telescopes attached directly to the lens of the glasses. These loupes are lighter than their flip-up counterparts and provide a better magnification because the telescopes are fixed in a way that is closer to the eye. TTL loupes fit more comfortably as they are custom-made for each individual. Declination angle is set in the factory, allowing the clinician to quickly adjust to the most comfortable body mechanics.

TTL loupes are not without a few disadvantages. For one thing, TTL loupes are more expensive than flip-up loupes. The cost rises higher in cases where the lens of the loupes is incorporated with the prescription of the glasses the clinician wears. If the clinician's prescription changes, the loupes have to be sent to the manufacturer to modify the lens, leaving the clinician unable to perform any procedure. Additionally, TTL loupes have to be removed when the clinician communicates with the patient, which can be quite inconvenient.

Flip-up Loupes

As the name suggests, the telescopes in the loupes can be easily flipped up as they are mounted on a hinge system. The easy "flipability" allows the clinician to communicate with the patient without any inconvenience. Moreover, flip-up loupes are less expensive than TTL loupes. Flip-up loupes are not custom-made and therefore can be shared between multiple operators; however, users need to adjust the declination angle to fit their needs. But in a case where the prescription lenses are incorporated into the loupes, only the operator for whom it was customized can use the loupe.

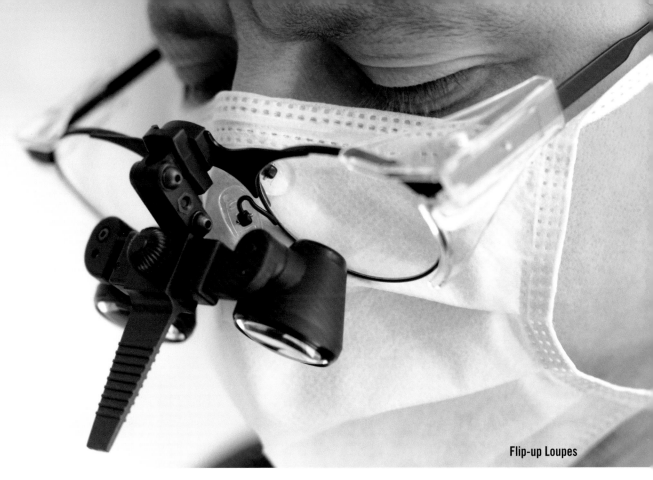

Flip-up Loupes

Another disadvantage is that because the flip-up loupe requires adjustment of the declination angle, the clinician might strain his eyes if the angle is not adjusted correctly. These loupes are also a bit uncomfortable because they are heavy. And, finally, due to the hinge system, the telescopes are mounted away from the eye, thus narrowing the field of view.

Galilean or Class II loupes are named after the 17th century astronomer Galileo Galilei. Galilean Loupes are lightweight, less expensive, and easy to use. They consist of three lenses, but have limited magnification in the range of 2.0X to 3.5X. A major drawback of the Galilean loupes is that the image is sharpest in the center and blurs towards the periphery.

Prismatic or Keplerian loupes or Class IV loupes are named after Johannes Kepler, the 17th century astronomer who developed the Keplerian Design. The prismatic loupe consists of a compound system of several lenses with a superior resolution throughout the field. However, they are heavier than Galilean loupes because of multiple lenses and longer telescopes.[48]

Summary

The objective of microsurgery is to remove dead space between tissues, appose tissues with adequate tension, and improve esthetic outcome. Appropriate microsurgical technique coupled with a combination of a properly selected needle and suture greatly contributes to the success of the procedure. It is very important for the clinicians to undergo proper training and practice because such procedures and techniques often require the operator to be familiar with visual feedback, as compared to the tactile feedback in macrosurgery. Various simulation models and labs are available to practice microsurgical techniques before applying it on patients. Periodontal microsurgery is a promising technique for the future of periodontics. For the clinicians, an initial investment in appropriate magnification can earn them great dividends later in their practice, as well as for their personal health.

References

1. Atiyeh BS, Rubeiz MT, Hayek SN. Aesthetic/Cosmetic surgery and ethical challenges. Aesthetic Plast Surg. 2008 Nov;32(6):829-39; discussion 840-1.

2. Kelleher MG, Djemal S, Lewis N. Ethical marketing in 'aesthetic' ('esthetic') or 'cosmetic dentistry'. Part 1. Dent Update. 2012 Jun;39(5):313-6, 318-20, 323-4 passim.

3. Kelleher MG, Djemal S, Lewis N. Ethical marketing in 'aesthetic' ('esthetic') or 'cosmetic dentistry' part 2. Dent Update. 2012 Jul-Aug;39(6):390-2, 394-6, 398-400 passim.

4. Kelleher MG, Djemal S, Lewis N. Ethical marketing in 'aesthetic' ('esthetic') or 'cosmetic dentistry'. Part 3. Dent Update. 2012 Sep;39(7):472-4, 476-8, 481-2 passim.

5. Ghiabi E, Taylor KL. Teaching methods and surgical training in North American graduate periodontics programs: exploring the landscape. J Dent Educ. 2010 Jun;74(6):618-27.

6. Balasundaram I, Aggarwal R, Darzi LA. Development of a training curriculum for microsurgery. Br J Oral Maxillofac Surg. 2010 Dec;48(8):598-606.

7. Tamai S. History of microsurgery--from the beginning until the end of the 1970s. Microsurgery. 1993;14(1):6-13.

8. Tamai S. History of microsurgery. Plast Reconstr Surg. 2009 Dec;124(6 Suppl):e282-94.

9. Apotheker H, Jako GJ. A microscope for use in dentistry. J Microsurg. 1981 Fall; 3(1):7-10.

10. Carr GB. Microscopes in endodontics. J Calif Dent Assoc. 1992 Nov; 20(11):55-61.

11. Tibbetts LS, Shanelec DA. An overview of periodontal microsurgery. Curr Opin Periodontol. 1994:187-93. Review.

12. Tibbetts LS, Shanelec D. Periodontal microsurgery. Dent Clin North Am. 1998 Apr; 42(2):339-59.

13. de Campos GV, Bittencourt S, Sallum AW, Nociti Júnior FH, Sallum EA, Casati MZ. Achieving primary closure and enhancing aesthetics with periodontal microsurgery. Pract Proced Aesthet Dent. 2006 Aug;18(7):449-54; quiz 456.

14. Reinhardt RA, Johnson GK, Tussing GJ. Root planing with interdental papilla reflection and fiber optic illumination. J Periodontol. 1985 Dec; 56(12):721-6.

15. Drisko CL, Killoy WJ. Scaling and root planing: removal of calculus and subgingival organisms. Curr Opin Dent. 1991 Feb;1(1):74-80. Review.

16. Leknius C, Geissberger M. The effect of magnification on the performance of fixed prosthodontic procedures. J Calif Dent Assoc. 1995 Dec;23(12):66-70.

17. Francetti L, Del Fabbro M, Testori T, Weinstein RL. Periodontal microsurgery: report of 16 cases consecutively treated by the free rotated papilla autograft technique combined with the coronally advanced flap. Int J Periodontics Restorative Dent. 2004 Jun;24(3):272-9.

18. Zuhr O, Fickl S, Wachtel H, Bolz W, Hürzeler MB. Covering of gingival recessions with a modified microsurgical tunnel technique: case report. Int J Periodontics Restorative Dent. 2007 Oct; 27(5):457-63.

19. Burkhardt R, Lang NP. Coverage of localized gingival recessions: comparison of micro- and macrosurgical techniques. J Clin Periodontol. 2005 Mar; 32(3):287-93.

20. Cortellini P, Tonetti MS. Microsurgical approach to periodontal regeneration. Initial evaluation in a case cohort. J Periodontol. 2001 Apr; 72(4):559-69.

21. Wachtel H, Schenk G, Böhm S, Weng D, Zuhr O, Hürzeler MB. Microsurgical access flap and enamel matrix derivative for the treatment of periodontal intrabony defects: a controlled clinical study. J Clin Periodontol. 2003 Jun; 30(6):496-504.

22. Fickl S, Thalmair T, Kebschull M, Böhm S, Wachtel H. Microsurgical access flap in conjunction with enamel matrix derivative for the treatment of intra-bony defects: a controlled clinical trial. J Clin Periodontol. 2009 Sep;36(9):784-90.

23. Chacha PB. Operating microscope, microsurgical instruments and microsutures. Ann Acad Med Singapore. 1979 Oct; 8(4): 371-81.

24. VanderKam V. Care of microvascular surgical instruments. Plast Surg Nurs. 1999 Spring;19(1):31-4. Review.

25. Hoyt RF Jr, Clevenger RR, McGehee JA. Microsurgical instrumentation and suture material. Lab Anim (NY). 2001 Oct;30(9):38-45. Review.

26. Hyland WT, Botens SR. The needle holder. Plast Reconstr Surg. 1980 Nov;66(5):763-5.

27. Owen ER. The microneedleholderscissors and the microforceps. Microsurgery. 1984;5(4): 213-7.

28. Kohno M, Segawa H, Nakatomi H, Sano K, Akitaya T, Takahashi T. Microsuture-tying forceps with attached scissors for bypass surgery. Surg Neurol. 2003 Nov;60(5):463-6.

29. Bao JY. Adjustable microforceps. J Reconstr Microsurg. 1991 Apr;7(2):139-41.

30. Qiu Y, Lin Y, Pang Y, Luo Q, Jiang J. Bipolar microscissors. Minim Invasive Neurosurg. 2004 Oct;47(5):316-8.

31. Cristante L. A set of coaxial microneurosurgical instruments. Neurosurgery. 1999 Dec;45(6):1492-3; discussion 1494.

32. Menovsky T, De Ridder D. A new flexible and 360° rotating shaft needle-holder for microneurosurgery: technical note. Minim Invasive Neurosurg. 2011 Oct;54(5-6):274-5.

33. Kazemi H, Rappel JK, Poston T, Hai Lim B, Burdet E, Leong Teo C. Assessing suturing techniques using a virtual reality surgical simulator. Microsurgery. 2010 Sep; 30(6):479-86.

34. Bateman GJ, Saha S, Pearson D. Contemporary periodontal surgery: 2. Surgical practice. Dent Update. 2008 Sep;35(7):470-2, 475-6, 478.

35. Belcher JM. A perspective on periodontal microsurgery. Int J Periodontics Restorative Dent. 2001 Apr;21(2):191-6. Review.

36. Takeishi M, Hirase Y, Kojima T. Microsurgical use of polydioxanone (PDS) suture: an experimental report. Microsurgery. 1992; 13(5):268-72.

37. Sun W, Wang Z, Qiu S, Li S. A practical microsurgical anastomosis knot-tying technique in the moist surgical field. Microsurgery. 2011 Jan;31(1):83-4.

38. Alghoul MS, Gordon CR, Yetman R, Buncke GM, Siemionow M, Afifi AM, Moon WK. From simple interrupted to complex spiral: a systematic review of various suture techniques for microvascular anastomoses. Microsurgery. 2011 Jan;31(1):72-80.

39. Ramdhian RM, Bednar M, Mantovani GR, Facca SA, Liverneaux PA. Microsurgery and telemicrosurgery training: a comparative study. J Reconstr Microsurg. 2011 Nov;27(9):537-42.

40. Christensen GJ. Magnification in dentistry: useful tool or another gimmick? J Am Dent Assoc. 2003 Dec;134(12):1647-50.

41. Syme SE, Fried JL, Strassler HE. Enhanced visualization using magnification systems. J Dent Hyg. 1997 Fall;71(5):202-6. Review.

42. van As G. Magnification and the alternatives for microdentistry. Compend Contin Educ Dent. 2001 Nov;22(11A):1008-12, 1014-6. Review.

43. Millar BJ. Focus on loupes. Br Dent J. 1998 Nov 28; 185(10):504-8.

44. Hsu PA, Cooley BC. Effect of exercise on microsurgical hand tremor. Microsurgery. 2003; 23(4):323-7.

45. Maillet JP, Millar AM, Burke JM, Maillet MA, Maillet WA, Neish NR. Effect of magnification loupes on dental hygiene student posture. J Dent Educ. 2008 Jan; 72(1):33-44.

46. Du LT, Wessels IF, Underdahl JP, Auran JD. Stereoacuity and depth perception decrease with increased instrument magnification: comparing a non-magnified system with lens loupes and a surgical microscope. Binocul Vis Strabismus Q. 2001;16(1):61-7.

47. Friedman MJ. Magnification in a restorative dental practice: from loupes to microscopes. Compend Contin Educ Dent. 2004 Jan; 25(1):48, 50, 53-5.

48. Mansueto MA, Overton JD. A clinician's guide to purchasing surgical loupes. TexDent J. 2007 Feb; 124(2):174-86.

Notes

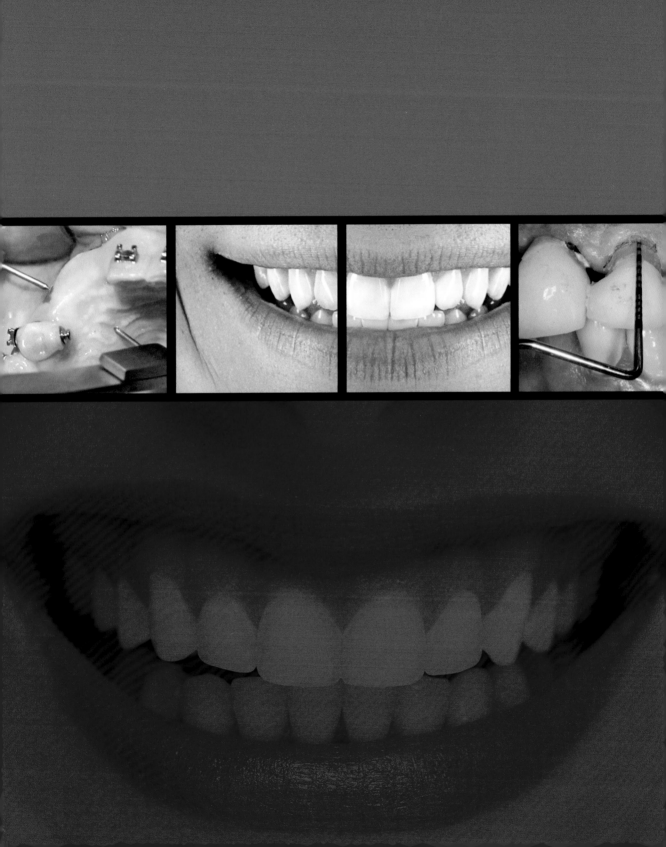

Improving Patients' Smiles: Crown-Lengthening Esthetics

4

The anterior maxillary region of dentition is the most important area for esthetics, dependent largely on the appearance of gingival tissues surrounding the teeth. Asymmetrical or distorted gingival tissues can significantly mar the harmonious appearance of natural or prosthetic dentition. Therefore, there are many treatment options available to enhance or improve the esthetics of an individual's smile. Crown lengthening, until relatively recently, was performed to provide adequate tooth structure for restorative purposes. However, with the growing trend of smile-enhancement therapies, and with more people striving for that perfect smile, crown-lengthening procedures have come to be widely accepted as legitimately esthetic-driven periodontal surgery. The procedure involves recontouring of both gingiva and supporting bone to expose more crown length, thus making the teeth and soft tissue appear optimally proportional. Before the clinician considers performing a crown-lengthening procedure, he or she should be aware of the relationship between hard and soft tissues, in addition to the definitive restorative or natural parameters to be achieved, as well as complications that could involve compromising the periodontium.[1-4]

Crown-lengthening procedures are indicated in mainly two conditions: to provide adequate tooth structure, and to help eliminate indications of a "gummy smile." "Gummy smile" refers to the condition where the teeth appear too small in relation to the gingival tissue,

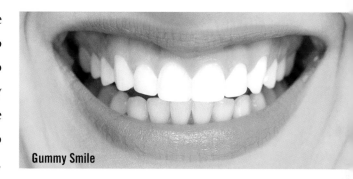

Gummy Smile

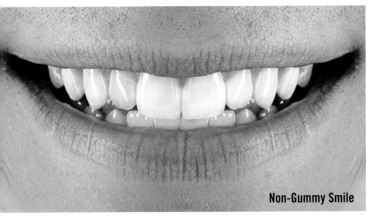
Non-Gummy Smile

and there is an excess of gingival display upon smiling. In general, it is acceptable for up to 2 mm of gingival tissue to be displayed upon a full smile.[5-8] Hence, a display of more than 2 mm of gingival tissue leads to excessive gingival display or "gummy smile." Healthy periodontal tissues are important in restoration and retention of prosthesis. Restorations that impinge on surrounding tissues can lead to periodontal inflammation and to altering the form and contour of gingival tissues. A clinician should educate himself or herself on what gingival biological width is acceptable,[9-11] what the consequences are if the width is altered, what lengthening of the clinical crown involves, and when such lengthening should be attempted.[12-16]

Crown-Lengthening Terminology

There are several important terminologies with which the clinician must be familiar before making any serious attempt at performing crown lengthening.

Clinical Crown of the Tooth

The distance from the level of marginal gingiva to the incisal edge or occlusal surface of the tooth is called the clinical crown of the tooth. It is the structure of the teeth that is most visible. Length of the clinical crown needs to be increased in cases of subgingival caries, subgingival crown fractures, and in cases where the tooth crown is too short for retention of restoration. A 2013 study concentrating on measuring the marginal

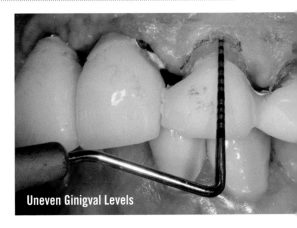
Uneven Ginigval Levels

adaptation of crowns and fixed dental prostheses concluded, "There was a substantial lack of consensus relating to marginal adaptation of various crown systems due to differences in testing methods and experimental protocols employed." The study also concluded that "using a combination of two measurement methods can be useful in verification of results."[17]

Biologic Width

The biologic width is the area of gingiva attached to the surface of the tooth, coronal to the alveolar bone. The dimensions were first described by Dr. A. W. Garguilo, Dr. F. Wentz, and Dr. B. Orban in 1961,[18] and later confirmed by Dr. J. S. Vacek and co-authors in 1994.[19] The following values were established: connective tissue attachment – 0.77 mm; epithelial attachment – 1.14 mm; depth of gingival sulcus – 1.34 mm. The mean value of biologic width is 3 mm. If there is less than 3 mm of distance from restoration margin to alveolar bone, the biologic width would be violated, thus leading to gingival inflammation.[20] Studies have shown the importance of measuring gingival biological width before and after crown-lengthening procedures. For example, a 2010 study evaluated "the positional changes of the periodontal tissues, particularly the biologic width, following surgical crown-lengthening in human subjects," determining that the biologic width in treated sites "was reestablished to its original vertical dimension by 6 months, [and] a consistent 2-mm gain of coronal tooth structure was observed at the 1-, 3- and 6-month examinations."[21]

Bone Sounding

Bone sounding is an important part of many surgical approaches, including crown lengthening. The clinician must determine the level of alveolar crest to decide the surgical approach and feasibility. Factors such as thickness of the gingival tissue layer and proximity of the alveolar bone are important considerations in crown-lengthening procedures. To determine the level of the alveolar bone, a measuring instrument is used to penetrate the mucosa until it reaches the underlying bone while the patient is under local anesthesia. A 2013 study tried to determine whether or not characteristics associated with bone sounding, gingival thickness, and related periodontal features might in fact be determined by the shapes of teeth.[22] The study included measurements of the height and width of maxillary central incisor crowns, the height of keratinized mucosa, the thickness of buccal gingiva, sulcus and bone-sounding depths, as well as the interproximal maxillary central papilla height. The 50 patients in the study were divided into three groups, based on tooth shape: triangular, square, or square-tapered. The significant statistical differences involved measurements of the keratinized mucosa, including the "bucco-lingual thickness and the height of the interproximal maxillary central papilla." Despite the fact that bone sounding differences were negligible, clinicians must remain cognizant of studies such as these,

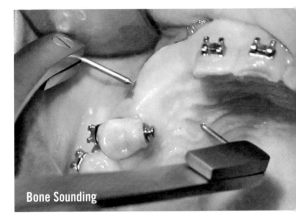

Bone Sounding

including those involving age and gender factors[23] to help aid them in determinations affecting crown-lengthening procedures.

Indications for Crown Lengthening

Crown lengthening is performed in cases of subgingival fracture,[24] subgingival caries,[25] root resorption,[26] unequal gingival levels, esthetically short crowns due to tooth wear, inadequate axial height for restoration retention, and altered passive eruption

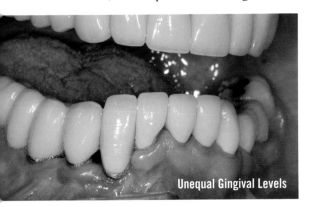

Unequal Gingival Levels

of a tooth, the last two factors being the most common indications.

Empirically, esthetic crown-lengthening procedures are performed in two types of clinical conditions—restorative cases and non-restorative cases—and the surgical approach for each differs significantly. In restorative cases, crown lengthening is performed prior to restoration, mainly to increase the axial length of the crown to strengthen anchoring of the restored teeth. In non-restorative cases, crown lengthening is an independent procedure used to enhance esthetics and is not associated with restorations.[27]

Crown Lengthening in Restorative Cases

The objective of crown lengthening in restorative cases is to increase the axial length by surgically moving the alveolar bone crest to a more apical position, thereby providing adequate tooth structure to anchor the restoration. It also helps to reestablish the new physiologic biologic width. Evidence suggests that the biologic width is genetically predetermined and tends to regrow to its predetermined height in relation to the bone, irrespective of the bone modification in crown lengthening.[18,19] Additionally, radiographic exploration techniques used to measure "the dentogingival unit on the buccal surfaces of anterior teeth, and to provide additional information on the dimensions of the dentogingival unit in humans" revealed "[a] statistically significant relationship... between free gingival width and thickness of connective [tissue] attachment, and the depth of the gingival sulcus," verifying the high variability in humans of "dimensions of the dentogingival unit."[28] In fact, more variability was discovered in "thickness of the bone crest, distance between CEJ and bone crest, and biologic width" than in the "thicknesses of both the connective tissue attachment and free gingiva."

Restorations without crown lengthening can violate biologic width and induce inflammatory changes in gingiva. An apically positioned flap combined with resective osseous surgery is performed for crown lengthening in cases of multiple contiguous teeth restoration in the upper anterior segment. A buccal flap is elevated and reflected apically to the mucogingival junction. If the crown lengthening involves palatal and interproximal aspects of the teeth being treated, a palatal flap can also be combined with a buccal flap. When designing the flap, the clinician should try to create thick and long surgical papillae. Upon healing, the papillae develop into a well-shaped gingival line with the presence of full papillae. Additionally, the clinician's reflecting the buccal flap apically to the mucogingival junction increases flap mobility and exposes the alveolar bone, which allows for the access necessary for recontouring of the bone. After the elevation of the buccal and palatal flaps, the clinician should remove the gingival tissue which is left in contact with the teeth and bone. Thereafter, osseous surgery is performed using a high-speed handpiece under copious water spray, burs, and chisels.

Osteoplasty is followed by ostectomy or bone removal to create a distance between the restoration margin and the alveolar crest. This distance should be at least 2 mm greater than the actual biologic width of the patient so as to accommodate the restorative margin if it tends to become displaced apically during final restorations. The flaps are sutured and temporary restorations are cemented. Sutures are removed at the end of the first operative week.

For crown lengthening of an isolated tooth planned for restoration, the clinician should be very careful when deciding the treatment approach. An inappropriate treatment modality may lead to an asymmetrical gingival line. Forced tooth eruption is the most common procedure involved. When performed with orthodontic extrusion, such a procedure exposes more tooth structure to the supragingival environment without changing the position of the gingival margin and the alveolar bone. Evidence suggests a positive outcome with atraumatic surgical extrusion with the clinician's use of a specially designed instrument (periotome).[29,30]

A 2010 review of crown-lengthening therapy examined "the rationale, basic surgical principles, contraindications and wound healing associated with periodontal crown-lengthening surgery."[11] Along with literature reviews, the authors examined both clinical studies and radiographic studies. The authors focused only on the literature which "pertained to the surgical exposure of the natural dentition to facilitate restorative therapy, esthetic concerns or both." The study found that "crown lengthening can be used for esthetic enhancement in the presence of delayed passive eruption." Furthermore, the study concluded that "for teeth with subgingival caries, fractures or both...[crown lengthening can] establish a biological width and, if needed, a ferrule length facilitating prosthetic management." The study notes that a variety of techniques are used in crown-lengthening surgery ("gingivectomy or gingivoplasty or apically positioned flaps, which may include osseous resection"), and that "[a]uthors of wound-healing investigations have reported that an average of 3 millimeters of supragingival soft tissue will rebound coronal to the alveolar crest and can take a minimum of three months to complete vertical growth." The clinical implications of the study warn clinicians that "final prosthetic treatment should wait at least three months and possibly up to six months for esthetically important areas, as the free gingival margin requires a minimum of three months to establish its final vertical position" and that "osseous resection could affect periodontal stability and may pose a contraindication to crown-lengthening therapy."[11]

Post-operatively, the factors that determine the outcome of the crown-lengthening procedure include the length of time between the surgical procedure and the placement of restorations, and the position of the gingival margin after the surgery. If the gingival margins recede after healing, the restorative margins may become positioned on the supragingival aspect, thereby exposing the restorative crown margins. A study suggests that there should be a time gap of six months after the surgery for the final preparation and impression making of the teeth.[31] There is evidence that demonstrates changes happening in gingival margins up to 12 months after osseous resection in crown-lengthening procedures.[32]

Crown Lengthening in Non-restorative Cases

Esthetic crown lengthening in non-restorative cases is usually performed to treat excessive display of gingival tissue. Excessive gingival display, or "gummy smile," can be due to three reasons; however, crown lengthening may not be the treatment of choice for all. The clinician should be extremely careful in diagnosing the cause and prescribing appropriate treatment.

"Gummy smile" may be due to a genetically predetermined skeletal deformity, in which the middle third of the face is vertically long, a condition usually associated with malocclusion. Surgical crown lengthening is not indicated in these patients as there is a skeletal deformity, and periodontal procedures may expose the roots. These cases should be treated with orthodontic procedures combined with orthognathic surgery in severe cases.

Short and/or hyper mobile lips are another cause of excessive gingival display. Dimensions of the lips and their range of movement are genetically predetermined. Little can be done to modify these dimensions. Therefore, crown lengthening may not be an appropriate treatment modality because it may lead to root exposure, again requiring restorative treatment.

A study describes the technique of repositioning the upper lip that limits the range of its motion; after the procedure, there is less display of gingiva upon smiling.[33] Another successful technique for lip repositioning involves "removing a strip of mucosa from maxillary buccal vestibule and creating a partial thickness flap between mucogingival junction and upperlip musculature, and suturing the lip mucosa [to the] mucogingival junction, resulting in a narrow vestibule and restricted muscle pull, thereby reducing gingival display."[34]

Excessive gingival display due to altered passive eruption of teeth is the most important indication of crown-lengthening procedure. In human beings, tooth eruption takes place in two phases: the active eruption phase, when there is movement of the teeth in the coronal direction, up to the point at which occlusal contacts are established; and the passive eruption phase, during which the gingival tissue and the alveolar bone margin move in the apical direction. The process of eruption usually finishes by the end of adolescence, with the gingival line located 1 mm to 3 mm coronally to the cementoenamel junction (CEJ), and the coronal end of the junctional epithelium being coincident with the CEJ. Altered passive eruption refers to incomplete or absent passive eruption in individuals due to reasons unknown and leads to the coronal margin of the alveolar bone located at less than 2 mm from or at the level of the CEJ. Thus, the gingival margin becomes positioned more coronally to the CEJ. These individuals have square-shaped clinical crowns, and they tend to display excessive gingival tissue upon smiling.

Crown Lengthening for Altered Passive Eruption

When performing crown lengthening for individuals with altered passive eruption, the clinician must determine the position of underlying bone in relation to the gingival tissue. Osseous resection is essential to placement of an apically positioned gingival margin; therefore, the technique that gives most access to the bone for osseous resection should be chosen. Periodontal flap surgery, by and large, is the most widely used technique. Gingivectomy is limited to cases where there is a wider zone of attached gingiva and is not used for cases where osseous resection is required. Crown lengthening for altered passive eruption is usually not associated with restoration, so procedures that decrease the height of interdental papillae should be prevented.

Fig 4-1 Clinical Crown Lengthening for Non-restorative Cases "Gummy Smile"

a

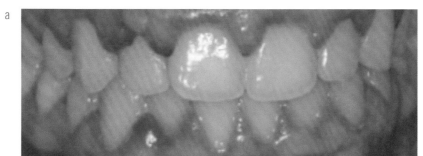

(a) Short clinical crowns due to excessive, hyperplastic gingiva.

b

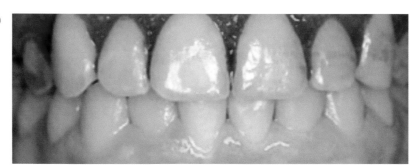

(b) Gingivectomy/ gingivoplasty of the maxillary teeth.

c

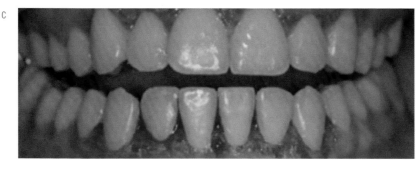

(c) Appearance of the mandibular teeth after removal of excess gingiva.

d

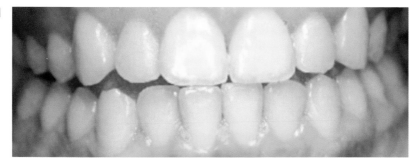

(d) Normal appearing clinical crowns after four weeks of healing. ■

Taking all these factors into consideration, the clinician is advised to elevate a buccal flap only and leave the interproximal papillae and the palatal tissue intact. Including the interproximal papillae and the palatal tissue in the flap may compromise the blood supply to these tissues and cause tissue shrinkage. Preservation of the interproximal papillae is mandatory to obtaining desirable final results in the esthetic region.[35-37]

As the foregoing discussion has shown, crown-lengthening procedures typically involve flap surgery, and as many studies suggest, may be associated with postoperative complications like infection, bleeding, inflammation, and changes in tissue position during the healing process.[38,39] These complications have adverse effects on the esthetic outcomes of the procedure.

Laser surgeries have been reported to cause less damage to the soft tissues and, thereby, enhance esthetic results. One study reports that use of an erbium laser offers a minimally-invasive alternative to osseous crown lengthening and minimizes the adverse side effects associated with conventional treatment.[40] Lee describes the use of 810 nm diode laser for periorestorative procedures in the anterior maxilla.[41] Another study describes that the use of an erbium laser treatment requiring minimal tissue displacement and flap preparation is limited to isolated papillae as necessary. Other advantages of using the laser for osseous crown lengthening include hemostasis, improved visualization, and fewer post-operative complications.[42] Indeed, Flax points out that "[d]entistry has seen a huge breakthrough with the introduction of a combination hard-soft tissue erbium wavelength, [and that]…[a]mong the many benefits of this technique are less invasive care and quicker healing responses."[43] Another study describes the advantages of traditional scalpel surgery instead of laser surgery, combined with depigmentation procedure.[44]

Classification and Treatment of Altered Passive Eruption

Delayed passive eruption conditions can be classified into three categories for differential diagnosis and appropriate treatment:[5,36,45-48]

Altered Passive Eruption Based on
Attached Gingiva-Crown Relationship

TYPE I: The gingival margin is coronal to the CEJ with a wide zone of attached gingiva. In these cases, gingivectomy can be performed for crown lengthening, provided 3 mm to 5 mm of attached gingiva is preserved.

TYPE II: The gingival margin is coronal to the CEJ, but the width of attached gingiva is normal. In these cases, apical positioning of the gingiva is performed for crown lengthening since the attached gingival width must be preserved.

Altered Passive Eruption Based on
Alveolar Crest and CEJ Relationship

SUBGROUP A: The underlying alveolar crest is located 1.5 mm to 2.0 mm apical to the CEJ. Crown lengthening is performed without osseous resection in these cases.

SUBGROUP B: The alveolar crest is at the CEJ. Crown lengthening requires 2 mm to 3 mm of osseous resection in these cases to establish the ideal biological width.

Altered Passive Eruption Based on the
Relationship between the Alveolar Crest Positions Relative to
the Anticipated Postsurgical Gingival Margin Level

This classification was first suggested by Dr. W. J. Lee (2004). The treatment approach for each type is different.[13,49-51]

TYPE I - ESTHETIC CROWN LENGTHENING: In this type, there is an adequate amount of gingiva coronal to the alveolar crest. Crown lengthening can be achieved by gingivectomy or gingivoplasty without the need of bone resection. Because there is sufficient gingival tissue present, surgery performed on the gingiva rarely violates the gingival margin. The surgery is best performed with the use of a laser device rather than a scalpel blade because incision with a scalpel blade makes the operative area bloody. Lasers also offer intraoperative hemostasis. The provisional restorations can be placed immediately if the procedure is managed well.

TYPE II - ESTHETIC CROWN LENGTHENING: Although the gingival tissue is normal and an osseous recontouring may not be required, any surgical intervention may violate the biological width. Therefore, a gingival excision should be followed by bone resection through elevation of the mucoperiosteal flap; the alveolar crest thus recontoured would help to reestablish the biologic width. The procedure can be performed in two stages because the gingival tissue reaction is not immediate.[49]

TYPE III - ESTHETIC CROWN LENGTHENING: In these cases, gingival tissue is inadequate, and repositioning the gingival margin will result in exposure of the osseous crest. The flap is repositioned coronally rather than apically in order to maximize tissue preservation and to allow the anticipated revisions to the gingival margin that will follow, once healing from the osseous surgery has been completed.[49] Evidence suggests that efforts should be made to use sutures that will approximate the papillae and reduce the risk of increased gingival embrasure spaces postsurgery.

TYPE IV - ESTHETIC CROWN LENGTHENING: This procedure is indicated in cases where there is an insufficient amount of attached gingiva and a gingival excision may not be feasible. An apically positioned mucoperiosteal flap is used in these cases.

Fig 4-2 **Classification and Treatment of Altered Passive Eruption**

a

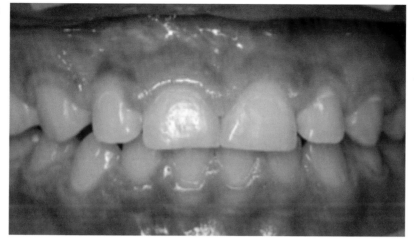

(a) Altered passive eruption classification Type I Subgroup A.

b

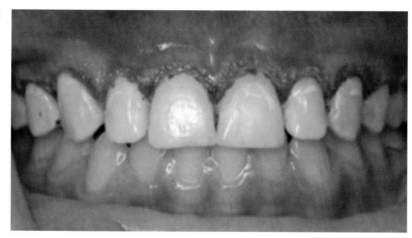

(b) Type I esthetic crown lengthening accomplished by performing gingivectomy/ gingivoplasty using a laser.

c

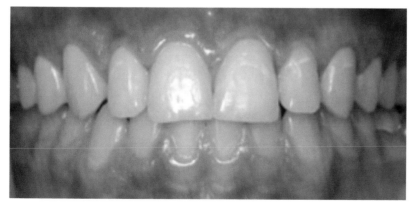

(c) Normal length clinical crowns after four weeks of healing. ■

Complications

As discussed earlier, the optimal biologic width is 3 mm. In response to any procedure that impinges on this width, the body tries to repair this dimension of 3 mm by resorbing the bone. The amount of bone resorbed depends upon the space needed for gingival attachment between restoration and alveolar bone. In addition, the periodontal ligament is also lost.[50] These changes may manifest themselves in different forms, depending upon the biotype of individual periodontium.[51]

There are two basic biotypes: thin periodontium (where thickness of attached gingiva is less than 1 mm and width is 3.5-5 mm with thin marginal bone) and thick periodontium (where thickness of attached gingiva is up to 1.3 mm, and width is 5 mm to 6 mm or more with thick marginal bone). In thin periodontal biotypes, the postoperative periodontal changes may lead to resorption of the alveolar crest and subsequent gingival recession. In thick periodontal biotypes, the periodontal changes may manifest themselves as chronic gingival inflammation. In both these conditions, the esthetic outcome of the procedure is compromised.

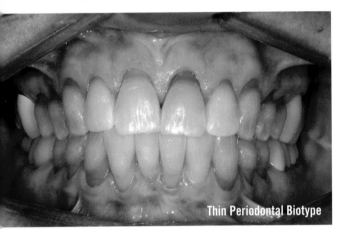

Thin Periodontal Biotype

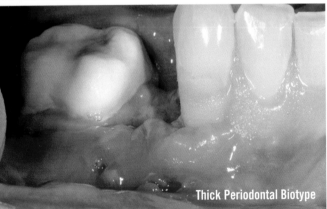

Thick Periodontal Biotype

In thin biotypes, bone resorption and gingival recession occur faster, and if proper hygiene of the area is performed optimally, then resolution of the gingival inflammation happens often. On the other hand, if proper hygiene is not performed, the gingival inflammation persists, bone further resorbs, and a periodontal pocket is formed. In thick biotypes, gingival recession is rare and bone loss is slow, but bone defects and unfavorable bone contour form more often. Subsequently, it may result in periodontal pockets, root caries, tooth mobility due to loss of tooth attachment apparatus, and tooth loss. Therefore, to avoid pathological changes and to predict treatment results more precisely, the clinician must strive to keep gingival biological width unaltered during teeth restoration.[52]

There are studies that show the changes that periodontal tissues undergo after crown lengthening.[53] For example, it was found that six weeks after surgery, attachment level and probing depth did not change. In such a case, the gingival margin established during the operation more or less matched the gingival margin after healing. In about 85 percent of cases, there was zero or minimal +1 mm changes of marginal gingival level between six weeks and six months. Gingival retraction of more than 1 mm occurred in about 12 percent of cases. Based on these studies, it is recommended that final restoration should be made no earlier than six weeks after operation, and because of possible retraction, it is recommended that the clinician wait longer in esthetic areas. It is also observed that the recovery of the epithelial basal membrane takes more than four weeks; therefore, dental treatment on the operative area should not be attempted before that.[32,54] Other complications after crown-lengthening procedures include unsatisfactory esthetics due to gingival retraction, distortion of gingival contour, possible loss of gingival papilla, interdental spaces, and clinical tooth crown longer than adjacent teeth.[55]

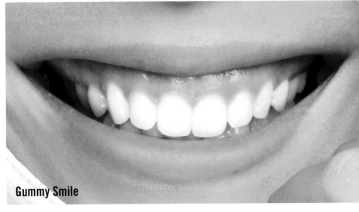
Gummy Smile

Summary

The crown-lengthening procedure in restorative cases can be used for multiple teeth and single tooth restorations; however, the approach differs for each. It is also a treatment of choice to treat cases of "gummy smile" or excessive gingival display caused by altered passive eruption. In these cases, the treatment modality should depend upon the etiology of altered passive eruption. The orthodontic extrusion approach and the minor periodontal surgical approach, when combined, give better results in an esthetic zone's short, clinical crowns by not compromising the periodontal support system of the extruded tooth or its adjacent teeth.

The decision of treatment modality for esthetic crown lengthening should be based on detailed diagnostic work on each case because the type of therapy selected by the clinician will have direct implications on the resulting esthetics.[56] The clinician should also have a good understanding of wound healing processes in soft tissues in order to help develop a new, symmetrical, and scalloped gingival line. On the whole, clinical crown-lengthening procedures should be coupled with osseous recontouring and gingival flaps for better esthetic outcomes.

References

1. Davarpanah M, Jansen CE, Vidjak FM, Etienne D, Kebir M, Martinez H. Restorative and periodontal considerations of short clinical crowns. Int J Periodontics Restorative Dent. 1998 Oct;18(5):424-33. Review.

2. Bitter RN. The periodontal factor in esthetic smile design--altering gingival display. Gen Dent. 2007 Nov; 55(7):616-22.

3. Cunliffe J, Grey N. Crown lengthening surgery--indications and techniques. Dent Update. 2008 Jan-Feb;35(1):29-30, 32, 34-5.

4. Fletcher P. Biologic rationale of esthetic crown lengthening using innovative proportion gauges. Int J Periodontics Restorative Dent. 2011 Sep-Oct;31(5):523-32.

5. Garber DA, Salama MA. The aesthetic smile: diagnosis and treatment. Periodontology 2000. 1996 11:18-28.

6. Silberberg N, Goldstein M, Smidt A. Excessive gingival display--etiology, diagnosis, and treatment modalities. Quintessence Int. 2009 Nov-Dec;40(10):809-18.

7. Gill DS, Naini FB, Tredwin CJ. Smile aesthetics. Dent Update. 2007 Apr;34(3): 152-4, 157-8.

8. Bidra AS. Three-dimensional esthetic analysis in treatment planning for implant-supported fixed prosthesis in the edentulous maxilla: review of the esthetics literature. J Esthet Restor Dent. 2011 Aug;23(4):219-36.

9. Wolffe GN, van der Weijden FA, Spanauf AJ, de Quincey GN. Lengthening clinical crowns--a solution for specific periodontal, restorative, and esthetic problems. Quintessence Int. 1994 Feb; 25(2):81-8.

10. Bateman GJ, Karir N, Saha S. Principles of crown lengthening surgery. Dent Update. 2009 Apr;36(3):181-2, 184-5.

11. Hempton TJ, Dominici JT. Contemporary crown-lengthening therapy: a review. J Am Dent Assoc. 2010 Jun;141(6):647-55. Review.

12. Ingberg JS, Rose LF, Coslet JG. The biologic width – a concept in periodontics and restorative dentistry. Alpha Omegan 1977; 70: 62-65.

13. Yeh S, Andreana S. Crown lengthening: basic principles, indications, techniques and clinical case reports. N Y State Dent J. 2004 Nov; 70(8):30-6.

14. Planciunas L, Puriene A, Mackeviciene G. Surgical lengthening of the clinical tooth crown. Stomatologija. 2006;8(3):88-95. Review.

15. Ziada H, Irwin C, Mullally B, Byrne PJ, Allen E. Periodontics: 5. Surgical crown lengthening. Dent Update. 2007 Oct;34(8):462-4, 467-8.

16. Oh SL. Biologic width and crown lengthening: case reports and review. Gen Dent. 2010 Sep-Oct;58(5):e200-5. Review.

17. Nawafleh NA, Mack F, Evans J, Mackay J, Hatamleh MM. Accuracy and Reliability of Methods to Measure Marginal Adaptation of Crowns and FDPs: A Literature Review. J Prosthodont. 2013 Jan 4.

18. Gargiulo AW, Wentz F, Orban B. Dimensions and relations of the dentogingival junction in humans. J Periodontol 1961; 32: 261-7.

19. Vacek JS, Gehr ME, Asad DA, Richardson AC, Giambarresi LI. The dimensions of the human dentogingival junction. Int J Periodontics Restorative Dent 1994; 14:154-65.

20. Carranza FA, Rapley JW, Kinder Hake S. Gingival inflammation. Carranza's clinical periodontology. 9th ed. 2002. Chap.16. p. 263-8.

21. Shobha KS, Mahantesha, Seshan H, Mani R, Kranti K. Clinical evaluation of the biological width following surgical crown-lengthening procedure: A prospective study. J Indian Soc Periodontol. 2010 Jul;14(3):160-7.

22. Stellini E, Comuzzi L, Mazzocco F, Parente N, Gobbato L. Relationships between different tooth shapes and patient's periodontal phenotype. J Periodontal Res. 2013 Feb 27.

23. Kuriakose A, Raju S. Assessment of thickness of palatal mucosal donor site and its association with age and gender. J Indian Soc Periodontol. 2012 Jul;16(3):370-4.

24. Hu WJ, Li LS, Zhang H. Root reshaping in combination of conservative osseous resection: a modified technique for surgical crown lengthening. Beijing Da Xue Xue Bao. 2008 Feb 18; 40(1):83-7.

25. Hempton TJ, Esrason F. Crown lengthening to facilitate restorative treatment in the presence of incomplete passive eruption. J Calif Dent Assoc. 2000 Apr; 28(4):290-1, 294-6, 298.

26. Reddy MS. Achieving gingival esthetics. J Am Dent Assoc. 2003 Mar;134(3):295-304; quiz 337-8.

27. Kao RT, Dault S, Frangadakis K, Salehieh JJ. Esthetic crown lengthening: appropriate diagnosis for achieving gingival balance. J Calif Dent Assoc. 2008 Mar; 36(3):187-91.

28. Alpiste-Illueca F. Dimensions of the dentogingival unit in maxillary anterior teeth: a new exploration technique (parallel profile radiograph). Int J Periodontics Restorative Dent. 2004 Aug;24(4):386-96.

29. Kim CS, Choi SH, Chai JK, Kim CK, Cho KS. Surgical extrusion technique for clinical crown lengthening: report of three cases. Int J Periodontics Restorative Dent. 2004 Oct; 24(5):412-21.

30. Blase D, Bercy P. An esthetic crown lengthening technic of the clinical crown. Rapid orthodontic extrusion. Rev Belge Med Dent. 1993; 48(3):9-28.

31. Rosenberg ES, Cho SC, Garber DA. Crown lengthening revisited. Compend Contin Educ Dent. 1999 20:527-32.

32. Pontoriero R, Carnevale G. Surgical crown lengthening: a 12-month clinical wound healing study. J Periodontol. 2001 Jul;72(7):841-8.

33. Rosenblatt A, Simon Z. Lip repositioning for reduction of excessive gingival display: a clinical report. Int J Periodontics Restorative Dent. 2006 Oct;26(5):433-7.

34. Gupta KK, Srivastava A, Singhal R, Srivastava S. An innovative cosmetic technique called lip repositioning. J Indian Soc Periodontol. 2010 Oct;14(4):266-9.

35. Nemcovsky CE, Artzi Z, Moses O. Pre-prosthetic clinical crown lengthening procedures in the anterior maxilla. Pract Proced Aesthet Dent. 2001 Sep; 13(7):581-8; quiz 589.

36. Camargo PM, Melnick PR, Camargo LM. Clinical crown lengthening in the esthetic zone. J Calif Dent Assoc. 2007 Jul; 35(7):487-98.

37. Silverstein LH, Kurtzman GM, Kurtzman D, Shatz PC, Szikman R. Placing dental implants and/or natural tooth restorations in the aesthetic zone: achieving proper gingival contours. Dent Today. 2007 Jul;26(7):129-30, 132-5; quiz 135, 128.

38. Powell CA, Mealey BL, Deas DE, McDonnell HT, Moritz AJ. Post-surgical infections: prevalence associated with various periodontal surgical procedures. J Periodontol. 2005 Mar;76(3):329-33.

39. Kois J. Altering gingival levels: The restorative connection. Part 1: Biologic variables. J Esthet Dent. 1994 6:3-9.

40. Brett Dyer. Minimally Invasive Osseous Crown-Lengthening Procedure Using an Erbium Laser: Clinical Case and Procedure Report. The Journal of Cosmetic Dentistry. 2008 23(4):72-78.

41. Lee EA. Laser-assisted gingival tissue procedures in esthetic dentistry. Pract Proced Aesthet Dent. 2006 Oct; 18(9): suppl 2-6.

42. Pozner JM, Goldberg DJ. Histologic effect of a variable pulsed Er:Yag laser. Dermatol Surg. 2000 26:733-736.

43. Flax HD. Soft and hard tissue management using lasers in esthetic restoration. Dent Clin North Am. 2011 Apr;55(2):383-402, x.

44. Roshna T, Nandakumar K. Anterior esthetic gingival depigmentation and crown lengthening: report of a case. J Contemp Dent Pract. 2005 Aug 15; 6(3):139-47.

45. Goldman HM, Cohen DW, Periodontal Therapy. 4th ed. St. Louis, CV Mosby, 1968.

46. Volhansky A, Cleaton-Jones P, Fatti LP, A three-year longitudinal study of the position of the gingival margin in man. J Clin Periodontol. 1979 6:231-7.

47. Tjan AHL, Miller GD, The JG, Some esthetic factors in a smile. J Prosthet Dent. 1984 51: 24-8.

48. Coslet JG, Vanarsdall R, Weisgold A, Diagnosis and classification of delayed passive eruption of dentogingival junction in the adult. Alpha Omegan. 1977 70:24-30.

49. Lee EA. Aesthetic crown lengthening: classification, biologic rationale, and treatment planning considerations. Pract Proced Aesthet Dent. 2004 Nov-Dec; 16(10):769-78.

50. Bensimon GC. Surgical crown-lengthening procedure to enhance esthetics. Int J Periodontics Restorative Dent 1999; 19: 332-41.

51. Wagenberg BD. Surgical tooth lengthening: biologic variables and esthetic concerns. J Esthet Dent 1998 10: 30-6.

52. Spear FM, Cooney JP. Periodontal-restorative interrelationships. Carranza's clinical periodontology. 9th ed. 2002., Chap.75. p. 949-64.

53. Müler HP, Eger T. Masticatory mucosa and periodontal phenotype: a review. Int J Periodontics Restorative Dent 2002; 2:173-83.

54. Padbury Jr. A., Eber R. & Wang H-L. Interactions between the gingiva and the margin of restorations. J Clin Periodontol 2003; 30: 379-85.

55. Brägger U, Launchenauer D, Lang NP. Surgical crown lengthening of the clinical crown. J Clin Periodontol 1992; 19: 58-63.

56. Häkkinen L, Uitto VJ, Larjava H. Cell biology of gingival wound healing. Periodontology 2000; 24: 127-52.

Notes

_____

_____

_____

_____

_____

_____

_____

_____

_____

_____

_____

_____

_____

_____

_____

_____

_____

_____

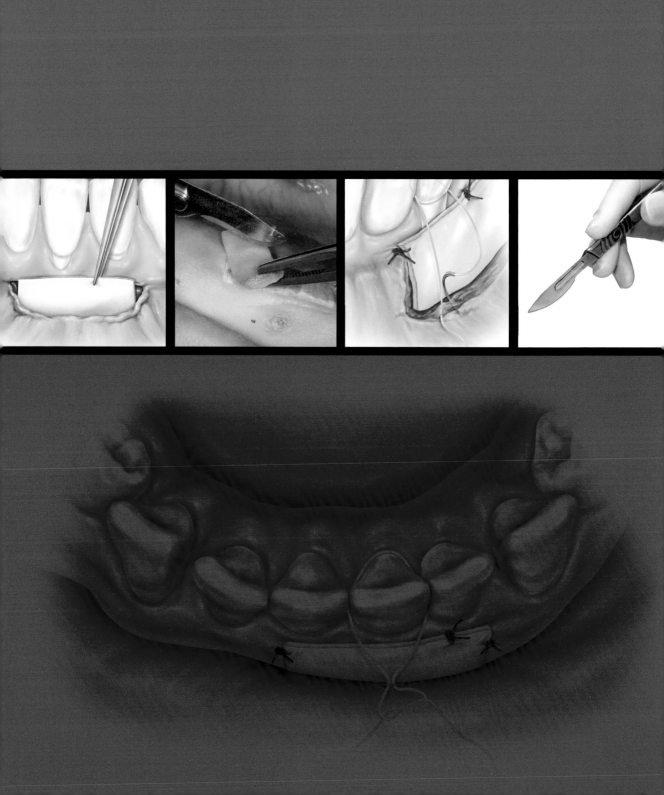

A free gingival graft is commonly used for treating gingival recessions and root exposures as well as to increase keratinized/attached gingiva, that portion of the gingival tissue that is thick, stippled, and firmly attached to the underlying periosteum, tooth, and bone. The procedure can be used to treat a single tooth or multiple teeth. The width of keratinized/attached gingiva varies in different areas of the mouth: it is greatest in the incisor region (4.5 mm–6.5 mm in the maxilla, 3.3 mm–3.9 mm in the mandible) and least in the 1st premolar area (1.9 mm in the maxilla, 1.8 mm in the mandible). A sufficient amount of attached gingival tissue is required for optimal periodontal function, health, and esthetics. Oral inflammation usually occurs in the areas where there is a lack of attached gingival tissue and less than optimal oral hygiene.

One example of the appropriate use of a free gingival graft is prior to a clinician's performing the facial orthodontic movement of a tooth which has minimal to no attached gingiva; in such cases, the clinician can use free gingival grafting to increase the width of the gingival tissue and to prevent recession of the gingival margin during or after the orthodontic treatment. In addition to increasing the width of keratinized and attached gingiva, free gingival grafting can also be used to treat severe physiologic gingival pigmentation,[1] though other methods for treating gingival pigmentation issues have also been documented, including electrosurgery, scalpel surgery, and surgical abrasion.[2] Graft thickness is one of the most important factors for the success of this procedure.[3-5] A minimum graft thickness of 1.5 mm to 2 mm is needed for a successful result. Additional factors that affect the outcome of the procedure include proper suturing techniques, adequate mechanical root preparation, and entrapment of a blood clot between the graft, the root surface, and adjacent soft-tissue recipient bed.

Limitations of free gingival grafting include the procedure's inability to achieve complete root coverage, the "tire patch" appearance of the healed site, and the need for a second surgical site to harvest the graft. Furthermore, a free gingival graft is not recommended in esthetic areas due to the "tire patch" appearance of the healed site; nor is the procedure recommended for root coverage of Miller Class III and Class IV recession defects or for coverage of tooth roots with narrow interproximal tissues due to the limited source of blood supply. Nevertheless, with the exception of such contraindications, for decades free gingival grafting has remained "a simple, predictable technique for increasing the zone of attached gingiva...[so] [d]entists interested in performing minor surgical procedures should include the free gingival graft in their armamentarium," provided that the clinician has considered a number of factors including "the width of the attached gingiva, the patient's age, recession history, oral hygiene practices, teeth involved, and dental records."[6]

History of Free Gingival Grafting

A free gingival graft is commonly used for treating gingival recessions. Gingival recession is the displacement of the gingival margin apical to the cementoenamel junction. The main causes of gingival recessions are restorations, trauma, inadequate oral hygiene, orthodontic movement, aberrant frenum pull, abnormal tooth position, bony dehiscence, thin marginal soft tissue, and bone loss secondary to periodontal disease.[7-20] Gingival recession occurs in more than 50% of the population.[21] Occurrence increases at age 13,[22-27] and it is estimated that by age 60, almost 90% of Americans will have at least one site with ≥1 mm of recession, and about 40% will have at least one site with ≥3 mm of gingival recession.[27]

In the absence of good oral hygiene, areas with untreated gingival recessions are at an increased risk for further recession. Prevention of further gingival recession is important to prevent further attachment loss and compromised function and esthetics.

Figure 5-1 **Free Gingival Graft Procedure**

a Incision at the mucogingival junction

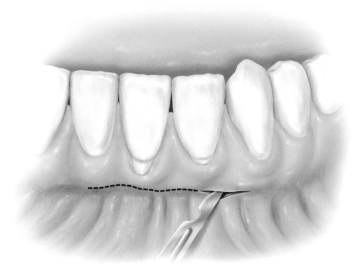

b Preparation of the recipient site ▼

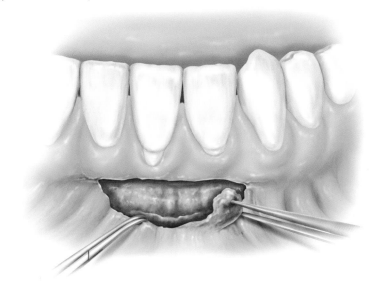

Figure 5-1 **Free Gingival Graft Procedure** (CONT.)

c Making a template as a guide to harvest the appropriate size graft

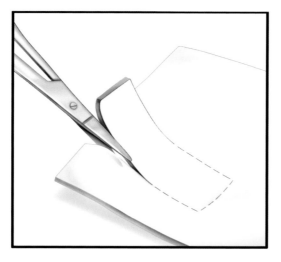

d Verifying the proper size of the needed graft with a template

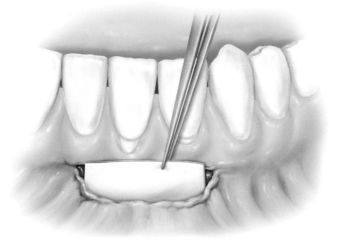

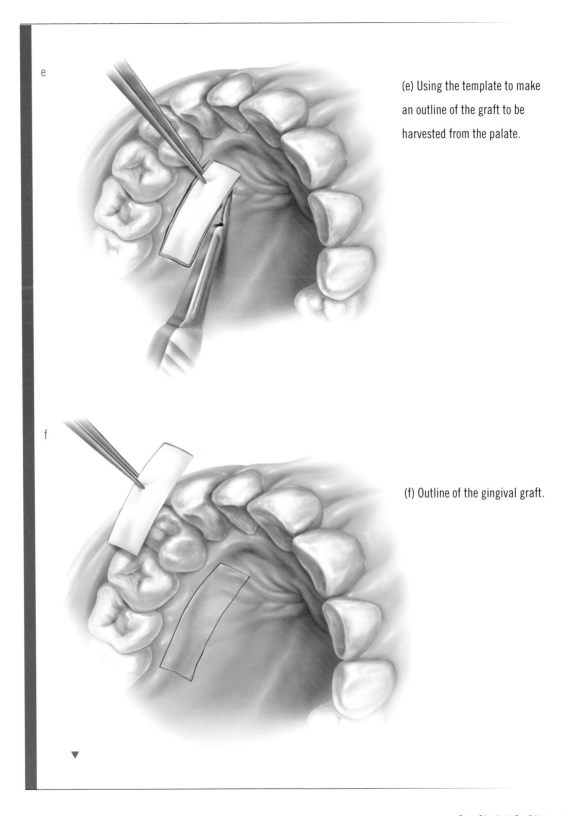

(e) Using the template to make an outline of the graft to be harvested from the palate.

(f) Outline of the gingival graft.

Figure 5-1 **Free Gingival Graft Procedure** (CONT.)

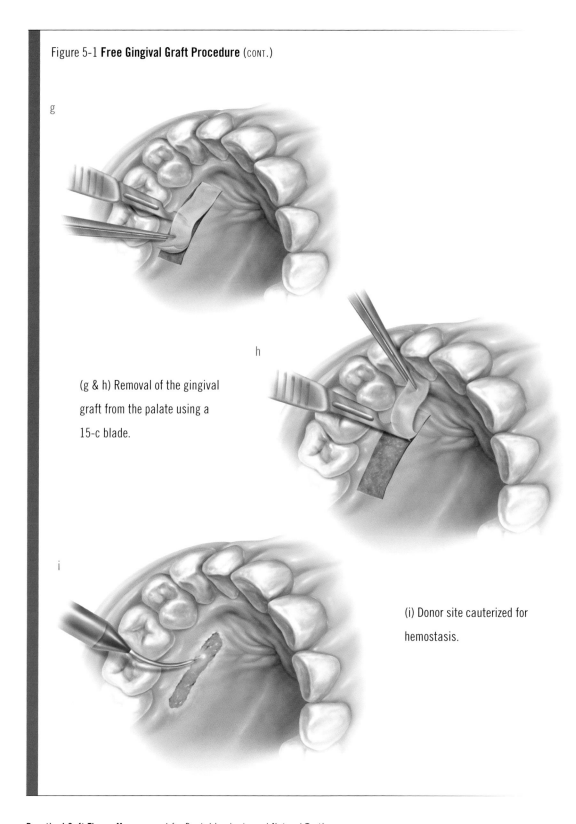

g

(g & h) Removal of the gingival graft from the palate using a 15-c blade.

h

(i) Donor site cauterized for hemostasis.

i

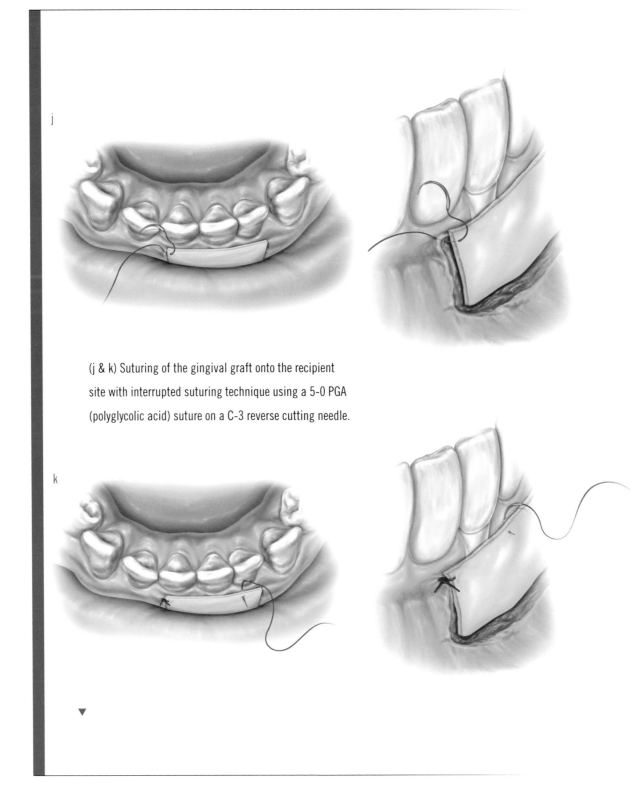

j

k

(j & k) Suturing of the gingival graft onto the recipient site with interrupted suturing technique using a 5-0 PGA (polyglycolic acid) suture on a C-3 reverse cutting needle.

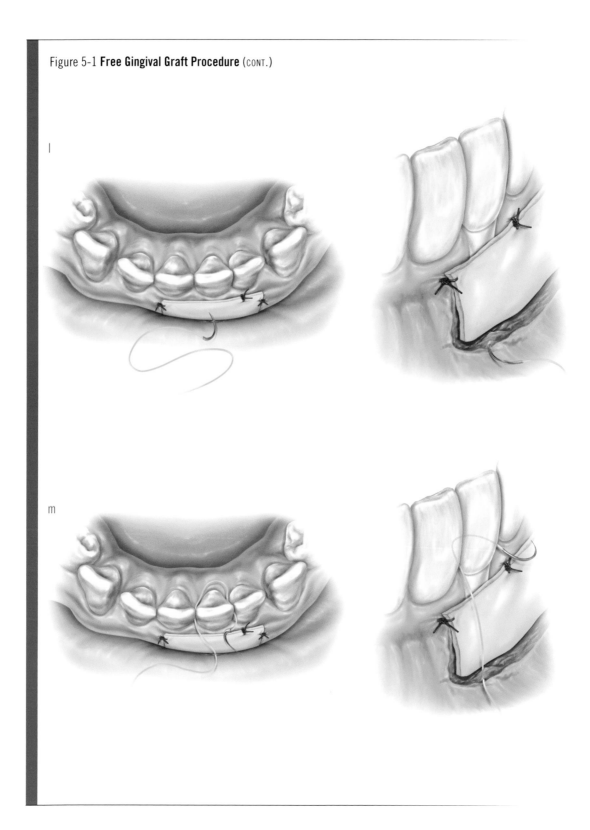

Figure 5-1 **Free Gingival Graft Procedure** (CONT.)

l

m

n

(l, m, n & o) Suturing of the free gingival graft onto the recipient site with a sling suture technique using a 4-0 PGA suture on a FS-2 reverse cutting needle. ■

o

Gingival recessions result in exposed root surfaces. Exposed root surfaces may be sensitive, are more susceptible to decay, and may be esthetically unappealing.

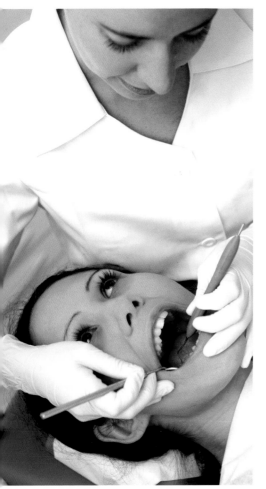

Free gingival grafting was first mentioned in 1963 by Dr. Hilding Bjorn, and it was later described by Sullivan and Atkins in 1968.[28] Studies conducted by Dordick et al., James and McFall, and Caffesse et al., reported the procedure to be an effective means of augmenting the gingival tissue.[29-32] Studies by Dorfman et al. demonstrated excellent predictability of free autogenous soft tissue graft in augmenting the zone of attached gingiva[33] and that non-grafted areas underwent further recessions compared to areas that were grafted.[34]

The procedure of free gingival grafting begins with preparation of the recipient site by supraperiosteal dissection; the epithelium, connective tissue, and muscle fibers are removed up to the level of the periosteum. The palate is usually the donor site from which the graft is harvested, and then grafted onto the recipient site. The ideal thickness of the graft should be at least between 0.75 mm to 1.25 mm, as suggested by studies performed by Soehren et al.[35] P.D. Miller found a thicker graft to be more appropriate for root coverage.[36]

Classification of Gingival Recession

Treatment of recession defects depends on the degree of recession. Gingival recessions can be classified in many ways. The ideal classification must take into consideration the important parameters that provide predictable guidelines to the clinician to help achieve complete root coverage.[17,37,38]

The classification provided by Sullivan and Atkins was based on the relation between vertical and horizontal defects and the relative importance of vertical and horizontal defect dimensions as predictors of final defect coverage. According to this classification, gingival recessions could be categorized as shallow narrow, shallow wide, deep narrow, and deep wide. This classification, although not widely used, still holds importance for clinicians performing complete root coverage. However, a more widely used classification was suggested by Miller using interproximal bone and soft tissue levels as determining factors in achieving complete root coverage.[17] Miller proposed that the level of marginal tissue recession in relation to the mucogingival junction and the level of the interproximal tissues are important predictors of procedure outcome.

According to Miller's classification, gingival recessions fall into one of the following four categories:

CLASS I - Marginal tissue recession of the gingival tissue does not extend to the mucogingival junction, and there is no loss of interdental bone or soft tissue.

CLASS II - Marginal tissue recession of the gingival tissue extends to or beyond the mucogingival junction, and there is no loss of interdental bone or soft tissue.

CLASS III - Marginal tissue recession of the gingiva extends to or beyond the mucogingival junction. In addition, there may be loss of interdental bone or soft tissue apical to the cementoenamel junction but coronal to the apical extent of the marginal tissue recession.

CLASS IV - Marginal tissue recession of the gingiva extends beyond the mucogingival junction, and there is a loss of interdental bone that extends to a level apical to the extent of marginal tissue recession.

According to this classification, complete root coverage is possible in Class I and Class II recession defects; however, only partial coverage can be expected with Class III defects. Class IV defects are not considered for free gingival grafting because root coverage may not be achieved.

Figure 5-2 **Step-by-Step Harvest of a Free Autogenous Gingival Graft on a Pig Jaw Model**

a

b

c

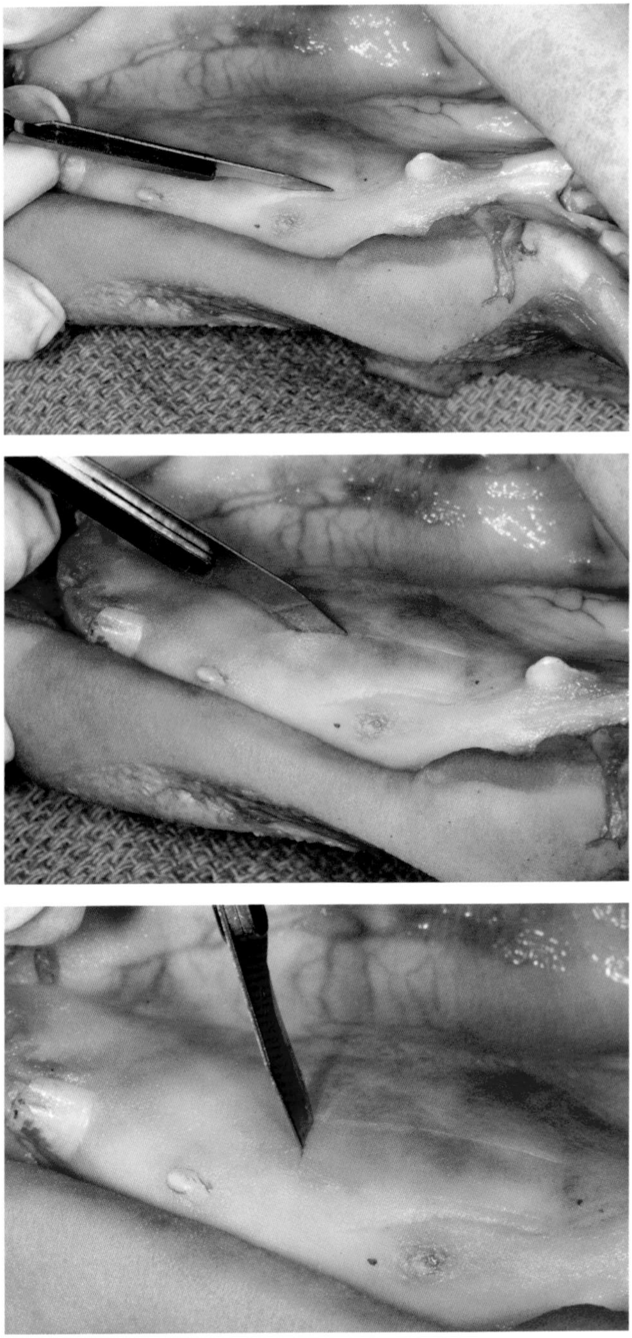

d

e

f

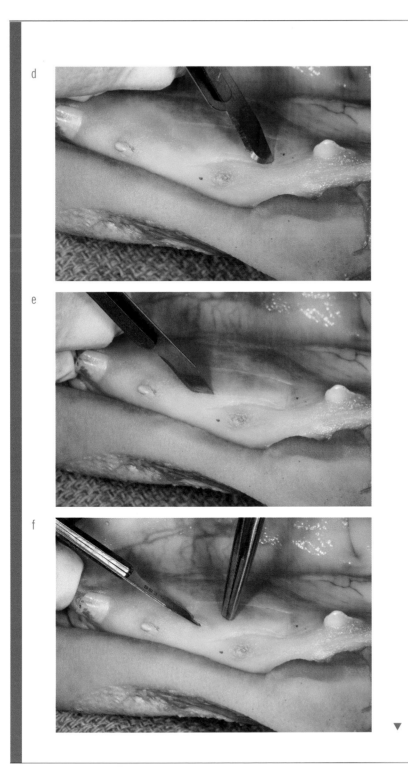

g

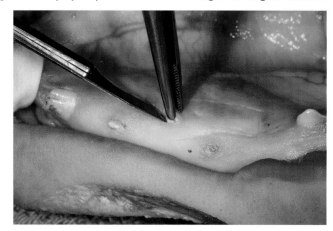

h

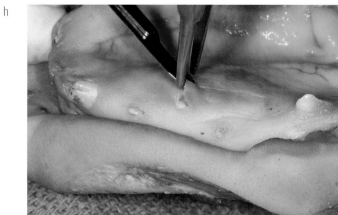

i

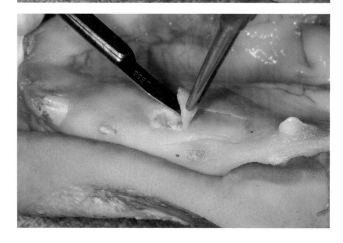

j

k

l

m

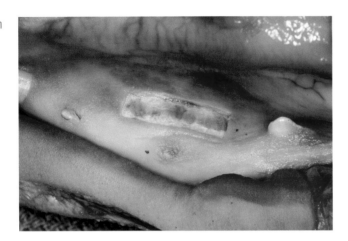

A 2010 study involving coverage of a denuded root in the lower molar area "with Miller Class III gingival recession" notes the "especially difficult" nature of such a grafting procedure, since "the recession has the additional complication of an inadequate zone of attached gingiva in association with frenal attachment;" the zone, however, was "successfully treated by a two-step procedure with an autogenous masticatory mucosal graft and a connective tissue graft."[39]

Smith suggested another classification which is unique in its thoroughness with respect to characterization of vertical and horizontal defect dimensions.[34] The new classification has a two figure Index of Recession, (F2-4*) in which the first digit refers to the proportional evaluation of the horizontal extent of gingival recession at the level of cementoenamel junction, and the second digit is the vertical extent of gingival recession from cementoenamel junction in millimeters. There is an asterisk that denotes involvement of the mucogingival junction. The prefixed F or L denotes whether gingival recession is facial or lingual to the involved root. The classification, however, does not provide predictive guidelines and is, therefore, most useful as an epidemiologic tool.

Techniques for Performing the Free Gingival Graft Procedure

Under local anesthesia, the recipient site is prepared by deepithelialization of the marginal gingiva and mucosa, and the exposed root is planed thoroughly with a Gracey curet (1-2, 5-6 or 7-8). A 1 mm-thick to 2 mm-thick free gingival graft is harvested from the palate opposite the premolar and first molar areas. The graft is sutured in place by means of interrupted sutures (5-0 polyglycolic acid sutures) at the coronal and apical corners. A noneugenol periodontal dressing is applied to both donor and recipient sites. Evidence suggests long-term stability (up to four years) for these treatment procedures.[40,41]

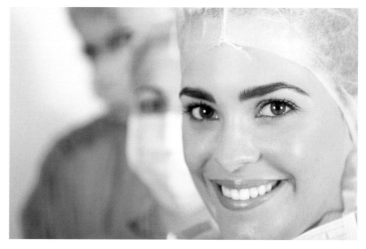

Although root coverage is not a primary goal of the free gingival graft procedure, it may occur when grafted tissue remains vital over the avascular zone of the root.[42] This condition occurs in cases of narrow recession (< 3 mm) as a result of bridging. Some root coverage may also result from another mechanism known as "creeping attachment," which was described by Goldman and Cohen as the "postoperative migration of the gingival marginal tissue in a coronal direction over portions of a previously denuded root."[43]

Several studies were conducted which reported that gingival grafts were more likely to revascularize and survive on an avascular root surface if they were comparatively thick.[36,44-49] The harvested free gingival graft should be at least 2 mm thick. Site preparation included butt joint margins between the papilla base and the graft at the level of the cementoenamel junction to facilitate graft revascularization.[36] A thick graft is found to be associated with good outcomes, but the procedure is technique sensitive. Revascularization of the graft is also found to be dependent on contact with an adequate amount of vascular base, 75% to 80%, which often requires a very large graft.[50,51]

The mean defect coverage in thick free gingival graft ranges from 39% to 100%.[46,52–56] After the procedure, final root exposure ranged from 0.0 to 1.8 mm, with a mean of 0.9 mm relative to mean initial recession of 3.2 mm. Two studies showed that 90% of the defect was covered 84% of the time.[46,53]

Variation of the Free Gingival Grafting Technique

In cases where a large area needs gingival augmentation, certain modified techniques can be adopted. The Strip Technique (Han et al.) and Vertical Strip Technique (Khoshkhoonejad et al.) are variations of the free gingival graft that can be used for areas involving three or more teeth.[57-59]

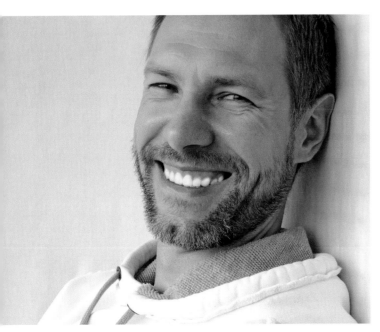

The Strip Technique maximally covers the recipient site with a graft while causing minimal trauma to the donor and/or recipient site. The technique requires a partial thickness flap with a stable periosteum. The apical mucosal border of the recipient site is sutured to the periosteum. The grafts from the donor site are harvested in 2 mm wide strips, transferred to the recipient site, and sutured.

For areas involving three or more teeth with shallow vestibule and short vertical alveolar bone height, the Modified Vertical Strip Technique is a good alternative to the free gingival graft procedure. In this technique, a wide and free gingival graft of about 7 mm to 9 mm is harvested from the palatal donor area and is divided longitudinally into two equal parts. The two pieces of graft are placed and fixed onto the recipient site and covered with a periodontal dressing. The division of the palatal gingival graft into two parts allows coverage of a wider recipient area. The study results showed significant increase in the width of attached gingiva with the use of less donor tissue.[60]

Creeping Attachment

Creeping attachment is the postoperative migration of the gingival marginal tissue in a coronal direction over portions of a previously denuded root. It is best observed in the mandibular anterior teeth with narrow areas of recessions.[43,61-66] Creeping attachments can be seen within one to twelve months after graft surgery with an average coverage of about 1 mm. However, creeping attachments may continue beyond the first postoperative year. The cases of creeping attachments reported in dental literature have usually involved unrestored mandibular anterior teeth in young adults.

Tissue Adhesives

Immobilization of the graft onto the recipient site is very important for revascularization of the tissue and growth of the gingiva. Tissue grafts are elastic and may be difficult to handle and immobilize. If immobilization is not performed properly, the graft may not adapt and would eventually undergo necrosis. Immobilization is usually accomplished through suturing, but the number of the sutures should be kept to a minimum to prevent unnecessary trauma to the graft tissue while still being sufficient to hold the graft in a stable and correct position. Suturing material may also cause foreign body reaction, which may damage the graft tissue.

Tissue adhesives were introduced as an alternative. Ardis introduced tissue adhesives in 1949.[67] In a study comparing butyl cyanoacrylates and silk sutures for immobilizing periodontal flaps, minimum edema and better gingival outcomes were noted with butyl cyanoacrylates.[68] In 1978, Hoxter introduced the concept of suture-free gingival grafting.[69] The concept was based on the fact that if the gingival graft is placed and fixed correctly on the recipient site, suturing may not be required. In the same year, Reatzke used tissue adhesives and reported 60% to 80% coverage of the localized root exposure with the palatal connective tissue.[70] Another study reported reduction of scar tissue formation by 38% with the use of tissue adhesives.[71] Tissue adhesives are hemostatic in nature, a characteristic which facilitates a blood-free area and better visual clarity for the procedure.

Epiglu is a commonly used cyanoacrylate-type tissue adhesive with numerous applications in periodontal surgeries. Many studies have suggested good clinical outcomes in graft surgeries with no adverse effects.[67-72] Epiglu is absorbed in the body and is eliminated via the lungs and urine. Some studies also confirmed that its products, namely Formaldehyde and Cyanoacetate, are not carcinogenic.[72,73]

Due to its strong bonding, hemostatic, and bacteriostatic properties, Epiglu facilitates healing within five to six days as compared to sutures that take seven to nine days to heal.[72-74]

A 2009 study compared the dimensional changes in free gingival grafts attached with ethyl cyanoacrylate and grafts attached with sutures.[75] The study included patients with gingival recession and an absence of keratinized mucosa, half of which (12) had free gingival grafts fixed with ethyl cyanoacrylate and the other half with sutures. A series of comparative criteria were evaluated over several time periods postoperatively, including immediately, and then from 15 days up to 90 days after surgery. The criteria of evaluation included "probing depth, clinical attachment level, gingival recession, and dimensional changes of height and width." Dimensional changes were similar for the two groups. The study concluded that "the thickness of the gingival graft tissue influenced the dimensional changes in the height of the grafts in the recipient bed (p < 0.047)...and that gingival grafts, thinner than 1 mm, showed a greater average height at the end of the study and with no significant changes regarding the total area of the graft." Most importantly, the study determined that "the modality of gingival graft fixation did not present any significant influence over the clinical parameters evaluated," and that "the use of ethyl cyanoacrylate did not alter the graft healing process, suggesting a possible alternative for free gingival graft fixation."[75]

Postoperative Instructions after Free Gingival Grafting

A periodontal dressing is placed on the recipient site to protect the area when the patient eats or brushes. An ice pack applied extraorally on the recipient site for the first 24 hours at 20-minute intervals will help minimize the swelling and bruising. The patient is advised to avoid drinking from a straw and spitting to minimize bleeding, especially from the donor site. The patient is placed on a cold and soft diet for the first 24 hours after surgery, and soft, regular temperature food for several days after. Smoking is strictly prohibited, and gentle light cleaning with a Q-tip dipped in alcohol-free chlorhexidine rinse twice a day is recommended.

A 2010 study concluded that "smoking alters FGG donor site wound healing by reducing immediate bleeding incidence and by delaying epithelialization, although it does not have discernible effects on postoperative FGG dimensional changes."[76]

Complications

Despite its simplicity and decades of predictability,[77] free gingival grafting is associated with a number of clinical complications,[78] including excessive bleeding from the donor site, failure of the graft to integrate, and esthetically unacceptable outcomes due to color mismatch of the donor tissue and the recipient site. Additionally, grafts may fail to integrate due to insufficient blood supply caused by wide areas of root exposure, improper graft adaptation, and premature graft movement. Vertical graft shrinkage can also affect the clinical outcomes of the free gingival graft procedure,[79] in addition to epithelial inclusion cysts and exostoses developing after the placement of a free gingival graft, which have also been reported.[80] The clinician considering root coverage of denuded tooth root surfaces should heed a 2005 study that compared histologic healing and clinical root coverage for free gingival grafts and other similar therapies (including pedicle flaps, subepithelial connective tissue grafts, acellular dermal matrix grafts, and guided tissue regeneration); this study concluded that subepithelial connective tissue grafts and guided tissue regeneration "should be considered the treatment of choice for root coverage.... [because] they are the most predictable with average root coverage as high as 98.9% and 92.3%, respectively."[82]

Summary

The free gingival graft is a predictable periodontal procedure to increase the amount of attached gingival tissue. However, achieving root coverage with this technique is often not very successful. The procedure is best suited for treating minor gingival recession. Care should be exercised in proper case selection, immobilization of the graft on the recipient site, and prevention of trauma to both the recipient and donor sites.

One of the most attractive features of this procedure is the high level of predictability in increasing the width of keratinized gingival tissue. While root coverage with the free gingival graft often does not produce successful results, these results might be improved by combining free gingival grafting with coronal repositioning of the augmented gingiva. Although the procedure is best suited for treating minor gingival recessions, the clinician should use his or her discretion when deciding the indications for the procedure. The factors to consider are the width of the attached gingiva, the patient's age, history of recession defect, hygiene practices, and the number of teeth involved. The choice of technique solely depends on the clinician's diagnosis of the recession defect and the clinician's experience in treating it.

References

1. Tamizi M, Taheri M. Treatment of severe physiologic gingival pigmentation with free gingival autograft. Quintessence Int. 1996 Aug;27(8):555-8.

2. Kasagani SK, Nutalapati R, Mutthineni RB. Esthetic depigmentation of anterior gingiva. A case series. N Y State Dent J. 2012 Apr;78(3):26-31.

3. Hatipoğlu H, Keçeli HG, Güncü GN, Sengün D, Tözüm TF. Vertical and horizontal dimensional evaluation of free gingival grafts in the anterior mandible: a case report series. Clin Oral Investig. 2007 Jun;11(2):107-13.

4. Wessel JR, Tatakis DN. Patient outcomes following subepithelial connective tissue graft and free gingival graft procedures. J Periodontol. 2008 Mar;79(3):425-30.

5. Thoma DS, Benić GI, Zwahlen M, Hämmerle CH, Jung RE. A systematic review assessing soft tissue augmentation techniques. Clin Oral Implants Res. 2009 Sep;20 Suppl 4:146-65.

6. Hall WB, Lundergan WP. Free gingival grafts. Current indications and techniques. Dent Clin North Am. 1993 Apr;37(2):227-42. Review.

7. Koke U, Sander C, Heinecke A, et al. A possible influence of gingival dimensions on attachment loss and gingival recession following placement of artificial crowns. Int J Periodontics Restorative Dent. 2003 Oct;23(5):439-45.

8. Khocht A, Simon G, Person P, Denepitiya JL. Gingival recession in relation to history of hard toothbrush use. J Periodontol. 1993 Sep;64(9):900-5.

9. Gorman WJ. Prevalence and etiology of gingival recession. J Periodontol. 1967 Jul-Aug;38(4):316-22.

10. Coatoam GW, Behrents RG, Bissada NF. The width of keratinized gingiva during orthodontic treatment: its significance and impact on periodontal status. J Periodontol. 1981 Jun;52(6):307-13.

11. Stoner JE, Mazdyasna S. Gingival recession in the lower incisor region of 15-year-old subjects. J Periodontol. 1980 Feb;51(2):74-6.

12. Ingervall B, Jacobsson U, Nyman S. A clinical study of the relationship between crowding of teeth, plaque and gingival condition. J Clin Periodontol. 1977 Aug;4(3):214-22.

13. Baker DL, Seymour GJ. The possible pathogenesis of gingival recession. A histological study of induced recession in the rat. J Clin Periodontol. 1976 Nov;3(4):208-19.

14. Gartrell JR, Mathews DP. Gingival recession. The condition, process, and treatment. Dent Clin North Am. 1976 Jan;20(1):199-213.

15. Sognnaes RF. Periodontal significance of intraoral frictional ablation. J West Soc Periodontol Periodontal Abstr. 1977; 25(3):112-21.

16. Hoag PM. Isolated areas of gingival recession: etiology and treatment. CDS Rev. 1979 May;72(5):27-34.

17. Smith RG. Gingival recession. Reappraisal of an enigmatic condition and a new index for monitoring. J Clin Periodontol. 1997 Mar;24(3):201-5. Review.

18. Prato GP, Rotundo R, Magnani C, Ficarra G. Viral etiology of gingival recession. A case report. J Periodontol. 2002 Jan;73(1):110-4.

19. Pradeep K, Rajababu P, Satyanarayana D, Sagar V. Gingival recession: review and strategies in treatment of recession. Case Rep Dent. 2012;2012:563421. doi: 10.1155/2012/563421. Epub 2012 Oct 2.

20. Chambrone L, Sukekava F, Araújo MG, Pustiglioni FE, Chambrone LA, Lima LA. Root coverage procedures for the treatment of localised recession-type defects. Cochrane Database Syst Rev. 2009 Apr 15;(2):CD007161. doi: 10.1002/14651858.CD007161.pub2. Review.

21. Kassab MM, Cohen RE. The etiology and prevalence of gingival recession. J Am Dent Assoc. 2003 Feb;134(2):220-5.

22. Löe H, Anerud A, Boysen H. The natural history of periodontal disease in man: prevalence, severity, and extent of gingival recession. J Periodontol. 1992 Jun; 63(6):489-95.

23. O'Leary TJ, Drake RB, Crump PP, Allen MF. The incidence of recession in young males: a further study. J Periodontol. 1971 May;42(5):264-7.

24. Tenenbaum H. A clinical study comparing the width of attached gingiva and the prevalence of gingival recessions. J Clin Periodontol. 1982 Jan;9(1):86-92.

25. Serino G, Wennström JL, Lindhe J, Eneroth L. The prevalence and distribution of gingival recession in subjects with a high standard of oral hygiene. J Clin Periodontol. 1994 Jan;21(1):57-63.

26. Oliver RC, Brown LJ, Löe H. Periodontal diseases in the United States population. J Periodontol. 1998 Feb;69(2):269-78.

27. Albandar JM, Kingman A. Gingival recession, gingival bleeding, and dental calculus in adults 30 years of age and older in the United States, 1988-1994. J Periodontol. 1999 Jan;70(1):30-43.

28. Sullivan HC, Atkins JH. Free autogenous gingival grafts. I. Principles of successful grafting. Periodontics. 1968 Jun;6(3):121-9.

29. Dordick B, Coslet JG, Seibert JS. Clinical evaluation of free autogenous gingival grafts placed on alveolar bone. Part I. Clinical predictability. J Periodontol. 1976 Oct;47(10):559-67.

30. James WC, McFall WT Jr. Placement of free gingival grafts on denuded alveolar bone. Part I: clinical evaluations. J Periodontol. 1978 Jun;49(6):283-90.

31. James WC, McFall WT Jr, Burkes EJ. Placement of free gingival grafts on denuded alveolar bone. Part II: microscopic observations. J Periodontol. 1978 Jun;49(6):291-300.

32. Caffesse RG, Burgett FG, Nasjleti CE, Castelli WA. Healing of free gingival grafts with and without periosteum. Part I. Histologic evaluation. J Periodontol. 1979 Nov; 50(11):586-94.

33. Dorfman HS, Kennedy JE, Bird WC. Longitudinal evaluation of free autogenous gingival grafts. J Clin Periodontol. 1980 Aug;7(4):316-24.

34. Dorfman HS, Kennedy JE, Bird WC. Longitudinal evaluation of free autogenous gingival grafts. A four year report. J Periodontol. 1982 Jun;53(6):349-52.

35. Soehren SE, Allen AL, Cutright DE, Seibert JS. Clinical and histologic studies of donor tissues utilized for free grafts of masticatory mucosa. J Periodontol. 1973 Dec;44(12):727-41.

36. Miller PD Jr. Root coverage using a free soft tissue autograft following citric acid application. Part 1: Technique. Int J Periodontics Restorative Dent. 1982;2(1):65-70.

37. Miller PD Jr. A classification of marginal tissue recession. Int J Periodontics Restorative Dent. 1985;5(2):8-13.

38. Volpe AR, Triratana T, Rustogi KN. Development of a system to assess visible and hidden gingival recession. J Clin Dent. 1991; 3 Suppl B:B1-5.

39. Park JB. A two-stage approach using an autogenous masticatory mucosal graft and an autogenous connective tissue graft to treat gingival recession: a case report. J Int Acad Periodontol. 2010 Apr;12(2):45-8.

40. Sullivan HC, Atkins JH. The role of free gingival grafts in periodontal therapy. Dent Clin North Am. 1969 Jan;13(1):133-48.

41. Oringer RJ, Iacono VJ. Current periodontal plastic procedures around teeth and dental implants. N Y State Dent J. 1999 Jun-Jul;65(6):26-31. Review.

42. Goldman HM, Cohen DW. Periodontal therapy. 5th ed. St. Louis: C.V. Mosby Co.; 1973. p. 715-8.

43. Mlinek A, Smukler H, Buchner A. The use of free gingival grafts for the coverage of denuded roots. J Periodontol. 1973 Apr;44(4):248-54.

44. Miller PD Jr. Root coverage using the free soft tissue autograft following citric acid application. II. Treatment of the carious root. Int J Periodontics Restorative Dent. 1983;3(5):38-51.

45. Miller PD Jr. Root coverage using the free soft tissue autograft following citric acid application. III. A successful and predictable procedure in areas of deep-wide recession. Int J Periodontics Restorative Dent. 1985; 5(2):14-37.

46. Miller PD Jr, Binkley LH Jr. Root coverage and ridge augmentation in Class IV recession using a coronally positioned free gingival graft. J Periodontol. 1986 Jun;57(6):360-3.

47. Holbrook T, Ochsenbein C. Complete coverage of the denuded root surface with a one-stage gingival graft. Int J Periodontics Restorative Dent. 1983;3(3):8-27.

48. Bertrand PM, Dunlap RM. Coverage of deep, wide gingival clefts with free gingival autografts: root planing with and without citric acid demineralization. Int J Periodontics Restorative Dent. 1988;8(1):64-77.

49. Goldstein M, Brayer L, Schwartz Z. A critical evaluation of methods for root coverage. Crit Rev Oral Biol Med. 1996;7(1):87-98. Review.

50. Breault LG, Fowler EB, Billman MA. Retained free gingival graft rugae: a 9-year case report. J Periodontol. 1999 Apr;70(4):438-40.

51. Müller HP, Eger T. Masticatory mucosa and periodontal phenotype: a review. Int J Periodontics Restorative Dent. 2002 Apr;22(2):172-83. Review.

52. Borghetti A, Gardella JP. Thick gingival autograft for the coverage of gingival recession: a clinical evaluation. Int J Periodontics Restorative Dent. 1990; 10(3):216-29.

53. Laney JB, Saunders VG, Garnick JJ. A comparison of two techniques for attaining root coverage. J Periodontol. 1992 Jan; 63(1):19-23.

54. Jahnke PV, Sandifer JB, Gher ME, Gray JL, Richardson AC. Thick free gingival and connective tissue autografts for root coverage. J Periodontol. 1993 Apr;64(4):315-22.

55. Paolantonio M, di Murro C, Cattabriga A, Cattabriga M. Subpedicle connective tissue graft versus free gingival graft in the coverage of exposed root surfaces. A 5-year clinical study. J Clin Periodontol. 1997 Jan;24(1):51-6.

56. Greenwell H, Bissada NF, Henderson RD, Dodge JR. The deceptive nature of root coverage results. J Periodontol. 2000 Aug;71(8):1327-37.

57. Han TJ, Takei HH, Carranza FA. The strip gingival autograft technique. Int J Periodontics Restorative Dent. 1993; 13(2):180-7.

58. Khoshkhoonejad A. A., Akbari S. Vertical strip gingival graft: a new technique for gingival augmentation. A pilot study. Journal of Dentistry, Tehran University of Medical Sciences 2004; Vol. 1, (2): 5-10.

59. Popova C, Boyarova T. Mucogingival surgery with free gingival graft (strip technique) for augmentation of the attached gingival tissues: report of three cases. Journal of IMAB - Annual Proceeding (Scientific Papers), 2007, book 2.

60. Bernimoulin JP, Lüscher B, Mühlemann HR. Coronally repositioned periodontal flap. Clinical evaluation after one year. J Clin Periodontol. 1975 Feb;2(1):1-13.

61. Livingston HL. Total coverage of multiple and adjacent denuded root surfaces with a free gingival autograft. A case report. J Periodontol. 1975 Apr;46(4):209-16.

62. Bell LA, Valluzzo TA, Garnick JJ, Pennel BM. The presence of "creeping attachment" in human gingiva. J Periodontol. 1978 Oct;49(10):513-7.

63. Pollack RP. Bilateral creeping attachment using free mucosal grafts. A case report with 4-year follow-up. J Periodontol. 1984 Nov;55(11):670-2.

64. de Castro LA, Vêncio EF, Mendonça EF. Epithelial inclusion cyst after free gingival graft: a case report. Int J Periodontics Restorative Dent. 2007 Oct;27(5):465-9.

65. Chambrone LA, Chambrone L. Bony exostoses developed subsequent to free gingival grafts: case series. Br Dent J. 2005 Aug 13; 199(3):146-9.

66. Echeverria JJ, Montero M, Abad D, Gay C. Exostosis following a free gingival graft. J Clin Periodontol. 2002 May; 29(5):474-7.

67. Ardis, A. U.S. patent number 2467927. 1949.

68. Binnie WH, Forrest JO. A study of tissue response to cyanoacrylate adhesive in periodontal surgery. J Periodontol. 1974 Aug;45:619-25.

69. Hoxter DL. The sutureless free gingival graft. J Periodontol. 1979 Feb;50(2): 75-78.

70. Raetzke PB. Covering localized areas of root exposure employing the "envelope" technique. J Periodontol. 1985 Jul;56(7):397-402.

71. Coover H, Joyner F, Shearer N. Chemistry and performance of cyanoacrylate adhesives. J Soc Plast Surg Eng. 1959;15:5.

72. Herod EL. Cyanoacrylate in dentistry. J Can Assoc. 1990 Apr;56(4): 331-34.

73. Fegler F, Fegler K. Results of a study with the tissue adhesive Epiglu. Munster, Germany 1993.

74. Paknejad M, Soleymani Shayesteh Y, Esmaielieh A. Free Gingival Grafting; Epiglu VS. Silk Thread Suturing: A Comparative Study. Journal of Dentistry, Tehran University of Medical Sciences, Tehran, Iran 2004; Vol. 1, No. 2.

75. Barbosa FI, Corrêa DS, Zenóbio EG, Costa FO, Shibli JA. Dimensional changes between free gingival grafts fixed with ethyl cyanoacrylate and silk sutures. J Int Acad Periodontol. 2009 Apr;11(2):170-6.

76. Silva CO, Ribeiro Edel P, Sallum AW, Tatakis DN. Free gingival grafts: graft shrinkage and donor-site healing in smokers and non-smokers. J Periodontol. 2010 May; 81(5):692-701.

77. Agudio G, Nieri M, Rotundo R, Cortellini P, Pini Prato G. Free gingival grafts to increase keratinized tissue: a retrospective long-term evaluation (10 to 25 years) of outcomes. J Periodontol. 2008 Apr;79(4):587-94.

78. Brasher WJ, Rees TD, Boyce WA. Complications of free grafts of masticatory mucosa. J Periodontol. 1975 Mar;46(3):133-8.

79. Efeoglu A, Demirel K. A further report of bony exostosis occurring as a sequel to free gingival grafts. Periodontal Clin Investig. 1994 Spring;16(1):20-2.

80. Visser H, Mausberg R. Free gingival grafts using a CO_2 laser: results of a clinical study. J Clin Laser Med Surg. 1996 Apr;14(2):85-8.

81. Hernández G, Lopez-Pintor RM, Arriba L, Torres J, De Vicente JC. Failure of free connective tissue grafts caused by recurrent herpes simplex virus type 1 infection. J Oral Maxillofac Surg. 2011 Jan;69(1):217-21.

82. Sedon CL, Breault LG, Covington LL, Bishop BG. The subepithelial connective tissue graft: part II. Histologic healing and clinical root coverage. J Contemp Dent Pract. 2005 May 15;6(2):139-50. Review.

Notes

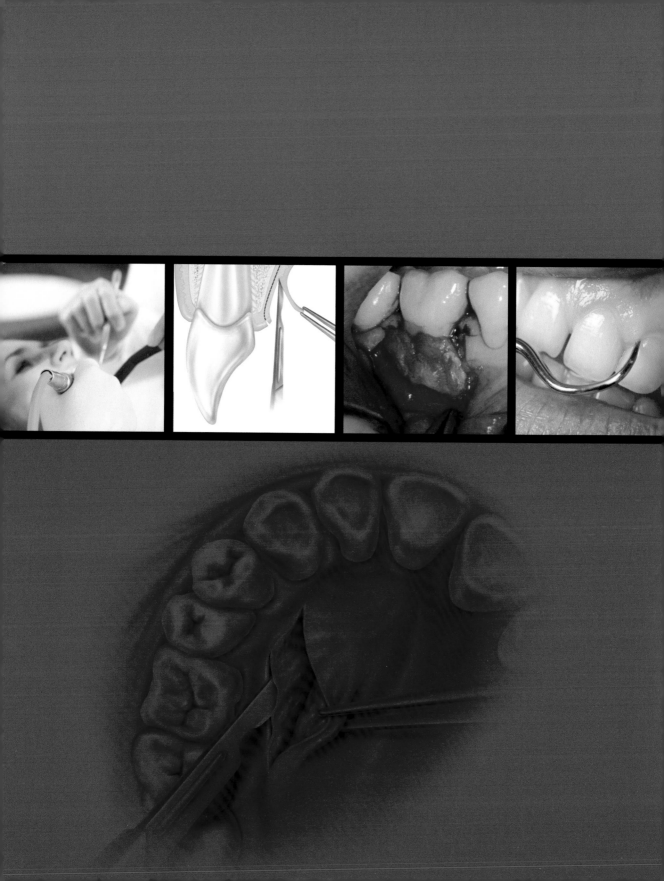

Subepithelial Connective Tissue Graft

The subepithelial connective tissue graft, a highly predictable procedure, was developed to overcome the esthetic limitations of the free gingival graft. The procedure involves removing a connective tissue layer from the donor site, usually the palate, leaving the overlying epithelial flap intact, thus helping to achieve primary closure and faster healing. The harvested connective tissue is then secured onto the recipient site and covered by a partial thickness flap. The resulting dual blood supply from the periosteum and overlying flap allows for better graft survival and integration, resulting in increased predictability of success. In addition to being associated with excellent esthetic outcomes, the subepithelial connective tissue graft procedure provides a smaller donor site wound and therefore can be used for treating both single and multiple-recession defects. However, this subepithelial connective tissue graft is very technique sensitive and surgically more demanding and time consuming than the free gingival graft. Thus, these challenges balance the advantages of the former procedure over the latter.

Histological evaluations of healing and revascularization of the subepithelial connective tissue graft have shown that the vascularization of the connective tissue graft originates from the periodontal plexus, supraperiosteal plexus, and overlying flap. A combination of epithelial downgrowth and connective tissue attachment is considered to be responsible for the attachment of the graft to the root surface.[1,2] The area of the hard palate (palatal to the premolars) is the most common site used to harvest the subepithelial connective tissue graft. When compared to other sites like the tuberosity region or an edentulous ridge, this area is associated with fewer complications.[1,3-13] Some studies have shown that the use of a freeze-dried connective tissue graft can effectively increase the zone of attached keratinized gingiva.[3] One study demonstrated that subepithelial connective tissue graft in conjunction with a coronally advanced flap is effective in covering multiple gingival recessions localized in the maxillary arch.[3] A 2013 study sought to examine the efficacy of using recombinant growth factor technology to facilitate the subepithelial connective tissue graft used in conjunction with coronally advanced flaps. The study concluded that "the addition of rhPDGF-BB appeared to improve early wound healing."[14] A 2012 study, by contrast, determined that plasma rich in growth factor did not appear to enhance the otherwise positive clinical outcome of subepithelial connective tissue grafting.[15] In some areas, however, such as the mandibular incisor region, root coverage may be quite a challenge due to a high frenum attachment, the presence of a shallow vestibule, and insufficient gingival tissue. These factors may compromise the blood supply and cause excessive flap tension. The close root proximity and thin interproximal bone in the mandibular incisor region result in the presence of little or no interdental papilla that can be used for flap design and suturing.

History of the Subepithelial Connective Tissue Graft

The connective tissue graft was first used by Edel, Broome, Taggart, and Donn to increase the width of keratinized gingiva.[16-18] Histological results of a study by Edel showed healed grafted sites with the characteristics of a fully keratinized tissue.[16] Two cases reported by Broome and Taggart using free autogenous connective tissue graft reported a clinically significant increase in the width of attached gingiva.[17,18] They also suggested in their reports that the primary flap at the donor site must have a broad base with adequate vascular supply to prevent subsequent necrosis and postoperative discomfort.

In 1985, Langer and Langer first described the subepithelial connective tissue graft technique to cover gingival recessions of both single and multiple adjacent teeth.[4] They employed a bilaminar technique, using a combination of connective tissue and epithelium harvested from the inside of a palatal flap and placed under a partial thickness flap over a denuded root. This process was designed specifically for wide multiple recessions frequently found in the maxilla. The palatal donor site healed

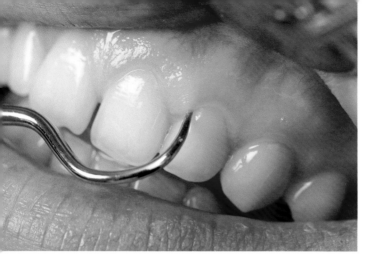

with less discomfort because of a smaller wound. The study reported achieving 2 mm to 6 mm of root coverage in 56 cases over four years with minimal sulcus depth and no recurrence of recession. It resulted in a closer color blend of the graft with adjacent tissue. This bilaminar procedure combines the features of the free gingival graft and the pedicle graft. In the latter procedure, the clinician grafts tissue not from the palate of the patient but from gingival area in close proximity to the root needing coverage. The flap (or "pedicle") from the patient with a good supply of gingiva is partially removed from the donor area site, so that it is still attached to the gingiva before the clinician sutures the flap into place to cover the exposed tooth root. Reatzk described a pouch procedure similar to Langer and Langer's technique but without vertical incisions. This technique involved excising some marginal tissue during the split thickness pouch preparation, followed by placement of the graft into the pouch. Surgical adhesive was used instead of sutures to immobilize the graft.[5-7]

The supraperiosteal envelope or "tunnel" and coronally positioned envelope were later described by Allen.[9,10] The free gingival graft procedure requires a large and thick graft for root coverage; by contrast, a connective tissue graft procedure shows effective root coverage with both thin and thick grafts when covered by a coronally positioned flap.[19] Many authors have reported a mean defect coverage ranging from 57% to 98%.[5,7, 8,10,20-22] For a mean initial recession of 3.7 mm, the achieved final root exposure after connective tissue grafting was reported to be 0.1 mm to 1.7 mm. Predictability data from studies demonstrated that 90% or greater defect coverage was achieved 68% of the time.[7,10,20,23-28]

Subepithelial Connective Tissue Graft Procedure

Despite the many techniques employed for subepithelial connective tissue grafting, the basic procedure remains the same in practice. It is performed in the following stages:

1. The recipient site is prepared by the clinician's planing and scaling the exposed root surfaces, and a split thickness flap is created.

2. The connective tissue graft is harvested from the palate. Parallel incisions are made to create an internal flap approximately 1.5 mm thick and of appropriate length for the recipient site, and from which the graft is removed by incising each end and the base internally. The trapdoor method involves raising a rectangular epithelial flap, removing the underlying connective tissue, and repositioning and suturing the epithelial flap.

3. The connective tissue graft is placed onto the recipient site and sutured.

4. The split thickness flap is sutured over the graft.

For deeper recessions, a coronally positioned flap can be raised to provide better coverage and to enhance blood supply to the graft.[29,30]

Nelson presented another modification of the technique called the subpedicle connective tissue graft, which was later modified by Harris.[6,7] The aim of these modifications was to increase the blood supply to the graft just over the root surface. Placing a double papilla flap over the recipient area was found to enhance the blood supply. Contrary to the approach used by Langer, this approach advocated the graft to be completely covered.

The "envelope technique" is another version of the connective tissue graft.[5] In this procedure, the connective tissue graft is obtained from the palate in such a way that only a narrow surface defect is created. The graft is then placed directly on the denuded root surface while its major part is inserted into an envelope that is created in the tissue around the denuded root surface with an undermining partial thickness incision so that the connective tissue graft completely covers the formerly exposed root area. The procedure showed average root coverage of 80%, of which 5% of the cases achieved total coverage. There was also a significant gain in keratinized gingiva. This procedure, however, is indicated only in cases of single tooth recession.

Vergara and Caffese demonstrated excellent root coverage and an increased amount of keratinized gingiva with the envelope technique. The complete root coverage mean was 85%, 65%, and 16% for recession Class I, II, and IV, respectively.[31] Becker and Becker suggested that the connected tissue graft can be simultaneously performed while treating other areas of the mouth with flap surgery.[32] Localized gingival recession was treated simultaneously with the surgical treatment of maxillary posterior region. This technique provides a conservative method for harvesting donor connective tissue and accomplishes the results of two separate surgical procedures at one time.

Ouhayoun, Khattab, and Serfaty conducted a study to determine the clinical use and histology of chemically separated connective tissue graft in the treatment of gingival recession.[33] A chemically separated connective tissue graft healed uneventfully similar to the surgically separated connective tissue graft. On histological evaluation, deep projections of epithelium into the connective tissue, with different morphological appearances, were observed. It was believed that these projections developed at the junction between the gingival flap and the transplanted connective tissue.

Harris described a technique for obtaining root coverage using the connective tissue graft and partial thickness double-pedicle graft.[34] After 12 weeks of treatment, it was found that mean root coverage could be accomplished in a predictable manner. Bruno presented some modifications of the original Langer and Langer technique for root coverage on areas of wide denudation.[11] He suggested that the mesiodistal length of the incision could be extended to provide easy access to the denuded root area without the use of vertical incisions. Two incisions were made following this technique without the use of vertical incisions at the palatal donor site to procure the connective tissue graft. This approach minimized the postoperative sequelae and promoted more rapid healing.

Bouchard compared the clinical and esthetic effects of two techniques of connective tissue graft for root coverage that differed with respect to the use of epithelial collar of the graft.[35] After a six month follow-up, it was found that both the procedures could accomplish root surface coverage in Class I and Class II recessions with reasonable esthetic results. It was concluded that removal of epithelial collar gives better esthetic results. However, when larger augmentation of keratinized tissue is required, the preferred technique is the connective tissue graft with the preserved epithelial collar.

A 2011 study by Ramakrishan and others concluded that "subepithelial connective tissue graft with embossed epithelium [can be] used to cover Miller's class II gingival recession in the upper right canine. They noted that the "embossed epithelium exactly fits the recession site and the connective tissue portion is tucked below the gingival margin of the recipient site." They also concluded that the "coronal advancement of flap is not needed...[and that a] [w]ider zone of attached gingiva at the recipient site was achieved by this technique."[36]

Allen, in a modification of Raetzke's technique, described the Tunnel or Supraperiosteal envelope technique made without horizontal or vertical incisions.[9] In sites with two adjacent recessions, a tunnel underneath the interproximal papilla is created and the connective tissue graft is drawn through the tunnel and sutured to the recipient bed. The technique permits conservation of existing gingiva, minimal surgical trauma to the recipient area, firm fixation of the connective tissue graft, and coverage of multiple adjacent areas of recession. The intimate coadaptation of the bilaminar soft tissue complex thus achieved may facilitate graft survival and postoperative blending of soft tissues.

Azzi and others described a surgical technique for simultaneous root coverage and papilla reconstruction.[37] A coronally positioned flap with subepithelial connective tissue was placed under the flap in the interdental area between the involved teeth. There was a gain of 4 mm soft tissue height interdentally with this technique. The authors suggested that the connective tissue graft would provide bulk and flap support and thus aid in maintaining a more coronal position of the papilla during healing.

Harris conducted a histological examination of the results obtained with a connective tissue graft combined with a partial thickness, double pedicle graft.[38] Two different healing patterns were observed. The first was characterized by a long junctional epithelial attachment that extended well beyond the original gingival margin and occasionally almost to the original bone level with minimal connective tissue adjacent to the tooth. The other pattern was a short junctional epithelium that stopped at the previously exposed root surface. There was connective tissue adjacent to the tooth with some isolated areas of epithelium. New bone growth and cementum

Figure 6-1 **Palatal Donor Site**

Epithelium

Connective Tissue

Adipose Tissue

Periosteum

Palatal Bone

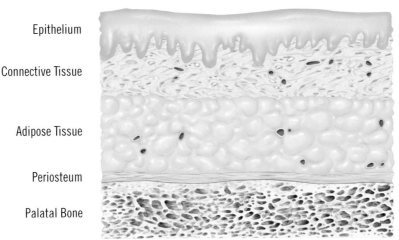

were also observed. The study concluded that though the procedure was successful clinically, it produced no true regeneration but instead healed only through repair.

One study described a surgical periodontal plastic procedure for the coverage of multiple adjacent gingival recessions. It involved creating a tunnel under the gingival tissue and using a sulcular incision beyond the mucogingival line but without raising the papillae. A large palatal connective tissue graft is introduced through this tunnel, covering the adjacent gingival recessions. It is sutured in such a way that it permits the graft to slip through the tunnel under the gingival tissues and also stabilizes the graft covering the recession. In 66.7% of the recessions treated, 100% root coverage was achieved. The procedure helps in coverage of multiple recessions with sufficient early healing and predictable root coverage.[8]

Riberiro and others described use of subepithelial connective tissue graft with the tunnel technique to treat multiple gingival recessions. They also described a technique used to enlarge the extension of the graft. The technique was effective in treatment of multiple recession defects and also resulted in an increase of the soft tissue volume and gain of keratinized tissue.[39] Tozum described the long-term results of root coverage with subepithelial connective tissue grafts and modified tunnel technique.[40] In cases where there is frenectomy expected, aberrant frenal attachments in the area of the recession should be eliminated 4 weeks to 6 weeks prior to grafting. Otherwise,

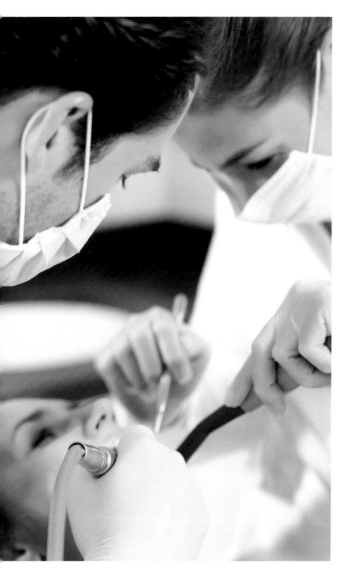

incisions made during the frenectomy could compromise blood flow to the flap and the success of the graft.[9] Langer and Langer also suggest removing cervical restorations to allow thorough scaling and root planing during the procedure.[41] One study described the use of an autogenous connective tissue graft soaked with platelet-rich plasma which was found to be effective in the treatment of shallow gingival recession.[42]

Root Conditioning

Root conditioning is an important part of the subepithelial connective tissue graft procedure. Similar to the practice in gingival grafting, roots are exposed to root conditioners before the clinician places the grafts. Langer and Langer suggested use of citric acid and tetracycline for root conditioning of endodontically-treated teeth or roots with a glass-like finish.[4,6] Generally, citric acid, tetracycline, and (more recently) Enamel Matrix Derivatives are applied to root surfaces before placement of the connective tissue. Current studies to evaluate the effectiveness of root conditioners have yielded mixed results.

Citric acid is the most widely-used root conditioner. Studies suggest that its use helps to remove microorganisms and their toxins, along with the smear layer. In addition, it is also thought to expose the collagen matrix and biologically active proteins and growth factors on the root that help in attachment of the graft.[43] A study completed by Register and Burdick indicated that citric acid accelerates soft tissue attachment to the root.[44]

Other studies also report that treatment with citric acid enhances development of connective tissue attachment. There is another school of thought which believes that citric acid has no contributory effect on roots. Caffesse and others and Bouchard and others found that root treatment with citric acid had no effect on root coverage.[45,46]

In one study, Miller suggested that citric acid for root treatment should be applied before incisions are made because it can compromise the blood supply of the graft by coagulation.[47] Tetracycline is another option for root conditioning. Studies reported that root conditioning with tetracycline inhibits microorganisms and collagenases, decreases bone resorption, enhances development of attachment gain, increases collagen formation, aids binding of fibronectin to dentin, and facilitates opening of the dentinal tubules.[48-53] However, in another study Labahn and others demonstrated that as compared to tetracycline, citric acid could induce larger dentinal tubules and deeper penetration.[54] Another study reported that tetracycline was not as effective as citric acid in demineralizing dentin.[55] Bouchard and others reported that tetracycline and citric acid had similar effects on subepithelial connective tissue grafts.[46] Erdinç and others demonstrated that tetracycline had no clinically noticeable benefits in subepithelial connective tissue grafting.[56] Zaman and others, in a study involving citric acid, EDTA, and tetracycline demonstrated that as compared to citric acid and EDTA, tetracycline had no effect on periodontal ligament cell attachment to root surfaces.[57]

Enamel matrix derivatives, or Emdogain, are another class of root conditioners. They are protein complexes consisting predominantly of amelogenins, secreted by ameloblasts during development of enamel, and are thought to be involved in cementogenesis.[58,59] A study undertaken by Hoang and others demonstrated that Emdogain regulates periodontal cell proliferation and migration. Some studies suggest that periodontal cells have the ability to differentiate into osteoblast-like and cementoblast-like cells that can contribute to periodontal regeneration.[60,61] However, the results from clinical studies have mostly yielded mixed results. Berlucchi and colleagues found that root conditioning with Emdogain showed results similar to other root conditioners.[62] One of the histological studies done by Rasperini and others demonstrated formation of woven bone and connective tissue fibers anchored in new cementum.[63] However, Carnio and others demonstrated that teeth treated by connective tissue and Emdogain resulted in periodontal regeneration in few regions; the majority of the regeneration was connective tissue adhesion to the root with minimal junctional epithelium.[64] These studies suggest the need for further research into the effectiveness and nature of healing demonstrated by root conditioners.

A 2010 study attempted to "evaluate and compare the outcome of gingival recession therapy using the subepithelial connective tissue graft with or without Er:YAG laser application for root surface biomodification." It concluded that "root surface conditioning with an Er:YAG laser does not enhance the results achieved when subepithelial connective tissue grafting was performed alone."[65] A similar study concluded that "the use of Nd:YAG laser as a root surface biomodifier negatively affected the outcome of root coverage with the subepithelial connective tissue graft."[66]

Preparation of the Recipient Site

Survival of the subepithelial connective tissue graft depends on its revascularization. The preparation of the recipient site, ideally, should enhance the blood supply to the graft so that necrosis of the graft is prevented. The site preparation should also aid in immobilization of the graft because movement of the graft can tear off the delicate vessels that form during the revascularization process. Various bilaminar procedures have been devised to help improve the blood supply of the recipient site. Langer and Calagna demonstrated the usefulness of subepithelial graft for ridge augmentation. The connective tissue graft, when combined with a pedicle graft, draws blood supply from connective tissue, the periosteum, and the overlying flap.[67] Later this technique was modified by Langer and Langer to be used for root coverage in areas with multiple recessions.[4] Mörmann and others reported that the gingival tissues receive the majority of their blood supply from an apical direction.[68] As a result, vertical releasing incisions are appropriate because such an approach may not interfere with the blood supply. However, in another study, Tarnow showed that the lateral blood supply was more important when tissues survived after the severing of the apico coronal blood supply.[69] Based on this study, the researchers concluded that vertical releasing incisions may compromise the lateral blood supply, and, therefore, the envelope flap is advantageous in preserving the blood supply.

In the studies with free gingival graft, Caffessee and others found that resorption of the denuded bone caused a significant delay in vascular proliferation.[70] The study suggested that the same condition may also be applicable for subepithelial connective tissue graft, and, therefore, a partial-thickness graft would be a better option; however, Nelson successfully included full-thickness flaps for root coverage in his study.[6]

Allen presented a technique employing a supraperiosteal envelope to cover multiple adjacent areas of recession. This technique allows conservation of existing gingiva with minimal surgical trauma to the recipient area, and the technique also helps in firm fixation of the connective tissue graft over single and multiple adjacent areas of recession. The technique involves creating a partial thickness supraperiosteal envelope located 3 mm to 5 mm lateral and apical to multiple adjacent recession defects. A tunnel is created apical to the papilla to keep the connective tissue graft tightly opposed to the denuded root. The ends of the graft are beveled, and a suture is placed in one end to help direct the graft through the tunnel.[9] Santarelli and colleagues performed a supraperiosteal tunnel with a vertical incision made from the distal corner of the base of the papilla to beyond the mucogingival junction to help in insertion and stabilization of a connective tissue autograft.[71]

Blanes and Allen combined the tunnel technique with lateral pedicle flaps to treat adjacent areas of recession. This approach combines the advantages of the tunnel technique with the increased blood supply and protection provided by pedicle flaps. Indications include adjacent Class I and Class II deep, wide recessions; however, the procedure may also be applied to Class III recessions.[8] A 2012 study by Zucchelli and others describes "a novel subepithelial connective tissue graft technique for soft tissue augmentation in Class III ridge defects." They describe an "in situ maintenance of a connective tissue 'platform' at the edentulous space, which facilitated the stabilization and suturing of the connective tissue grafts used for soft tissue augmentation." They note that they were able to obtain sufficient graft thickness "by doubling the width of a de-epithelialized free gingival graft that was subsequently folded on itself." Nine months after the initial surgery, the soft tissue was contoured at pontic level "with a bur and filling the space with flowable composite resin applied above the pontic." They explain that one year and two months after surgery, the concluding phase for a prosthesis began with the "reproduction of the anatomical cementoenamel junction in the provisional and definitive restorations...to improve the soft tissue emergence profile," resulting, finally, in "soft tissue augmentation of 5 mm in the vertical and 4 mm in the horizontal dimension." The noteworthy element of this study and technique is that it accomplished "horizontal and vertical soft tissue augmentation in a single surgical step."[72] Tözüm reported that creating a partial-thickness envelope lateral to the recession and a full-thickness envelope apical to the recession helps to maintain the integrity of critical gingival blood vessels by securing them within the flap.[73]

Harvesting Grafts from Donor Sites

The donor sites used for harvesting connective tissue grafts are the palate, the maxillary tuberosity, and edentulous ridges. The most common donor site is the palate. Some anatomical considerations should be kept in mind when the clinician harvests the graft. Clinicians should be aware that the thickest tissue on the palate is found from the mesial line angle of the palatal root of the first molar to the distal line angle of the canine. When harvesting the graft, the clinician should avoid the area of the greater and lesser palatine nerves and vessels. This includes the area 7 mm to 17 mm from the cementoenamel junction of the maxillary premolars, depending on the height of the palatal vault. The greater and lesser palatine nerves and vessels forming the neurovascular bundle pass through a bony groove anterior to the foramen from which they emerge. By palpating the groove, the clinician can indicate the approximate location of the nerve and vessels. It is recommended to limit incisions distal of the canine to avoid damaging the greater palatine nerve and artery.[74] Song and others concluded in a 2008 study involving computerized tomography to measure the thickness of the posterior palatal masticatory mucosa that "the palatal masticatory mucosa thickness increased from the canine to premolar region but decreased at the first molar region and increased again in the second molar region, with the thinnest area at the first molar region and the thickest at the second premolar region." They also noted that "the canine to premolar region seems to be the most appropriate donor site that contains a uniformly thick mucosa. Computerized tomography can be considered an alternative method for the measurement of palatal soft tissue thickness."[75]

Figure 6-2 **Harvesting Graft from the Palatal Donor Site**

a

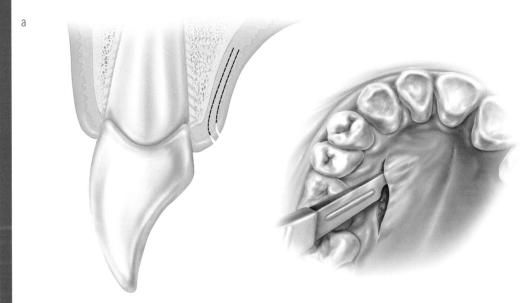

(a) Palatal incisions are made to create an internal flap approximately 1.5mm thick.

b

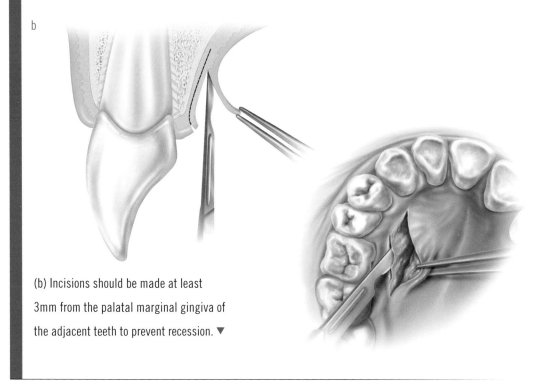

(b) Incisions should be made at least
3mm from the palatal marginal gingiva of
the adjacent teeth to prevent recession. ▼

Figure 6-2 **Harvesting Graft from the Palatal Donor Site** (CONT.)

c

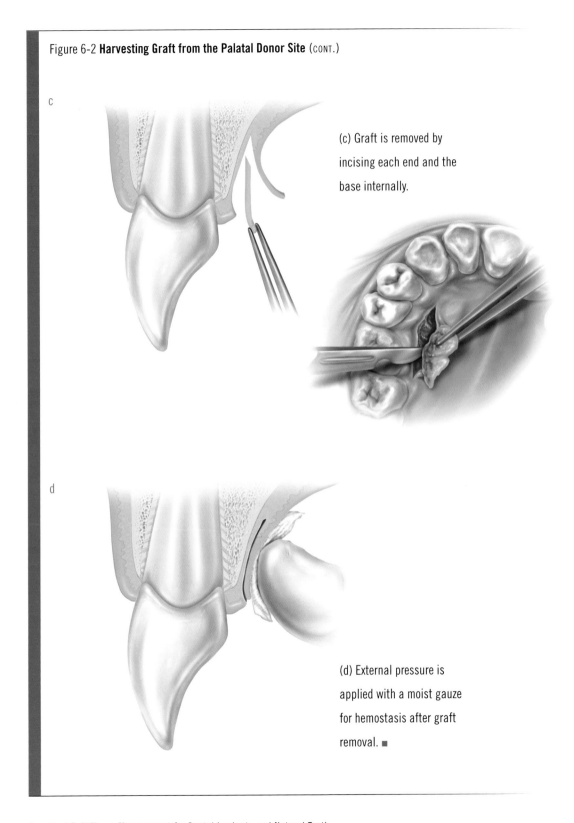

(c) Graft is removed by incising each end and the base internally.

d

(d) External pressure is applied with a moist gauze for hemostasis after graft removal. ■

Reiser and others described the anatomy of the palatal donor site providing the subepithelial connective tissue graft.[76] It was found that variations in the size and shape of the hard palate affect the dimensions of the donor tissue harvested as well as the location of the greater palatine neurovascular bundles. They classified the palatal vaults according to height as high, average, and shallow. Reiser and his colleagues reported that local anesthesia of the palate was associated with very few complications in terms of permanent anesthesia, paresthesia, or serious hemorrhage.[76] Infiltration into the graft tissue should be avoided as it may cause vasoconstriction in the graft, thereby affecting the outcome.[77] One study also suggested that the graft should be placed within 60 seconds of harvesting for better outcomes.[78]

Many types of flap designs are described for harvesting the connective tissue graft. Edel was the first to describe the trap door technique, in which no epithelium is removed from the palate. In this technique, the free gingival graft knife is used with the cutting shoe reversed to elevate a partial thickness trap door. Thereafter, a connective tissue flap is removed from underneath the trap door by pulling the knife mesially. A releasing incision at the mesial edge is given to release the graft.[16]

Langer and Langer developed the parallel incision method to harvest the graft.[4] Incisions are made 10 mm to 12 mm deep into the palate with vertical releases at the mesial and distal extent of the incision. An incision at the base of the connective tissue between the parallel incisions frees the graft from the palatal bone. Raetzke described a technique similar to this, where the incisions were made deep, just above the bone, thus creating a wedge of connective tissue.[5] In a comparative study of trap door and parallel-incision harvesting techniques, Harris found that both resulted in significant root coverage. However, if the trap door sloughed, it caused considerable morbidity.[78] The parallel incision method produced less patient discomfort, a smaller wound at one week postoperatively, and a more uniform graft, which was easier to use clinically. The study demonstrated that the parallel incision method meets more of the goals of an ideal technique for harvesting a connective tissue graft than the free gingival graft knife method.

Figure 6-3 **Subepithelial Connective Tissue Graft Case #1: Mandibular Incisor**

a

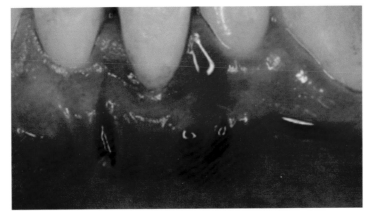

(a) Vertical incisions on the mesial and distal of the recipient site.

b

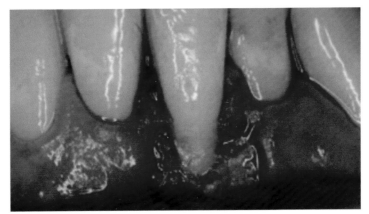

(b) Root preparation of the mandibular incisor after flap reflection.

c

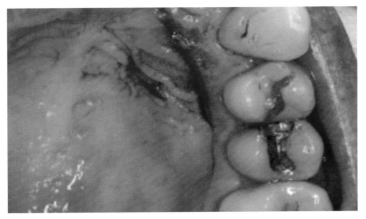

(c) Horizontal incision to harvest the connective tissue from the palate.

d

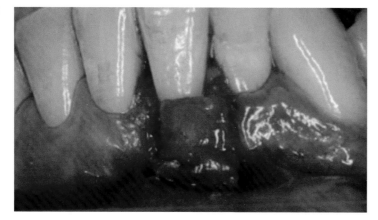

(d) Positioning of the harvested connective tissue graft onto the recipient site.

e

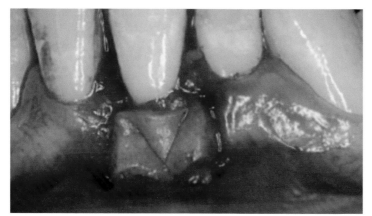

(e) Initial stabilization of the donor tissue onto the recipient site with a sling suture.

f

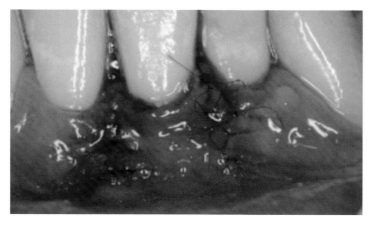

(f) Overlying flap coronally repositioned and stabilized with interrupted sutures.

▼

g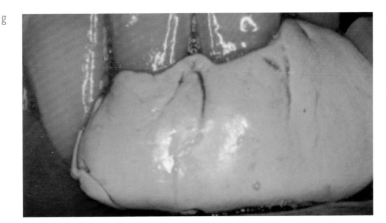

(g) Non-eugenol periodontal dressing placed to protect the surgical site

h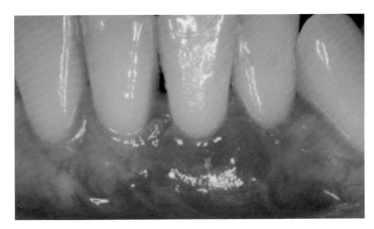

(h) Grafted site after 12 weeks of healing. ■

Hurzeler described and demonstrated a new and simplified surgical approach to harvest subepithelial connective tissue graft from the palate.[77] Only a single incision parallel to the gingival graft margin was used to access the donor site for graft preparation and graft harvesting of variable sizes and thickness. No band of epithelium was removed with the connective tissue graft, thereby facilitating healing of palatal donor site by primary intention. Postoperatively, no stents or hemostatic agents were required to cover the donor area.

Harvesting a graft may be difficult in patients having a thin palate. In these cases, Bosco and Bosco described a surgical approach to the harvesting of subepithelial connective tissue grafts. After the clinician raises a partial-thickness flap, a graft composed of epithelium and connective tissue is removed from the palate. The connective tissue layer of the graft is removed and used for root coverage, and the superficial layer consisting of epithelium is placed back at the donor site to facilitate healing.[79] Hirsch reported obtaining graft tissue from the maxillary tuberosity during pocket reduction therapy.[80]

Some authors suggest maintaining the epithelial collar of the graft while others suggest removing it; however, the decision should be based on the extent of keratinized gingiva at the recipient site. In a comparative study of two groups, one with de-epithelialized graft and the other with maintained epithelium, Bouchard found that both groups achieved comparable root coverage. The group with retained epithelial collar showed considerable increase in keratinized tissue but fewer aesthetically-acceptable outcomes.[35] One study even reported that there is a potential for development of a gingival cyst when the epithelium is left intact.[81]

Classification of Incision Designs

In 2002, Liu and Weisgold proposed a classification for incision design relative to the donor site preparation for subepithelial connective tissue grafting.[82] The study aimed to help determine the most effective incision or flap design to harvest the donor tissue. The classification is based upon the following factors:

- The graft size required by the recipient site
- The anatomy of the palatal vault, which is divided into high, average, and shallow
- Primary or secondary intention healing of the donor site[78]
- Blood supply for the overlying flap
- Postoperative discomfort
- The possibility of an exostosis[76]

- Use of sutures, stents, or hemostatic agents, and

- Visibility of the procedure.

The incision design classification is as follows:

Class I (One incision line)

This incision can be used in any connective tissue graft from the palatal site, and the technique can be applied to varying palatal forms. The advantages include a single incision line that heals with primary intention, enhanced blood supply for the overlying flap, and reduced patient discomfort. Additionally, this technique may not require sutures, stent, or hemostatic agents. However, this technique reduces visibility of the donor site during graft preparation and is challenging for the clinician to execute.

Class II (Two incision lines; L shape)

This simpler technique is used to avoid the greater palatine artery and nerve. The advantages include smaller incision with sufficient visibility as well as moderate blood supply for the overlying flap. However, the two incision lines may compromise the blood supply from the donor site.

Class III (Three incision lines; U shape)

This technique is used when there is a concern for the underlying anatomy and a need for a larger amount of tissue. The advantages include greater visibility and easy execution. But due to more incision lines, there could be a compromise of the blood supply from the donor site, more postoperative pain, and the requirement of more sutures.

Subclassification (Horizontal Incision)

TYPE A (One horizontal incision): These types of graft designs are used when the connective tissue graft needs to be without an epithelium covering and when a graft length larger than two premolars is needed. This incision type can be applied to different palatal forms and can be used in areas of minimal tissue depth.

Type B (Two horizontal incisions): This type of incision design is used when the palatal tissue is sufficient, the required graft needs to be harvested with epithelium, and the graft is planned to be partially exposed at the recipient site.

Complications

Despite the many benefits of subepithelial connective tissue graft procedure, many clinicians find that the procedure is associated with increased morbidity related to the donor site.[83] It causes discomfort to the patient because of postsurgical pain and the risk of bleeding from the donor area.[84] This procedure may not be applicable to patients who have a thin and friable gingiva. Studies suggest that the patients with thin palatal mucosa are not suitable candidates for connective tissue graft procedures.[85]

In rare cases, subepithelial connective tissue graft procedure may give rise to cysts and exostosis. Breault reported a case of a gingival cyst developing secondarily to a subepithelial connective tissue graft placed 15 months previously. A slightly raised form, soft tissue mass located in the alveolar mucosa was observed adjacent to the site of the previous connective tissue graft. On histological examination, it was concluded that the cyst resulted from the implanted epithelial remnants of the previously placed subepithelial connective tissue graft.[81] One study also mentions the formation of exostosis following a subepithelial connective tissue graft.[86] Vastardis and Yukna reported development of soft tissue abscess following subepithelial connective tissue graft for root coverage.[87] Parashis and Tatakis reported epithelial cell discharge as a late complication of the subepithelial connective tissue graft procedure.[88] It is also noteworthy that root coverage with connective tissue grafts appears to be negatively associated with cigarette smoking.[89]

Figure 6-4 Subepithelial Connective Tissue Graft Case # 2: Mandibular molar

a

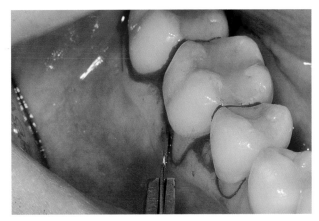

(a) Intrasulcular incision around the facial of the mandibular molar.

b

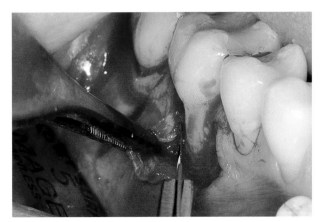

(b) Mesial and distal vertical releasing incisions.

c

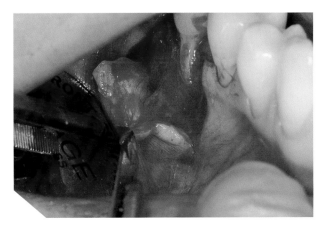

(c) Periosteal releasing incision done to be able to coronally reposition the overlying flap without tension.

d

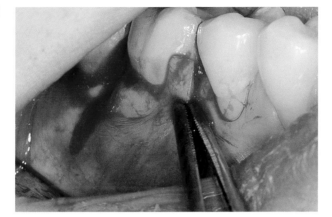

(d) Verification of a tension-free flap.

e

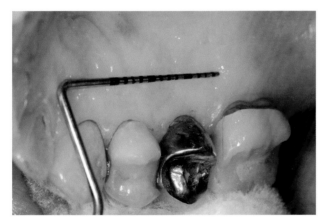

(e & f) A periodontal probe is used to measure the proper horizontal and vertical dimensions of the graft. ▼

f

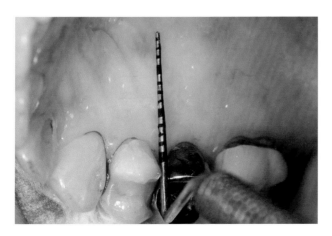

g

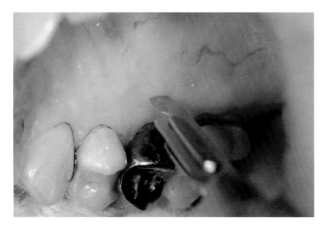

(g) The first incision on the palatal donor site is made perpendicular to the long axis of the teeth and at least 3mm apical to the palatal marginal gingiva.

h

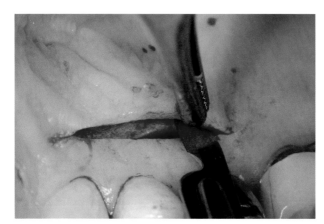

(h) The second incision is made parallel to the long axis of the teeth.

i

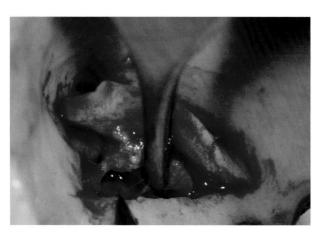

(i) The connective tissue is removed from the palate after incising each end and the base internally

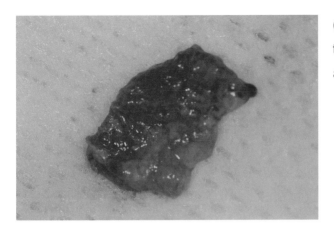

j

(j) Harvested connective tissue of sufficient size and thickness.

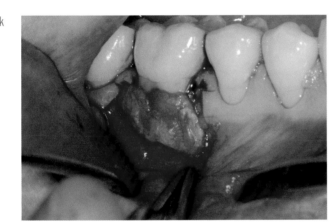

k

(k) Donor connective tissue positioned onto the prepared recipient site.

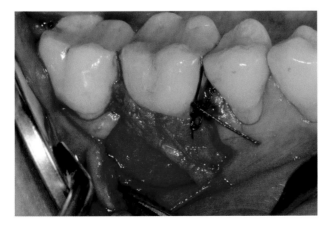

l

(l) A sling suture is used to adapt and stabilize the donor connective tissue onto the recipient site.

▼

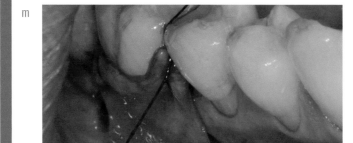

(m) Overlying flap is coronally repositioned tension free and stabilized with sling and interrupted sutures. ■

Summary

Subepithelial connective tissue grafting is an effective method for root coverage for single and multiple recession defects. The technique yields better esthetic outcomes but requires technical expertise in graft harvesting and graft placement. Among the various approaches available, the choice of technique depends upon the clinician's skill and experience, as well as various patient factors. The complications associated with subepithelial connective tissue grafting are few, but the clinician should take every precaution to prevent them. The postoperative instructions and medications after the procedure are the same as those after free gingival grafting.

References

1. Guiha R, el Khodeiry S, Mota L, Caffesse R. Histological evaluation of healing and revascularization of the subepithelial connective tissue graft. J Periodontol. 2001 Apr;72(4):470-8.

2. Goldstein M, Boyan BD, Cochran DL, Schwartz Z. Human histology of new attachment after root coverage using subepithelial connective tissue graft. J Clin Periodontol. 2001 Jul;28(7):657-62.

3. Langer B, Calagna LJ. The subepithelial connective tissue graft. A new approach to the enhancement of anterior cosmetics. Int J Periodontics Restorative Dent. 1982;2(2):22-33.

4. Langer B, Langer L. Subepithelial connective tissue graft technique for root coverage. J Periodontol. 1985 Dec;56(12):715-20.

5. Raetzke PB. Covering localized areas of root exposure employing the "envelope" technique. J Periodontol. 1985 Jul;56(7):397-402.

6. Nelson SW. The subpedicle connective tissue graft. A bilaminar reconstructive procedure for the coverage of denuded root surfaces. J Periodontol. 1987 Feb;58(2):95-102.

7. Harris RJ. The connective tissue and partial thickness double pedicle graft: a predictable method of obtaining root coverage. J Periodontol. 1992 May;63(5):477-86.

8. Blanes RJ, Allen EP. The bilateral pedicle flap-tunnel technique: a new approach to cover connective tissue grafts. Int J Periodontics Restorative Dent. 1999 Oct;19(5):471-9.

9. Allen AL. Use of the supraperiosteal envelope in soft tissue grafting for root coverage. I. Rationale and technique. Int J Periodontics Restorative Dent. 1994 Jun;14(3):216-27. Review.

10. Allen AL. Use of the supraperiosteal envelope in soft tissue grafting for root coverage. II. Clinical results. Int J Periodontics Restorative Dent. 1994 Aug;14(4):302-15.

11. Bruno JF. Connective tissue graft technique assuring wide root coverage. Int J Periodontics Restorative Dent. 1994 Apr;14(2):126-37.

12. Oliver MJ. Multiple denuded root surfaces. Complete coverage with a one-stage, subepithelial connective tissue graft. Oral Health. 1987 Apr;77(4):51-8.

13. Zabalegui I, Sicilia A, Cambra J, Gil J, Sanz M. Treatment of multiple adjacent gingival recessions with the tunnel subepithelial connective tissue graft: a clinical report. Int J Periodontics Restorative Dent. 1999 Apr;19(2):199-206.

14. Rubins RP, Tolmie PN, Corsig KT, Kerr EN, Kim DM. Subepithelial connective tissue graft with growth factor for the treatment of maxillary gingival recession defects. Int J Periodontics Restorative Dent. 2013 Jan-Feb;33(1):43-50.

15. Lafzi A, Faramarzi M, Shirmohammadi A, Behrozian A, Kashefimehr A, Khashabi E. Subepithelial connective tissue graft with and without the use of plasma rich in growth factors for treating root exposure. J Periodontal Implant Sci. 2012 Dec;42(6):196-203.

16. Edel A. Clinical evaluation of free connective tissue grafts used to increase the width of keratinised gingiva. J Clin Periodontol. 1974;1(4):185-96.

17. Bromme, W.C., Taggart, E. J. Free autogenous connective tissue grafting. A Report of two cases. J Periodontol. 1976;47:480-85.

18. Donn BJ Jr. The free connective tissue autograft: a clinical and histologic wound healing study in humans. J Periodontol. 1978 May;49(5):253-60.

19. Zucchelli G, Amore C, Sforza NM, Montebugnoli L, De Sanctis M. Bilaminar techniques for the treatment of recession-type defects. A comparative clinical study. J Clin Periodontol. 2003 Oct;30(10):862-70.

20. Tinti C, Parma-Benfenati S. The free rotated papilla autograft: a new bilaminar grafting procedure for the coverage of multiple shallow gingival recessions. J Periodontol. 1996 Oct;67(10):1016-24.

21. Jahnke PV, Sandifer JB, Gher ME, Gray JL, Richardson AC. Thick free gingival and connective tissue autografts for root coverage. J Periodontol. 1993 Apr;64(4):315-22.

22. Paolantonio M, di Murro C, Cattabriga A, Cattabriga M. Subpedicle connective tissue graft versus free gingival graft in the coverage of exposed root surfaces. A 5-year clinical study. J Clin Periodontol. 1997 Jan;24(1):51-6.

23. Levine RA. Covering denuded maxillary root surfaces with the subepithelial connective tissue graft. Compendium. 1991 Aug;12(8): 568, 570, 572 passim.

24. Jepsen K, Heinz B, Halben JH, Jepsen S. Treatment of gingival recession with titanium reinforced barrier membranes versus connective tissue grafts. J Periodontol. 1998 Mar;69(3):383-91.

25. Müller HP, Stahl M, Eger T. Root coverage employing an envelope technique or guided tissue regeneration with a bioabsorbable membrane. J Periodontol. 1999 Jul; 70(7):743-51.

26. Tal H, Moses O, Zohar R, Meir H, Nemcovsky C. Root coverage of advanced gingival recession: a comparative study between acellular dermal matrix allograft and subepithelial connective tissue grafts. J Periodontol. 2002 Dec;73(12):1405-11.

27. Goldstein M, Nasatzky E, Goultschin J, Boyan BD, Schwartz Z. Coverage of previously carious roots is as predictable a procedure as coverage of intact roots. J Periodontol. 2002 Dec;73(12):1419-26.

28. Goldstein M, Nasatzky E, Goultschin J, Boyan B, Schwartz Z. Coverage of carious roots by a subepithelial connective tissue graft. Am J Dent. 2002 Jun;15(3):143-8.

29. Allen EP. Pedicle flaps, gingival grafts, and connective tissue grafts in aesthetic treatment of gingival recession. Pract Periodontics Aesthet Dent. 1993 Jun-Jul;5(5):29-38, 40; quiz 40.

30. Miller PD Jr. Root coverage grafting for regeneration and aesthetics. Periodontol 2000. 1993 Feb;1:118-27. Review.

31. Vergara JA, Caffesse RG. Localized gingival recessions treated with the original envelope technique: a report of 50 consecutive patients. J Periodontol. 2004 Oct;75(10):1397-403.

32. Becker BE, Becker W. Use of connective tissue autografts for treatment of mucogingival problems. Int J Periodontics Restorative Dent. 1986;6(1):88-94.

33. Ouhayoun JP, Khattab R, Serfaty R, Feghaly-Assaly M, Sawaf MH. Chemically separated connective tissue grafts: clinical application and histological evaluation. J Periodontol. 1993 Aug;64(8):734-8.

34. Harris RJ. The connective tissue with partial thickness double pedicle graft: the results of 100 consecutively-treated defects. J Periodontol. 1994 May;65(5):448-61.

35. Bouchard P, Etienne D, Ouhayoun JP, Nilvéus R. Subepithelial connective tissue grafts in the treatment of gingival recessions. A comparative study of 2 procedures. J Periodontol. 1994 Oct;65(10):929-36.

36. Ramakrishnan T, Kaur M, Aggarwal K. Root coverage using epithelial embossed connective tissue graft. Indian J Dent Res. 2011 Sep-Oct;22(5):726-8.

37. Azzi R, Etienne D, Sauvan JL, Miller PD. Root coverage and papilla reconstruction in Class IV recession: a case report. Int J Periodontics Restorative Dent. 1999 Oct;19(5):449-55.

38. Harris RJ. Human histologic evaluation of root coverage obtained with a connective tissue with partial thickness double pedicle graft. A case report. J Periodontol. 1999 Jul; 70(7):813-21.

39. Ribeiro FS, Zandim DL, Pontes AE, Mantovani RV, Sampaio JE, Marcantonio E. Tunnel technique with a surgical maneuver to increase the graft extension: case report with a 3-year follow-up. J Periodontol. 2008 Apr;79(4):753-8.

40. Tözüm TF. Root coverage with subepithelial connective tissue grafts and modified tunnel technique. An evaluation of long-term results. N Y State Dent J. 2006 Jun-Jul;72(4):38-41.

41. Langer L, Langer B. The subepithelial connective tissue graft for treatment of gingival recession. Dent Clin North Am. 1993 Apr;37(2):243-64. Review.

42. El-Dessouky HF, Ibrahim SA, Sadek HS. Clinical comparison of the effect of subepithelial connective tissue graft and collagen membrane with the adjunct use of platelet rich plasma in root coverage procedures. Egyptian Dental Journal. 2007 Jan;53 (377): 396.

43. Lowenguth RA, Blieden TM. Periodontal regeneration: root surface demineralization. Periodontol 2000. 1993 Feb;1:54-68. Review.

44. Register AA, Burdick FA. Accelerated reattachment with cementogenesis to dentin, demineralized in situ. II. Defect repair. J Periodontol. 1976 Sep;47(9):497-505.

45. Caffesse RG, De LaRosa M, Garza M, and others Citric acid demineralization and subepithelial connective tissue grafts. J Periodontol. 2000 Apr; 71(4):568-72.

46. Bouchard P, Nilveus R, Etienne D. Clinical evaluation of tetracycline HCl conditioning in the treatment of gingival recessions. A comparative study. J Periodontol. 1997 Mar;68(3):262-9.

47. Miller PD Jr. Root coverage using the free soft tissue autograft following citric acid application. II. Treatment of the carious root. Int J Periodontics Restorative Dent. 1983;3(5):38-51.

48. Genco RJ. Antibiotics in the treatment of human periodontal diseases. J Periodontol. 1981 Sep;52(9):545-58. Review.

49. Ingman T, Sorsa T, Suomalainen K, Halinen S, Lindy O, Lauhio A, Saari H, Konttinen YT, Golub LM. Tetracycline inhibition and the cellular source of collagenase in gingival crevicular fluid in different periodontal diseases. A review article. J Periodontol. 1993 Feb;64(2):82-8. Review.

50. Gomes BC, Golub LM, Ramamurthy NS. Tetracyclines inhibit parathyroid hormone-induced bone resorption in organ culture. Experientia. 1984 Nov 15;40(11):1273-5.

51. Christersson LA, Norderyd OM, Puchalsky CS. Topical application of tetracycline-HCl in human periodontitis. J Clin Periodontol. 1993 Feb;20(2):88-95.

52. Terranova VP, Franzetti LC, Hic S, DiFlorio RM, Lyall RM, Wikesjö UM, Baker PJ, Christersson LA, Genco RJ. A biochemical approach to periodontal regeneration: tetracycline treatment of dentin promotes fibroblast adhesion and growth. J Periodontal Res. 1986 Jul;21(4):330-7.

53. Isik AG, Tarim B, Hafez AA, Yalçin FS, Onan U, Cox CF. A comparative scanning electron microscopic study on the characteristics of demineralized dentin root surface using different tetracycline HCl concentrations and application times. J Periodontol. 2000 Feb;71(2):219-25.

54. Labahn R, Fahrenbach WH, Clark SM, Lie T, Adams DF. Root dentin morphology after different modes of citric acid and tetracycline hydrochloride conditioning. J Periodontol. 1992 Apr;63(4):303-9.

55. Sterrett JD, Simmons J, Whitford G, Russell CM. Tetracycline demineralization of dentin: the effects of concentration and application time. J Clin Periodontol. 1997 Jul;24(7):457-63.

56. Erdinç M, Efeoglu A, Demirel K. Clinical evaluation of the effect of tetracycline hydrochloride root conditioning during flap surgery. Periodontal Clin Investig. 1995 Spring;17(1):6-9.

57. Zaman KU, Sugaya T, Hongo O, Kato H. A study of attached and oriented human periodontal ligament cells to periodontally diseased cementum and dentin after demineralizing with neutral and low pH etching solution. J Periodontol. 2000 Jul;71(7):1094-9.

58. Slavkin HC. Towards a cellular and molecular understanding of periodontics. Cementogenesis revisited. J Periodontol. 1976 May;47(5):249-55. Review.

59. Brookes SJ, Robinson C, Kirkham J, Bonass WA. Biochemistry and molecular biology of amelogenin proteins of developing dental enamel. Arch Oral Biol. 1995 Jan;40(1):1-14. Review.

60. Davidson D, McCulloch CA. Proliferative behavior of periodontal ligament cell populations. J Periodontal Res. 1986 Jul;21(4):414-28.

61. Mariotti A, Cochran DL. Characterization of fibroblasts derived from human periodontal ligament and gingiva. J Periodontol. 1990 Feb;61(2):103-11.

62. Berlucchi I, Francetti L, Del Fabbro M, Testori T, Weinstein RL. Enamel matrix proteins (Emdogain) in combination with coronally advanced flap or subepithelial connective tissue graft in the treatment of shallow gingival recessions. Int J Periodontics Restorative Dent. 2002 Dec;22(6):583-93.

63. Rasperini G, Silvestri M, Schenk RK, Nevins ML. Clinical and histologic evaluation of human gingival recession treated with a subepithelial connective tissue graft and enamel matrix derivative (Emdogain): a case report. Int J Periodontics Restorative Dent. 2000 Jun;20(3):269-75.

64. Carnio J, Camargo PM, Kenney EB, Schenk RK. Histological evaluation of 4 cases of root coverage following a connective tissue graft combined with an enamel matrix derivative preparation. J Periodontol. 2002 Dec;73(12):1534-43.

65. Dilsiz A, Aydin T, Yavuz MS. Root surface biomodification with an Er:YAG laser for the treatment of gingival recession with subepithelial connective tissue grafts. Photomed Laser Surg. 2010 Aug;28(4):511-7.

66. Dilsiz A, Aydin T, Canakci V, Cicek Y. Root surface biomodification with Nd:YAG laser for the treatment of gingival recession with subepithelial connective tissue grafts. Photomed Laser Surg. 2010 Jun;28(3):337-43.

67. Langer B, Calagna L. The subepithelial connective tissue graft. J Prosthet Dent. 1980 Oct;44(4):363-7.

68. Mörmann W, Meier C, Firestone A. Gingival blood circulation after experimental wounds in man. J Clin Periodontol. 1979 Dec; 6(6):417-24.

69. Tarnow DP. Semilunar coronally repositioned flap. J Clin Periodontol. 1986 Mar;13(3):182-5.

70. Caffesse RG, Burgett FG, Nasjleti CE, Castelli WA. Healing of free gingival grafts with and without periosteum. Part I. Histologic evaluation. J Periodontol. 1979 Nov; 50(11):586-94.

71. Santarelli GA, Ciancaglini R, Campanari F, Dinoi C, Ferraris S. Connective tissue grafting employing the tunnel technique: a case report of complete root coverage in the anterior maxilla. Int J Periodontics Restorative Dent. 2001 Feb;21(1):77-83.

72. Zucchelli G, Mazzotti C, Bentivogli V, Mounssif I, Marzadori M, Monaco C. The connective tissue platform technique for soft tissue augmentation. Int J Periodontics Restorative Dent. 2012 Dec;32(6):665-75.

73. Tözüm TF. A promising periodontal procedure for the treatment of adjacent gingival recession defects. J Can Dent Assoc. 2003 Mar;69(3):155-9. Review.

74. Studer SP, Allen EP, Rees TC, Kouba A. The thickness of masticatory mucosa in the human hard palate and tuberosity as potential donor sites for ridge augmentation procedures. J Periodontol. 1997 Feb; 68(2):145-51.

75. Song JE, Um YJ, Kim CS, Choi SH, Cho KS, Kim CK, Chai JK, Jung UW. Thickness of posterior palatal masticatory mucosa: the use of computerized tomography. J Periodontol. 2008 Mar;79(3):406-12.

76. Reiser GM, Bruno JF, Mahan PE, Larkin LH. The subepithelial connective tissue graft palatal donor site: anatomic considerations for surgeons. Int J Periodontics Restorative Dent. 1996 Apr;16(2):130-7.

77. Hürzeler MB, Weng D. A single-incision technique to harvest subepithelial connective tissue grafts from the palate. Int J Periodontics Restorative Dent.1999 Jun;19(3):279-87.

78. Harris RJ. A comparison of two techniques for obtaining a connective tissue graft from the palate. Int J Periodontics Restorative Dent. 1997 Jun;17(3):260-71.

79. Bosco AF, Bosco JM. An alternative technique to the harvesting of a connective tissue graft from a thin palate: enhanced wound healing. Int J Periodontics Restorative Dent. 2007 Apr;27(2):133-9.

80. Hirsch A, Attal U, Chai E, Goultschin J, Boyan BD, Schwartz Z. Root coverage and pocket reduction as combined surgical procedures. J Periodontol. 2001 Nov;72(11):1572-9.

81. Breault LG, Billman MA, Lewis DM. Report of a gingival "surgical cyst" developing secondarily to a subepithelial connective tissue graft. J Periodontol. 1997 Apr; 68(4):392-5.

82. Liu CL, Weisgold AS. Connective tissue graft: a classification for incision design from the palatal site and clinical case reports. Int J Periodontics Restorative Dent. 2002 Aug;22(4):373-9.

83. Aichelmann-Reidy ME, Yukna RA, Evans GH, Nasr HF, Mayer ET. Clinical evaluation of acellular allograft dermis for the treatment of human gingival recession. J Periodontol 2001 Aug; 72(8):998-1005.

84. Paolantonio M, Dolci M, Esposito P, D'Archivio D, Lisanti L, Di Luccio A, Perinetti G. Subpedicle acellular dermal matrix graft and autogenous connective tissue graft in the treatment of gingival recessions: a comparative 1-year clinical study. J Periodontol 2002 Nov; 73 (11):1299-307.

85. Muller HP, Eger T. Masticatory mucosa and periodontal phenotype: a review. Int J Periodontics Restorative Dent 2002 Apr; 22(2):172-83.

86. Corsair AJ, Iacono VJ, Moss SS. Exostosis following a subepithelial connective tissue graft. J Int Acad Periodontol. 2001Apr; 3(2):38-41.

87. Vastardis S, Yukna RA. Gingival/soft tissue abscess following subepithelial connective tissue graft for root coverage: report of three cases. J Periodontol. 2003 Nov; 74(11):1676-81.

88. Parashis AO, Tatakis DN. Subepithelial connective tissue graft for root coverage: a case report of an unusual late complication of epithelial origin. J Periodontol. 2007 Oct; 78(10):2051-6.

89. Erley KJ, Swiec GD, Herold R, Bisch FC, Peacock ME. Gingival recession treatment with connective tissue grafts in smokers and non-smokers. J Periodontol. 2006 Jul; 77(7):1148-55.

Notes

_____

_____

_____

_____

_____

_____

_____

_____

_____

_____

_____

_____

_____

_____

Notes

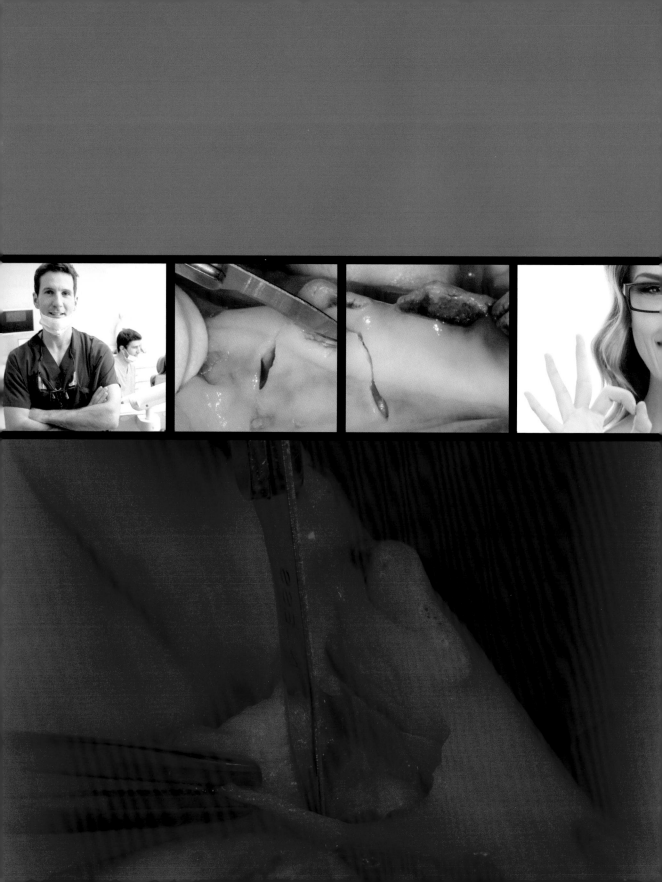

Pedicle Grafts: Rotational Flaps, Double-Papilla Procedures, and Coronally Advanced Flaps

A pedicle graft is an improved technique for covering gingival recessions and root defects. The basic objective of a pedicle graft is to cover the exposed root surface with a flap from the closest adjoining area. The pedicle graft is contiguous and not free, as in the case of gingival grafts. Because the root surfaces to be treated are avascular, it is very important that the soft tissue grafted on the defect should have a blood supply. Pedicle grafts are preferred to gingival grafts because they contain their own blood supply at the base. This blood supply helps the graft to survive by nourishing the graft, and the blood supply promotes revascularization across the recipient site.

Pedicle grafts for root coverage are divided into rotational flaps and advanced flaps. The types of rotational flaps include the laterally positioned flap, the obliquely positioned flap, and double papillae flaps. The advanced flaps include coronally positioned flaps and semilunar flaps. Combinations of these techniques with other root coverage techniques have been found to be useful. Compared to gingival grafts, pedicle grafts provide superior tissue augmentation, aesthetics, and root coverage. Both partial and full thickness grafts are used as the indications warrant.

The decision to use pedicle grafts is based on the presence of a sufficient amount of keratinized tissue—either adjacent or apical to the defect—which can be used as a donor site. There is, however, a risk of recession at the donor site of the flap. An edentulous area can also be used as a donor site, preferably in cases where gingival tissue on the facial surfaces of two or three consecutive teeth is not adequate for a donor site.

History of Pedicle Grafts

The pedicle graft was first introduced by Grupe and Warren in 1956, when they used a laterally positioned pedicle graft to cover exposed root surfaces.[1] However, the procedure resulted in formation of denuded osseous surfaces. To prevent this complication, Grupe modified the technique in 1966.[2] Thereafter, the technique was evaluated by many investigators, and the studies found the success of this root coverage procedure to be in the range of 69% to 72%.[3-5] Svoboda and Sheridan described a technique in which vertical releasing incisions were used to modify the basic pedicle graft procedure in the treatment of localized gingival recession.[6]

The different types of techniques derived from the basic laterally positioned flap to help minimize the donor site include the double papilla graft and the obliquely rotated graft.[7-10]

Another important pedicle graft technique, called the coronally positioned graft, was introduced by Bernimoulin and colleagues, and was used as a second stage procedure with a free gingival graft.[11] The current surgical approach for the coronally positioned flap alone often follows the previously described technique although other variations are also used.[12-18]

Lateral Sliding Flaps/Laterally Positioned Flaps

The term "lateral sliding flap" was first introduced by Grupe and Warren. The term now generally refers to the laterally positioned pedicle graft.[1] The original sliding flap was a full-thickness flap which gradually became a split-thickness flap at the mucogingival junction.[1] In the lateral sliding flap technique, a full-thickness flap is raised from the adjacent root tissue and then positioned laterally and sutured to cover the exposed root surface. Since this technique was associated with risk of recession at the donor site, the authors recommended not including the marginal soft tissue on the donor tooth. In addition, a split thickness flap instead of a full-thickness flap was used to reduce the potential risk of dehiscence at the donor tooth from exposure of the alveolar buccal plate.

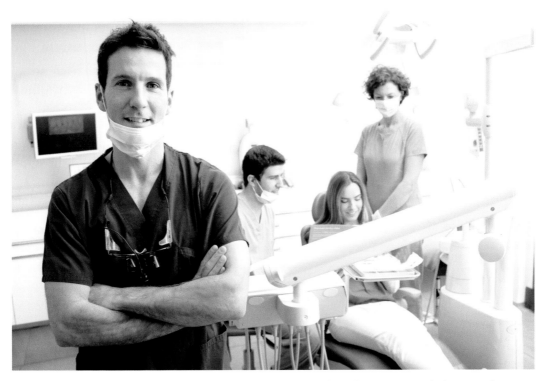

Laterally positioned grafts are indicated in isolated recession defects. Adequate width of keratinized tissue in the donor site is a necessary prerequisite for the procedure. Laterally positioned grafts are contraindicated in cases of multiple recession defects, inadequate keratinized tissue, and in areas with shallow vestibule since these factors may adversely affect the outcome of the procedure. During the procedure, the recipient bed lateral to the exposed root is prepared, from the margin of the gingival tissue to the base of the vestibule. An appropriately wide flap is raised and transposed laterally to cover the exposed root and the recipient bed. The flap is then firmly sutured over the recipient bed and the root. The main advantages of this technique are that it is technically easy and requires less time. The outcome of the procedure is esthetically optimal because there is a good color match of the tissues. Additionally, the procedure causes less discomfort to patients since there is no secondary surgical site from which donor tissue was harvested.

Staffileno reported that the laterally positioned grafts for isolated recession defects on mandibular teeth often left recession at the donor site.[19] To prevent recession defects, clinicians modified the technique, proposing that the marginal tissue at the donor site be left intact. This modified technique is applicable to sites with an adequate amount of keratinized tissue at the donor site.[2] Other techniques were also used to prevent gingival recession at the donor site, including covering the donor site with a free gingival graft after lateral positioning or using an edentulous area as the donor site.[20,21] The use of an edentulous area as a donor site is optimal where the gingiva of two to three teeth adjacent to the defect is inadequate.[22] A partial-thickness flap is developed and positioned around the involved teeth, and the interdental papillary tissues are placed over the buccal surfaces of the affected teeth.[23]

Oliveira and colleagues used the pedicle graft to cover the root surface exposed due to excision of a lesion, such as a pyogenic granuloma. The recipient and donor sites both showed good healing without any reported recurrence.[24] Zucchelli and others evaluated the effectiveness of a modified surgical approach of the laterally positioned flap for the treatment of an isolated type of recession defect.[25] The modification involved a laterally positioned coronally advanced flap and was found to be effective in treating isolated gingival recessions. Some authors also proposed a stimulated osteoperiosteal laterally positioned flap in areas which have an adequate thickness of facial bone. In addition to root coverage, this technique also helped in bone gain.[26,27] According to the authors, a needle is used to penetrate and slightly elevate the periosteum at multiple sites in a pincushion fashion. This procedure is completed approximately three weeks prior to flap elevation in order to stimulate osteoblasts into proliferating and producing osteoids. The proliferation and production of osteoids peaks at three weeks after the initial procedure. Thereafter, an osteoperiosteal flap consisting of the periosteum and stimulated osseous layer is elevated and positioned laterally to cover the recession defect.

Studies on a laterally positioned flap show that such a procedure brings about a defect coverage ranging from 61% to 74% with a mean for all studies of 67%.[4,5,28,29]

Therefore, the procedure is not very successful for accomplishing root coverage. Final root exposure reported from studies ranged from 0.8 mm to 1.8 mm, with a mean of 1.3 mm relative to mean initial recession of 3.9 mm.

Other Rotational Flaps

In addition to the laterally positioned flap, there are other flaps classified as rotational flaps. These are the double papilla repositioned flap, the oblique rotated flap, the rotation flap, and the papilla rotation flap.[8-10,30,31] Some authors have suggested that the free rotated papilla autograft should also be included with this group despite the fact that it uses a coronally positioned flap to cover the defect produced by excising the papilla and placing it over the recession defect.[32]

The papilla flaps involve taking tissue from the papilla and moving it to the mid-facial area. The prerequisite of any papilla procedure is the presence of a wide donor papilla. Because the donor tissue involves papilla and not the mid-facial tissue, there is a minimal risk of facial recession on the adjacent tooth. Unfortunately, no studies have examined the predictability of this technique. In general, rotational flaps from the papilla have not been systematically evaluated. This lack of evaluation may be due to the limited indications for their use.

Oblique Rotated Graft

In 1965, Pennel and colleagues described the oblique rotated graft.[10] The procedure, also known as papilla rotation graft, is used in cases where the gingival tissue amount at the donor site is not adequate for a laterally positioned pedicle graft, but there is a wide papilla adjacent to the recession defect.[31] The technique involves covering the exposed root by raising a partial-thickness flap and rotating it obliquely. The procedure is associated with good esthetic results, but is applicable only in a few cases.

Double-Papilla Repositioned Flap

Cohen and Ross proposed a double papilla repositioned flap to cover defects in which an insufficient amount of gingiva is present or in which there is an inadequate amount of gingiva in an adjacent area for a lateral sliding flap.[8] This is a modification of the oblique rotated flap, with use of papillae on both sides of a tooth with a denuded root. The papillae from each side of the tooth are reflected and rotated over the mid-facial aspect of the recipient tooth and sutured. The technique provides dual blood supply to the tissues and causes denudation of only the interdental bone. However, it may cause pulling of the sutures and tearing of the gingival papilla, which may lead to poor predictability.[8,33,34]

Coronally Positioned Flap Technique

The coronally positioned pedicle graft is found by most clinicians to be a relatively simple and predictable procedure. Furthermore, it is associated with good esthetic outcomes.[35] The technique involves repositioning of the gingiva. In 1971, Bjorn proposed displacing a free gingival graft laterally over an exposed root after one month of grafting.[36] The use of coronally positioned grafts was first described by Bernimoulin and colleagues as a two-stage procedure, with the coronally positioned graft procedure following a free gingival graft procedure. The authors raised a coronally positioned flap six months after the free gingival graft.[11] Allen and Miller termed the technique as "coronally positioned flap."[14] The "semilunar coronally repositioned flap" is another modification of coronally positioned flap, described by Tarnow.[13] These techniques require the donor sites to be apical rather than lateral to the recession defect.

The coronally positioned flap (Fig. 7-1) is an alternative to lateral transposition of soft tissue pedicle grafts. The prerequisites of the procedure include shallow crevicular depths on the proximal surfaces and approximately normal interproximal bone heights, tissue heights within 1 mm of cementoenamel junction on adjacent teeth, and reduction of any root prominence within the plane of the adjacent alveolar bone.[11] The coronally positioned flap can be used for the treatment of single or multiple recessions.

The first stage involves placing a free autogenous soft-tissue graft apical to an area of denuded root. The flap is then positioned coronally after healing. In the second phase of the procedure, a split thickness flap is developed with mesial and distal vertical releasing incisions. The flap is sutured 0.5 mm to 1 mm coronal to the cementoenamel junction and covered with a periodontal dressing.[37]

Huang and Wang introduced a modified incision design and a suturing technique called the "sling and tag" suturing technique to enhance the results of coronally positioned flap for root coverage.[38] Another study demonstrated that minimal flap tension does not influence recession reduction after three months when shallow

Figure 7-1 **Coronally Positioned Flap Technique** (Porcine Model)

a

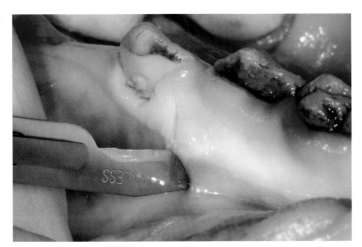

(a) Vertical releasing incision initiated apical to the mucogingival junction in an apico-coronal direction.

b

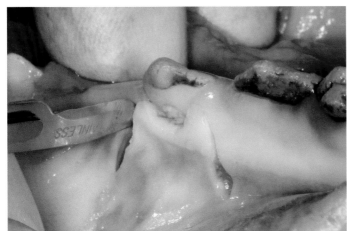

(b) Mesial and distal vertical releasing incisions accomplished in a convergent apico-coronal direction to provide the flap with a wide base for adequate blood supply.

c

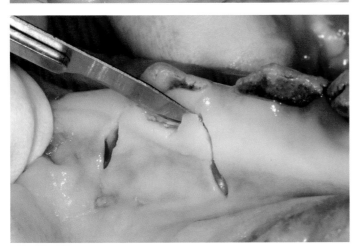

(c & d) Intrasulcular incision on the facial connecting the two vertical releasing incisions. ▼

Figure 7-1 **Coronally Positioned Flap Technique** (Porcine Model, CONT.)

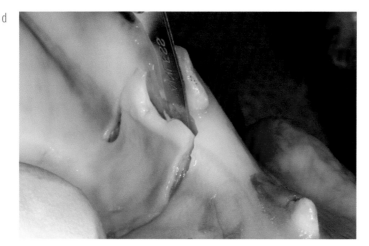

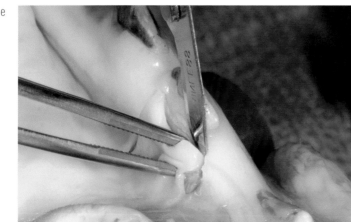

(e) Full-thickness flap reflected using a sharp dissection technique.

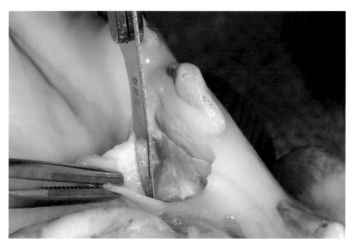

(f) Full-thickness flap reflection extended just pass the mucogingival junction.

▼

Figure 7-1 **Coronally Positioned Flap Technique** (Porcine Model, CONT.)

g

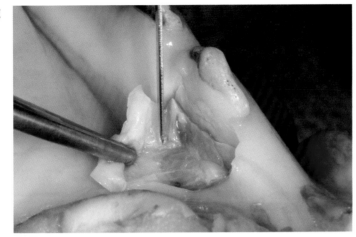

(g) Visualization of the periosteum prior to split-thickness flap dissection.

h

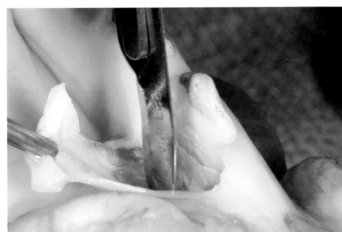

(h) Flap coronally advanced after adequate release of the periosteum. ■

recessions are treated by means of coronally positioned flap. The results suggested that the higher the flap tension, the lower the recession reduction.[39]

Some authors have suggested that the coronally positioned flap is a predictable means of root coverage under defined conditions.[14,40] These conditions include shallow recession of ≤4 mm, Miller Class I recession, keratinized tissue width ≥3 mm, and gingival thickness of ≥1 mm. One study attributes success primarily to marginal thickness alone, which the authors reported should be ≥0.8 mm.[18] It was found that a coronally positioned flap is a predictable procedure to treat Miller's Class I mucogingival defects.

Among all the factors studied, initial gingival thickness was the most significant factor associated with complete root coverage.[41]

In one study, Saletta and others demonstrated that the root coverage following coronally positioned flap procedure is not significantly correlated to papilla dimension. However, complete root coverage is significantly more frequent in sites with lower height of the adjacent papilla.[42]

A study that assessed the effect of thickness of the flap on root coverage when gingival recessions were treated using a coronally advanced flap found that there was a direct relation between flap thickness and recession reduction.[18] A more recent report indicates that a smaller, thinner graft may work as well as a larger, thicker graft as long as the site is completely covered by a coronally positioned flap.[43]

Some other studies reported slightly better results for sites that received polishing alone compared to those receiving root planing and flaps sutured with no tension compared to those with tension.[39,44] Pini Prato and others investigated whether the post-surgical location of gingival margin relative to the cementoenamel junction can influence the recession reduction and complete root coverage following coronally advanced flap procedure. The study showed that the location of the gingival margin relative to the cementoenamel junction following coronally positioned flap procedure seems to affect complete root coverage.[45] It has been shown that greater root coverage is associated with greater coronal displacement of the flap margins. For example, Modica and others reported mean root coverage of 55% to 99% for coronally positioned graft. When compared to connective tissue grafting, such grafting was more acceptable to patients since it does not require a donor site.[46]

Some authors compared coronally positioned flaps with lateral sliding flaps for treatment of localized gingival recessions.[47,48] During the six-month follow-up, both techniques yielded satisfactory outcomes with similar types of tissue coverage, sulcus depths, or gains of attached gingiva. However, the donor site of the lateral sliding flap had a recession of 1 mm, while there were no recessions noted at the coronally positioned flap donor site.

Allen and Miller described coronally positioned flaps as a single-stage technique for the treatment of shallow marginal recession. The procedure resulted in complete root coverage in 84% of the sites, with a mean root coverage gain of 3.2 mm. In a similar study, Harris reported a 98% success rate of root coverage in Class I defects.[14,49]

Another type of coronally positioned flap is the double lateral bridging flap, which combines the Edlan-Mejchar vestibuloplasty procedure with a coronally positioned flap to cover the root defect without increasing the amount of keratinized tissue.[12] A unique modification of the coronally positioned flap technique involves oblique incisions in the papillae, which is then rotated coronally. The technique is indicated for shallow recessions.[50]

Studies that considered flap thickness or keratinized tissue width as criteria for selecting the appropriate technique reported improved root coverage.[14,40,51] Collectively, there are general conclusions that multiple defects should be covered with a long-span coronally positioned flap. Sites with thick margins can be treated with the coronally positioned flap alone while the sites that have thin margins require additional connective tissues. Studies show mean defect coverage ranging from 50% to 98% with a mean for all studies of 78%.[14-16,18,39,42,44,46,51-58]

A 2012 ten-year follow-up study noted that the treatment for most gingival recessions is subepithelial connective tissue grafts; nevertheless, using an enamel matrix derivative has also yielded good results. The study concluded that treatment with either enamel matrix derivative and coronally advanced flap, or connective tissue graft and coronally advanced flap "for Miller Class I and II GR defects appears stable, clinically effective, and similar to each other on all measured parameters."[59] A 2012 randomized controlled study concluded that although the subepithelial connective tissue graft "is considered the gold standard for the treatment of gingival recession defects," the two techniques not only "have comparable clinical effectiveness, but PPG [periosteal pedicle graft] is superior to SCTG [subepithelial connective tissue graft] in terms of patient-centred outcomes, reflecting improved patient comfort and overall patient satisfaction."[60] One of the clinicians in that comparative study had earlier demonstrated that the PPG technique "can be successfully used for the treatment of multiple gingival recession defects."[61]

A 2007 study that evaluated effectiveness of a modification of the coronally advanced flap procedure for the treatment of isolated recession type defects in the upper jaw found that the modified coronally advanced surgical technique was effective in the treatment of isolated gingival recession in the upper jaw.[26] The frontal approach of the coronally advanced flap has been found to be effective for the treatment of multiple gingival recessions affecting the anterior teeth in patients with aesthetic demands, and these results are found to be successful both in terms of root coverage and increase in keratinized tissue height.[62]

Harris and Harris reported that coronally positioned pedicle graft with inlaid margins is a simple and predictable method to cover exposed root surfaces in shallow recession areas.[40] The procedure results in excellent final color and tissue contours of the grafts. While the outcome of a coronally advanced flap is not affected by its combination with platelet-rich plasma, the combination with enamel matrix derivative has shown mixed results. Del Pizzo and others, and Berlucchi and colleagues, in respective studies, found that the addition of enamel matrix derivative to coronally positioned flap technique did not affect root coverage outcomes.[63-65]

However, another study done by Cueva and others that compared differences in clinical parameters of root coverage procedures using coronally advanced flaps with and without enamel matrix derivative showed that application of enamel matrix derivative to denuded root surfaces receiving coronally advanced flaps significantly increased the percentage of root coverage compared to coronally advanced flaps without the use of enamel matrix derivative.[66] A 2011 study by Gamal and colleagues attempted to determine the "levels of platelet-derived growth factor-BB in gingival crevicular fluid during the early stages of healing for sites treated by marginal periosteal pedicle graft as an autogenous guided tissue membrane compared to that of the control open flap debridement." The study concluded that "[p]eriosteal coverage of periodontal defects is not associated with a significant increase in PDGF-BB levels."[67]

In situations with only shallow recession defects, the semi-lunar coronally positioned flap offers an alternative approach. It was originally presented in 1907 and reappeared in the literature in the 1980s. Described by Tarnow, this procedure involves an incision being placed along the curvature of the free margin of the gingiva and extending into the papillae, staying at least 2 mm from the tip of the papilla on either side.[13] The incision is made apically in such a way that the apical portion of the created flap rests on the bone after repositioning the flap. The scalpel blade is then inserted intramuscularly, and the gingiva which lies coronal to the initial incision is advanced over the exposed root. The split-thickness flap is then raised and repositioned; light pressure is applied on the flap to immobilize it. The advantage of the procedure includes less tension on the flap, no shortening of the vestibule, no reflection of the papillae, and, consequently, no esthetic compromise and no suturing. This technique may be useful in covering exposed crown margins.

Haghighat described a modification of this technique, which was found useful in cases where previous attempts for root coverage with soft tissue autografts resulted in residual recession defects on adjacent teeth and in patients with thick gingival tissue that would be amenable to partial thickness dissection. The technique also provides better control over flap repositioning.[68]

The use of semilunar coronally repositioned flap combined with Epiglu has been reported to provide excellent root coverage, especially in anterior and premolar teeth with shallow defects.[69] A 2009 study by Sorrentino and Tarnow describes a technique for performing a frenectomy simultaneously with a coronally repositioned gingiva for root coverage over the maxillary central incisors. The authors explain that "the surgical technique used to treat the areas of recession involved making semilunar incisions over the maxillary central incisors that blended into a frenectomy" and that "[c]omplete root coverage was achieved over the maxillary central incisors that initially presented with 2 mm of recession on the facial surface." They further note that this case confirms "the possibility of applying a combined semilunar coronally repositioned flap with a frenectomy...[when] maxillary central incisors were impinged upon by a broad aberrant frenum, probed </=3 mm, and presented with Miller Class I mucogingival defects."[70]

The Combination of Pedicle Grafts with Other Techniques

The pedicle grafts have been combined with other techniques in an attempt to improve root coverage outcomes.

Combination with Free Gingival Graft

Harvey combined a free gingival graft with a coronally positioned flap. The technique was not widely accepted since it involved an additional surgical procedure, increased treatment time and cost, and was limited to narrow defect only. The technique was also associated with gingival recession and bone loss at the donor site with subsequent root exposure.[71,72]

The combination of pedicle graft with a free gingival graft was a two-step procedure wherein the free gingival graft first augmented the zone of keratinized tissue, followed by a coronally positioned flap about two months later. According to Bernimoulin and colleagues, the flap design included new papilla tips located apical to the original tip by a distance equal to the millimeters of recession.[11] In some cases, the free gingival graft may heal as scar tissue, and then for coronal repositioning, the flap has to be raised through sharp rather than blunt dissection. This series of events can cause thinning or perforation of the flap. Studies show mean defect coverage ranging from 36% to 71% with a mean for all studies of 61%.[11,73-76]

Combination with Connective Tissue Graft

Nelson used a connective tissue graft placed over the denuded root surface, followed by a double pedicle graft that partially exposed the connective tissue graft.[33] The mean root coverage was 88% for recession defects of 7 mm to 10 mm, 92% for recession defects of 4 mm to 6 mm, and 100% for recessions less than 3 mm. Harris modified this technique by using a split-thickness pedicle graft instead of double pedicle graft.[34] The mean coverage was found to be 97%. The results were aging confirmed in a group of 100 patients.[49]

In their study, Wennström and Zucchelli compared a coronally positioned flap alone to its combination with connective tissue graft.[51] It was found that the combination

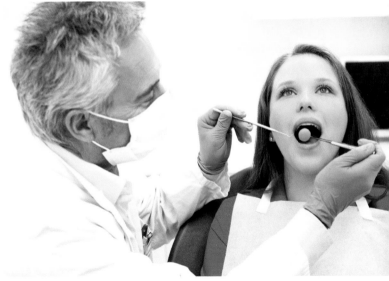

group had higher success rate of root coverage than the group that underwent coronally positioned flap alone. Harris observed two histologically different healing patterns in patients treated with a connective tissue graft combined with a partial thickness double pedicle graft.[77] A long junctional epithelium attachment was found to extend well beyond the original gingival margin and occasionally almost to the original bone level with minimal connective tissue adjacent to the tooth. The other was a short junctional epithelium that stopped at the previously exposed root surface. The authors concluded that though the procedure was successful clinically, it produced no true regeneration but healing by repair.

Blanes and Allen described a tunnel procedure with double lateral pedicle flaps to cover a connective tissue graft.[78] The objective was to compensate for the lack of blood supply that is associated with the tunnel technique in deep or wide adjacent recession. The technique was found to yield predictable success in adjacent class I and class II deep-to-wide recessions and can also be applied to mild class III recessions.

Mele and others described a bilaminar technique consisting of a connective tissue graft covered by a coronally advanced pedicle flap to treat a deep cervical abrasion associated with a recession-type defect. The connective tissue graft was placed inside the root concavity to compensate for the abrasion space and to prevent soft tissue flap collapse internally. It was found that the graft, by acting as a biologic filler, stabilized the covering flap and helped restore a correct tooth emergence profile.[79]

Milano proposed a new single-step mucogingival surgical technique for root coverage consisting of two flaps. A partial thickness epithelial connective tissue flap was designed to cover a second connective tissue double papilla flap positioned directly on the root surface. The procedure does not need a second donor site and results in good esthetic outcomes.[53] Carvalho attempted root coverage at adjacent multiple gingival recessions using a modified coronally positioned flap associated with the subepithelial connective tissue graft. The technique was found to be effective and predictable in root coverage at multiple adjacent gingival recessions associated with increased width of keratinized tissue.[80]

Francetti proposed a microsurgical technique to avoid a second surgical site when treating isolated gingival recessions with the combination of coronally advanced flap and a free connective tissue graft. Gingival recessions were covered with a coronally advanced flap associated with a connective tissue graft harvested from one adjacent papilla whose dimensions matched those of the exposed root area. The procedure demonstrated excellent root coverage without requiring a second surgical site.[81]

A combination of apically positioned flap, closed eruption technique, and a modified double pedicle graft has been used to uncover impacted teeth.[82] Based on their study, Harris and colleagues proposed that when clinicians are treating defects more than 3 mm deep, they should consider using the connective tissue graft with a double pedicle graft or a connective tissue graft with a tunneling procedure and a laterally positioned pedicle flap rather than the connective tissue graft with a coronally positioned flap. Additionally, when treating multiple defects at a time, clinicians should consider using the connective tissue graft with a double pedicle or connective tissue graft with a tunneling procedure and a laterally positioned pedicle rather than the connective tissue graft with a coronally positioned flap. In cases where an increased amount of keratinized tissue is desired, the connective tissue graft with a double pedicle may be the best procedure to use.[83]

A comparative study of double pedicle bilateral flap, coronally repositioned flap in combination with connective tissue graft, and coronally advanced flap in combination with guided tissue regeneration using collagen membranes showed that latter two procedures are mostly predictable and enable the stable coverage of gingival recession during a five-year observation period.[84]

Nemcovsky and other researchers conducted a study to evaluate the clinical efficacy of a coronally advanced flap procedure with the additional use of enamel matrix protein derivative to treat gingival recession and to compare this procedure to the subpedicle connective tissue graft procedure. It was found that the connective tissue graft procedure was superior to the coronally positioned flap procedure with the addition of enamel matrix proteins derivative in the percentage of coverage and increase in width of keratinized tissue.[85]

Another study comparing the combination of guided tissue regeneration with a bioabsorbable polylactic acid softened with citric acid ester membrane and the connective tissue graft combined with a coronally positioned pedicle graft without vertical incisions found the technique of connective tissue graft combined with a coronally positioned pedicle graft superior in terms of increasing the amount of keratinized tissue.[86]

A comparative study conducted by Matarasso to assess combinations of regenerative therapy using a resorbable polylactic acid membrane with double papilla flap procedure and coronally repositioned flap found both combinations to be effective in reducing recessions and probing depths. The group treated with double papilla flap procedure showed a significant increase in the amount of keratinized gingiva.[17] Some preclinical studies also indicate similar results obtained with guided tissue regeneration and coronally advanced flap procedure.[87]

Summary

The pedicle graft is an excellent surgical technique to treat isolated recession defects. The blood supply at the base of the gingiva results in better revascularization of the graft onto the recipient site and enhances the healing process. As a result, the outcomes are predictable in terms of width of gingival attachment and root coverage. The flap to cover the defect is taken from the adjoining area; thus, the esthetics are not compromised as in the case of free gingival grafts. In addition there is no need for a second donor site. However, because of the consistent results achieved with subepithelial connective tissue grafts, the use of pedicle grafts alone to treat recession defects has declined. Various combinations are now used to improve the pedicle technique further and bring about better root coverage.

References

1. Grupe HE, Warren RF, Jr. Repair of gingival defect by sliding flap operation. J. Periodontol. 1956;27:92-95.

2. Grupe HE. Modified technique for the sliding flap operation. J Periodontol. 1966 Nov-Dec;37(6):491-5.

3. McFall WT Jr. The laterally repositioned flap--criteria for success. Periodontics. 1967 Mar-Apr;5(2):89-92.

4. Smukler H. Laterally positioned mucoperiosteal pedicle grafts in the treatment of denuded roots. A clinical and statistical study. J Periodontol. 1976 Oct;47(10):590-5.

5. Guinard EA, Caffesse RG. Treatment of localized gingival recessions. Part I. Lateral sliding flap. J Periodontol. 1978 Jul;49(7):351-6.

6. Svoboda PJ, Sheridan PJ. A modification of the pedicle graft in the treatment of gingival recession. Oral Surg Oral Med Oral Pathol. 1984 Feb;57(2):143-6.

7. Gartrell JR, Mathews DP. Gingival recession. The condition, process, and treatment. Dent Clin North Am. 1976 Jan;20(1):199-213.

8. Cohen DW, Ross SE. The double papillae repositioned flap in periodontal therapy. J Periodontol. 1968 Mar;39(2):65-70.

9. Ross SE, Crosetti HW, Gargiulo A, Cohen DW. The double papillae repositioned flap--an alternative. I. Fourteen years in retrospect. Int J Periodontics Restorative Dent. 1986; 6(6):46-59.

10. Pennel BM, Higgason JD, Towner JD, King KO, Fritz BD, Salder JF. Oblique rotated flap. J Periodontol. 1965 Jul-Aug;36:305-9.

11. Bernimoulin JP, Lüscher B, Mühlemann HR. Coronally repositioned periodontal flap. Clinical evaluation after one year. J Clin Periodontol. 1975 Feb;2(1):1-13.

12. Marggraf E. A direct technique with a double lateral bridging flap for coverage of denuded root surface and gingiva extension. Clinical evaluation after 2 years. J Clin Periodontol. 1985 Jan;12(1):69-76.

13. Tarnow DP. Semilunar coronally repositioned flap. J Clin Periodontol. 1986 Mar;13(3):182-5.

14. Allen EP, Miller PD Jr. Coronal positioning of existing gingiva: short term results in the treatment of shallow marginal tissue recession. J Periodontol. 1989 Jun;60(6):316-9.

15. Romanos GE, Bernimoulin JP, Marggraf E. The double lateral bridging flap for coverage of denuded root surface: longitudinal study and clinical evaluation after 5 to 8 years. J Periodontol. 1993 Aug;64(8):683-8.

16. Trombelli L, Scabbia A, Wikesjö UM, Calura G. Fibrin glue application in conjunction with tetracycline root conditioning and coronally positioned flap procedure in the treatment of human gingival recession defects. J Clin Periodontol. 1996 Sep;23(9):861-7.

17. Matarasso S, Cafiero C, Coraggio F, Vaia E, de Paoli S. Guided tissue regeneration versus coronally repositioned flap in the treatment of recession with double papillae. Int J Periodontics Restorative Dent. 1998 Oct;18(5):444-53.

18. Baldi C, Pini-Prato G, Pagliaro U, Nieri M, Saletta D, Muzzi L, Cortellini P. Coronally advanced flap procedure for root coverage. Is flap thickness a relevant predictor to achieve root coverage? A 19-case series. J Periodontol. 1999 Sep;70(9):1077-84.

19. Staffileno H. Management of gingival recession and root exposure problems associated with periodontal disease. Compend Contin Educ Dent 1964;November:111-120.

20. Robinson RE. Utilizing an edentulous area as a donor site in the lateral repositioned flap. Periodontics 1964;2:79-85.

21. Irwin RK. Combined use of the gingival graft and rotated pedicle procedures: case reports. J Periodontol. 1977 Jan;48(1):38-40.

22. Corn H. Edentulous area pedicle grafts in mucogingival surgery. Periodontics 1964;2:229-42.

23. Hattler AB. Mucogingival surgery--utilization of interdental gingiva as attached gingiva by surgical displacement. Periodontics. 1967 May-Jun;5(3):126-31.

24. Oliveira TM, Greghi SL, Taveria LA, Santos CF, Machado MA, Silva SM. Surgical removal of an oral pyogenic granuloma and subsequent root coverage with a pedicle graft. J Dent Child (Chic). 2008 Jan-Apr;75(1):55-8.

25. Zucchelli G, Cesari C, Amore C, Montebugnoli L, De Sanctis M. Laterally moved, coronally advanced flap: a modified surgical approach for isolated recession-type defects. J Periodontol. 2004 Dec;75(12):1734-41. Erratum in: J Periodontol. 2005 Aug;76(8):1425.

26. de Sanctis M, Zucchelli G. Coronally advanced flap: a modified surgical approach for isolated recession-type defects: three-year results. J Clin Periodontol. 2007 Mar;34(3):262-8.

27. Smukler H, Goldman HM. Laterally repositioned "stimulated" osteoperiosteal pedicle grafts in the treatment of denuded roots. A preliminary report. J Periodontol. 1979 Aug;50(8):379-83.

28. Caffesse RG, Espinel MC. Lateral sliding flap with a free gingival graft technique in the treatment of localized gingival recessions. Int J Periodontics Restorative Dent. 1981;1(6):22-9.

29. Espinel MC, Caffesse RG. Comparison of the results obtained with the laterally positioned pedicle sliding flap-revised technique and the lateral sliding flap with a free gingival graft technique in the treatment of localized gingival recessions. Int J Periodontics Restorative Dent. 1981;1(6):30-7.

30. Patur B. The rotation flap for covering denuded root surfaces - a closed wound technique. J Periodontol. 1977 Jan;48(1):41-4.

31. Leis HJ, Leis SN. The papilla rotation flap. J Periodontol. 1978 Aug;49(8):400-2.

32. Tinti C, Parma-Benfenati S. The free rotated papilla autograft: a new bilaminar grafting procedure for the coverage of multiple shallow gingival recessions. J Periodontol. 1996 Oct;67(10):1016-24.

33. Nelson SW. The subpedicle connective tissue graft. A bilaminar reconstructive procedure for the coverage of denuded root surfaces. J Periodontol. 1987 Feb;58(2):95-102.

34. Harris RJ. The connective tissue and partial thickness double pedicle graft: a predictable method of obtaining root coverage. J Periodontol. 1992 May;63(5):477-86.

35. Brustein DD. Cosmetic periodontics-coronally repositioned pedicle graft. Dent Surv. 1970 Jul;46(7):22-5.

36. Björn H. Coverage of denuded root surfaces with a lateral sliding flap. Use of free gingival grafts. Odontol Revy. 1971;22(1):37-44.

37. Maynard JG Jr. Coronal positioning of a previously placed autogenous gingival graft. J Periodontol. 1977 Mar;48(3):151-5.

38. Huang LH, Wang HL. Sling and tag suturing technique for coronally advanced flap. Int J Periodontics Restorative Dent. 2007 Aug;27(4):379-85.

39. Pini Prato G, Pagliaro U, Baldi C, Nieri M, Saletta D, Cairo F, Cortellini P. Coronally advanced flap procedure for root coverage. Flap with tension versus flap without tension: a randomized controlled clinical study. J Periodontol. 2000 Feb;71(2):188-201.

40. Harris RJ, Harris AW. The coronally positioned pedicle graft with inlaid margins: a predictable method of obtaining root coverage of shallow defects. Int J Periodontics Restorative Dent. 1994 Jun;14(3):228-41.

41. Huang LH, Neiva RE, Wang HL. Factors affecting the outcomes of coronally advanced flap root coverage procedure. J Periodontol. 2005 Oct;76(10):1729-34.

42. Saletta D, Pini Prato G, Pagliaro U, Baldi C, Mauri M, Nieri M. Coronally advanced flap procedure: is the interdental papilla a prognostic factor for root coverage? J Periodontol. 2001 Jun;72(6):760-6.

43. Zucchelli G, Amore C, Sforza NM, Montebugnoli L, De Sanctis M. Bilaminar techniques for the treatment of recession-type defects. A comparative clinical study. J Clin Periodontol. 2003 Oct;30(10):862-70.

44. Pini-Prato G, Baldi C, Pagliaro U, Nieri M, Saletta D, Rotundo R, Cortellini P. Coronally advanced flap procedure for root coverage. Treatment of root surface: root planning versus polishing. J Periodontol. 1999 Sep;70(9):1064-76.

45. Pini Prato GP, Baldi C, Nieri M, Franseschi D, Cortellini P, Clauser C, Rotundo R, Muzzi L. Coronally advanced flap: the post-surgical position of the gingival margin is an important factor for achieving complete root coverage. J Periodontol. 2005 May;76(5):713-22.

46. Modica F, Del Pizzo M, Roccuzzo M, Romagnoli R. Coronally advanced flap for the treatment of buccal gingival recessions with and without enamel matrix derivative. A split-mouth study. J Periodontol. 2000 Nov;71(11):1693-8.

47. Guinard EA, Caffesse RG. Treatment of localized gingival recessions. Part III. Comparison of results obtained with lateral sliding and coronally repositioned flaps. J Periodontol. 1978 Sep;49(9):457-61.

48. Caffesse RG, Guinard EA. Treatment of localized gingival recessions. Part IV. Results after three years. J Periodontol. 1980 Mar;51(3):167-70.

49. Harris RJ. The connective tissue with partial thickness double pedicle graft: the results of 100 consecutively-treated defects. J Periodontol. 1994 May;65(5):448-61.

50. Zucchelli G, De Sanctis M. Treatment of multiple recession-type defects in patients with esthetic demands. J Periodontol. 2000 Sep;71(9):1506-14.

51. Wennström JL, Zucchelli G. Increased gingival dimensions. A significant factor for successful outcome of root coverage procedures? A 2-year prospective clinical study. J Clin Periodontol. 1996 Aug;23(8):770-7.

52. da Silva RC, Joly JC, de Lima AF, Tatakis DN. Root coverage using the coronally positioned flap with or without a subepithelial connective tissue graft. J Periodontol. 2004 Mar; 75(3):413-9.

53. Milano F. A combined flap for root coverage. Int J Periodontics Restorative Dent. 1998 Dec;18(6):544-51.

54. Amarante ES, Leknes KN, Skavland J, Lie T. Coronally positioned flap procedures with or without a bioabsorbable membrane in the treatment of human gingival recession. J Periodontol. 2000 Jun;71(6):989-98.

55. Hägewald S, Spahr A, Rompola E, Haller B, Heijl L, Bernimoulin JP. Comparative study of Emdogain and coronally advanced flap technique in the treatment of human gingival recessions. A prospective controlled clinical study. J Clin Periodontol. 2002 Jan;29(1):35-41.

56. Lins LH, de Lima AF, Sallum AW. Root coverage: comparison of coronally positioned flap with and without titanium-reinforced barrier membrane. J Periodontol. 2003 Feb;74(2):168-74.

57. McGuire MK, Nunn M. Evaluation of human recession defects treated with coronally advanced flaps and either enamel matrix derivative or connective tissue. Part 1: Comparison of clinical parameters. J Periodontol. 2003 Aug;74(8):1110-25.

58. Woodyard JG, Greenwell H, Hill M, Drisko C, Iasella JM, Scheetz J. The clinical effect of acellular dermal matrix on gingival thickness and root coverage compared to coronally positioned flap alone. J Periodontol. 2004 Jan;75(1):44-56.

59. McGuire MK, Scheyer ET, Nunn M. Evaluation of human recession defects treated with coronally advanced flaps and either enamel matrix derivative or connective tissue: comparison of clinical parameters at 10 years. J Periodontol. 2012 Nov;83(11):1353-62.

60. Mahajan A, Bharadwaj A, Mahajan P. Comparison of periosteal pedicle graft and subepithelial connective tissue graft for the treatment of gingival recession defects. Aust Dent J. 2012 Mar;57(1):51-7.

61. Mahajan A. Treatment of multiple gingival recession defects using periosteal pedicle graft: a case series. J Periodontol. 2010 Oct;81(10):1426-31.

62. Zucchelli G, De Sanctis M. The coronally advanced flap for the treatment of multiple recession defects: a modified surgical approach for the upper anterior teeth. J Int Acad Periodontol. 2007 Jul;9(3):96-103.

63. Huang LH, Neiva RE, Soehren SE, Giannobile WV, Wang HL. The effect of platelet-rich plasma on the coronally advanced flap root coverage procedure: a pilot human trial. J Periodontol. 2005 Oct;76(10):1768-77.

64. Del Pizzo M, Zucchelli G, Modica F, Villa R, Debernardi C. Coronally advanced flap with or without enamel matrix derivative for root coverage: a 2-year study. J Clin Periodontol. 2005 Nov;32(11):1181-7.

65. Berlucchi I, Francetti L, Del Fabbro M, Basso M, Weinstein RL. The influence of anatomical features on the outcome of gingival recessions treated with coronally advanced flap and enamel matrix derivative: a 1-year prospective study. J Periodontol. 2005 Jun;76(6):899-907.

66. Cueva MA, Boltchi FE, Hallmon WW, Nunn ME, Rivera-Hidalgo F, Rees T. A comparative study of coronally advanced flaps with and without the addition of enamel matrix derivative in the treatment of marginal tissue recession. J Periodontol. 2004 Jul; 75(7):949-56.

67. Gamal AY, El-Shal OS, El-Aasara MM, Fakhry EM. Platelet-derived growth factor-BB release profile in gingival crevicular fluid after use of marginal periosteal pedicle graft as an autogenous guided tissue membrane to treat localized intrabony defects. J Periodontol. 2011 Feb;82(2):272-80.

68. Haghighat K. Modified semilunar coronally advanced flap. J Periodontol. 2006 Jul;77(7):1274-9.

69. M. Jahangirnezhad. Semilunar coronally repositioned flap for the treatment of gingival recession with and without tissue adhesives: A pilot study. Journal of Dentistry, Tehran University of Medical Sciences, Tehran, Iran. 2006; Vol: 3, No 1.

70. Sorrentino JM, Tarnow DP. The semilunar coronally repositioned flap combined with a frenectomy to obtain root coverage over the maxillary central incisors. J Periodontol. 2009 Jun;80(6):1013-7.

71. Harvey PM. Management of advanced periodontitis. I. Preliminary report of a method of surgical reconstruction. N Z Dent J. 1965 Jul;61(285):180-7.

72. Langer B, Langer L. Subepithelial connective tissue graft technique for root coverage. J Periodontol. 1985 Dec;56(12):715-20.

73. Caffesse RG, Guinard EA. Treatment of localized gingival recessions. Part II. Coronally repositioned flap with a free gingival graft. J Periodontol. 1978 Jul;49(7):357-61.

74. Matter J. Free gingival graft and coronally repositioned flap. A 2-year follow-up report. J Clin Periodontol. 1979 Dec;6(6):437-42.

75. Liu WJ, Solt CW. A surgical procedure for the treatment of localized gingival recession in conjunction with root surface citric acid conditioning. J Periodontol. 1980 Sep;51(9):505-9.

76. Tenenbaum H, Klewansky P, Roth JJ. Clinical evaluation of gingival recession treated by coronally repositioned flap technique. J Periodontol. 1980 Dec;51(12):686-90.

77. Harris RJ. Human histologic evaluation of root coverage obtained with a connective tissue with partial thickness double pedicle graft. A case report. J Periodontol. 1999 Jul; 70(7):813-21.

78. Blanes RJ, Allen EP. The bilateral pedicle flap-tunnel technique: a new approach to cover connective tissue grafts. Int J Periodontics Restorative Dent. 1999 Oct;19(5):471-9.

79. Mele M, Zucchelli G, Montevecchi M, Checchi L. Bilaminar technique in the treatment of a deep cervical abrasion defect. Int J Periodontics Restorative Dent. 2008 Feb;28(1):63-71.

80. Carvalho PF, da Silva RC, Cury PR, Joly JC. Modified coronally advanced flap associated with a subepithelial connective tissue graft for the treatment of adjacent multiple gingival recessions. J Periodontol. 2006 Nov; 77(11):1901-6.

81. Francetti L, Del Fabbro M, Testori T, Weinstein RL. Periodontal microsurgery: report of 16 cases consecutively treated by the free rotated papilla autograft technique combined with the coronally advanced flap. Int J Periodontics Restorative Dent. 2004 Jun;24(3):272-9.

82. Sunil S, Avinash BS, Prasad D, Jagadish L. A modified double pedicle graft technique and other mucogingival interceptive surgeries for the management of impacted teeth: a case series. Indian J Dent Res. 2006 Jan-Mar;17(1):35-9.

83. Harris RJ, Miller LH, Harris CR, Miller RJ. A comparison of three techniques to obtain root coverage on mandibular incisors. J Periodontol. 2005 Oct;76(10):1758-67.

84. Dominiak M, Konopka T, Lompart H, Kubasiewicz P. Comparative research concerning clinical efficiency of three surgical methods of periodontium recessions treatment in five-year observations. Adv Med Sci. 2006;51 Suppl 1:18-25.

85. Nemcovsky CE, Artzi Z, Tal H, Kozlovsky A, Moses O. A multicenter comparative study of two root coverage procedures: coronally advanced flap with addition of enamel matrix proteins and subpedicle connective tissue graft. J Periodontol. 2004 Apr;75(4):600-7.

86. Harris RJ. A comparison of 2 root coverage techniques: guided tissue regeneration with a bioabsorbable matrix style membrane versus a connective tissue graft combined with a coronally positioned pedicle graft without vertical incisions. results of a series of consecutive cases. J Periodontol. 1998 Dec;69(12):1426-34.

87. Lee EJ, Meraw SJ, Oh TJ, Giannobile WV, Wang HL. Comparative histologic analysis of coronally advanced flap with and without collagen membrane for root coverage. J Periodontol. 2002 Jul;73(7):779-88.

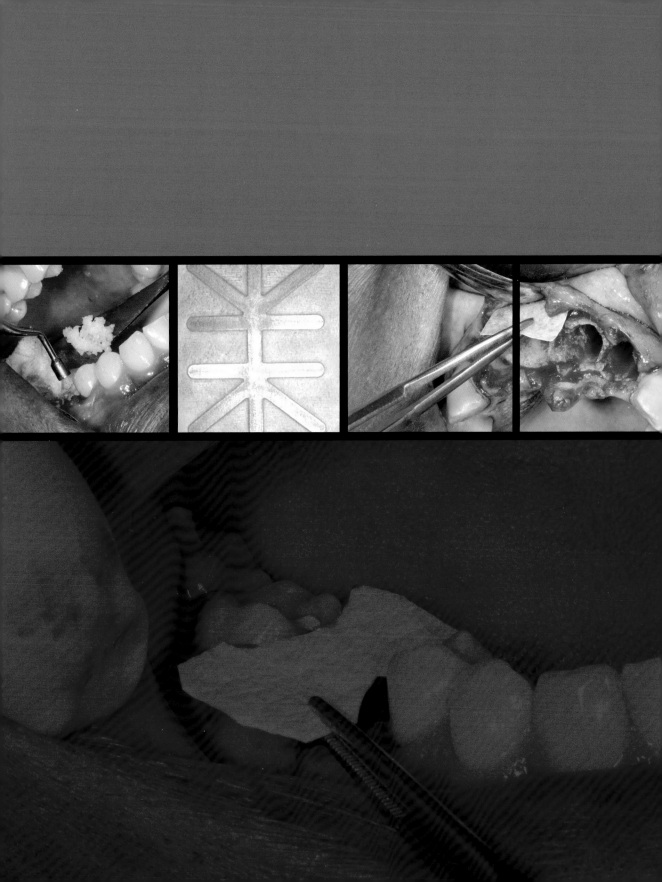

Guided Tissue/Bone Regeneration

8

Using microporous membranes as selective cell barriers, clinicians employ guided tissue regeneration to treat deficient periodontium. Such membrane barriers allow only certain types of cells to enter the area of the defect and then to regenerate into specific tissues. The method can be used to regenerate both soft and hard tissues. Initially, the technique of guided tissue regeneration was used in periodontal surgery to treat bony defects. The main objective was to enhance the tissue and to allow for the regeneration of new bone around teeth with bony defects due to periodontal disease. The technique is also widely used for root coverage and gingival recessions, helping to improve the shape and contour of the area, thereby enhancing esthetics.

Guided tissue regeneration is often referred to as "repopulating" the periodontium by guiding the periodontal ligament progenitor cells to regenerate specific cells. The contact between the root and the soft tissue is blocked by synthetic membranes or collagen membranes used as barriers. These barriers help to create a space for regeneration and enable the periodontal ligament progenitor cells to regenerate specific cells at desired places. This procedure is the method of choice for treating bone defects caused by periodontal diseases which cannot be treated by a conservative approach or through pharmacotherapy.

Guided tissue regeneration (GTR) is the term used for regeneration of lost bone and periodontium around natural teeth while guided bone regeneration (GBR)(Figs. 8-1 and 8-2) is used to describe the procedure to preserve and/or regenerate bone around extraction sockets (Fig. 8-4) or edentulous spaces in preparation for implant placement and to regenerate bone defects around implants during and after placement (Fig. 8-5).

History of Guided Tissue Regeneration

Guided tissue regeneration is not new to medicine. It was introduced by Hurley and others in 1959 for orthopedic indications.[1] The basic principles of the procedure were described in 1976 by Melcher, who identified the role of blocking the unwanted cells from the wound tissues to allow regeneration of selective cells.[2] The applications of guided tissue regeneration in periodontology was not identified until the 1980s, when research began involving the procedure for regenerating alveolar bone to treat alveolar bone defects.

Nyman, Lindhe, Karring, and Ryland, and later Gottlow and Wennström were the first to use barrier membranes in the oral cavity for guided tissue regeneration to reduce gingival pocket depths. This procedure emerged as an alternative to the resective surgical procedures.[3-5] Later, Tinti and colleagues used the technique to cover

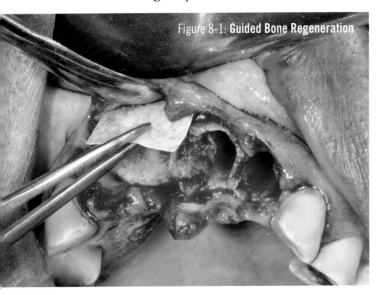

Figure 8-1: **Guided Bone Regeneration**

root defects and to reestablish a connective tissue attachment to exposed root surfaces.[6,7] Pini Prato and colleagues used guided tissue regeneration for the simultaneous treatment of osseous defects, exposed roots, and mucogingival problems. Their study also showed superiority of guided tissue regeneration over mucogingival surgeries.[8] Cortellini and others analyzed the histology of the new attachment following the treatment of gingival recession by guided tissue regeneration.[9] It was found that the technique is independent of the width of the surrounding keratinized gingiva and can be applicable in single recessions.

For years, research has focused on identifying the optimal substance for barrier membranes, one that satisfies the criteria for successful periodontal treatment, including "biocompatibility, occlusivity, spaciousness, clinical manageability and the appropriate integration with the surrounding tissue."[10] Studies have focused on different

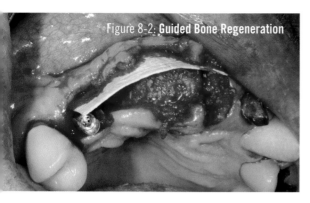

Figure 8-2: **Guided Bone Regeneration**

resorbable and non-resorbable membranes exhibiting a variety of characteristics. The ideal membrane still eludes clinicians. Clinicians must weigh the advantages and disadvantages of the different types of membranes, and most clinicians agree that "[a] thorough understanding of the benefits and limitations inherent to various materials in specific clinical applications will be of great value and aid in the selection of an optimal membrane for guided bone regeneration."[10]

In their 2011 study, Gentile, Chiono, and others succinctly summarize the basic conflict between barriers that offer stable mechanical properties but low biocompatibility versus membranes that are biocompatible but mechanically unstable: "The polyester-based membranes are biodegradable, permit a single-stage procedure, and have higher manageability than non-resorbable membranes; however, they have shown poor biocompatibility. In contrast, membranes based on natural materials, such as collagen, are biocompatible but are characterized by poor mechanical properties and stability due to their early degradation."[11] Some studies have focused on titanium mesh membranes due to their "superb mechanical properties."[10] Others have concentrated on single-stage membranes that offer various degrees of complementary mechanical stability and biocompatibility.[11] In a study published in 2012, Bottino, Thomas, and others "hypothesized that the next generation of guided tissue and guided bone regeneration (GTR/GBR) membranes for periodontal tissue engineering will be a biologically active, spatially designed and functionally graded nanofibrous biomaterial that closely mimics the native extracellular matrix (ECM)." These clinicians speculate that "hydrogels in combination with scaffold materials [offer] a promising approach for periodontal tissue engineering."[12] In another 2012 study, Dimitriou, Mataliotakis, and others conclude that "[a]lthough there are a few promising preliminary human studies, before clinical applications can be recommended, future research should aim to establish the 'ideal' barrier membrane and delineate the need for additional bone grafting materials aiming to 'mimic' or even accelerate the normal process of bone formation. Reproducible results and long-term observations with barrier membranes in animal studies, and particularly in large animal models, are required as well as well-designed clinical studies to evaluate their safety, efficacy and cost-effectiveness."[13]

Basic Principles of Guided Tissue Regeneration

Wang and Boyapati proposed "The PASS Principle" to describe the physiological processes involved in regeneration and the factors affecting it.[14] The Principle holds true for regeneration of both bone and soft tissues. These important elements for tissue regeneration are:

- **PRIMARY WOUND CLOSURE** ("to ensure undisturbed and uninterrupted wound healing")

- **ANGIOGENESIS** ("to provide necessary blood supply and undifferentiated mesenchymal cells")

- **SPACE MAINTENANCE/CREATION** ("to facilitate adequate space for bone ingrowth")

- **STABILITY OF THE WOUND AND IMPLANT** ("to induce blood clot formation and uneventful healing events").[14]

Primary closure of the wound is important to help the tissue heal undisturbed and uninterrupted. Additionally, primary closure promotes the second principle, that is, angiogenesis. Revascularization is necessary to provide the required nourishment to the growing undifferentiated tissues. Lack of blood supply may have adverse effects on regeneration of tissues. Creating a space is required for providing room to the growing tissues; equally important is maintaining the created space until the tissues have fully differentiated. The surgical wound needs to be stable to promote blood clot formation, thereby helping the wound to heal uneventfully.

Guided Tissue Regeneration Technique

In the guided tissue regeneration procedure, a trapezoidal, full-thickness flap is created approximately 3 mm above the margin of the root defect. The barrier membrane (Fig. 8-3) to be used is shaped to a convex form and modified as per the size of the defect to be covered. The root surface is reshaped to a concave form to create a space between the root surface and the barrier membrane. The membrane is then sutured over the exposed root. The flap raised earlier is coronally positioned to cover the barrier membrane and is sutured.

In general, periodontal procedures cause epithelium to migrate faster along the root surface, thereby inhibiting the periodontal ligament and bone from regenerating in the defects. To prevent epithelium migration, the clinician places a barrier over the treated root surface, which not only prevents migration of epithelium but also allows selective repopulation of the exposed root surface.[4,15,16] The barrier creates an environment that stabilizes blood clotting and helps cells from the periodontal ligament to repopulate the debrided root surface and to form a new periodontal attachment.[5]

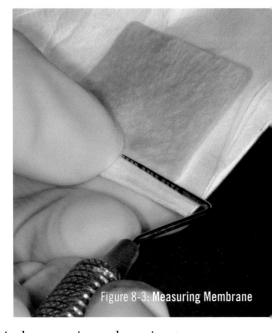

Figure 8-3: Measuring Membrane

In a 1994 study, Tinti and Vincezi reported mean root coverage of 74%, with more than 100% improvement in the width of keratinized gingiva.[17] Guided tissue regeneration routinely results in good esthetic outcomes and restoration of the lost periodontal attachment.[18] In addition, such a procedure does not require a second surgical site as a tissue donor site. However, there are certain disadvantages to the technique. The procedure is relatively expensive and requires two surgeries if a nonresorbable membrane is used. The membrane exposure, if it occurs, may result in a poor outcome. It was also found that the surgery outcome following guided tissue regeneration in gingival recession defects is impaired in cigarette smokers.[20] Villar and Cochran concluded in a 2010 study that while "[q]uantitative analysis of clinical outcomes after guided tissue regeneration suggests that this therapy is a successful and predictable procedure to treat narrow intrabony defects and class II mandibular furcations, ...[guided tissue regeneration] offers limited benefits in the treatment of other types of periodontal defects."[21]

Figure 8-4 **GBR for Bone Regeneration and Preservation Around a Molar Extraction Socket**

a
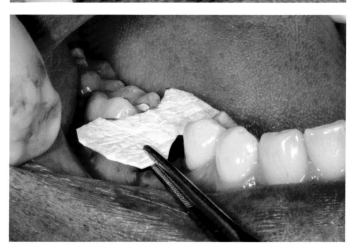

(a) Measuring and trimming of resorbable membrane.

b
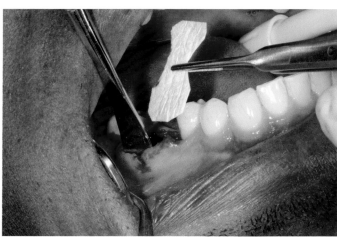

(b) Verification of the proper size and shape of the membrane for the site.

c

(c & d) Half of the membrane inserted underneath the buccal flap.

d

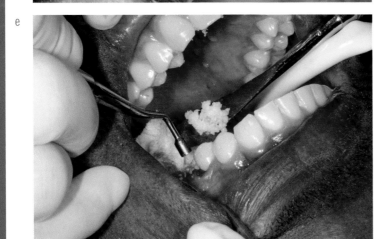

e

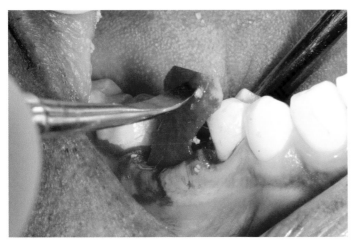

f

(e) Extraction socket packed with freeze dried bone allograft (FDBA).

(f & g) Remaining half of the membrane placed over and tucked underneath the lingual flap. ▼

g

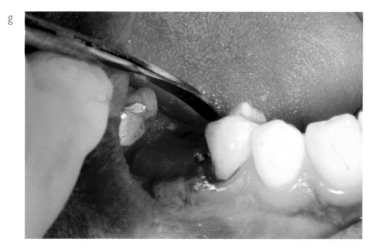

h

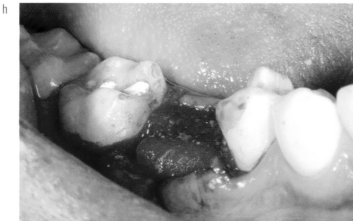

(h) Membrane in place prior to tension free primary closure. ■

Trombelli and colleagues reported that treatment of buccal gingival recession using guided tissue regeneration procedure plus tetracycline root demineralization and fibrin-fibronectin glue application results in a consistent and predictable improvement of mucogingival defects.[22] These results were further confirmed in a split mouth clinical trial.[23] A combination of tetracycline HCl root demineralization, fibrin sealing system application, guided tissue regeneration procedure, and coronal sliding flap operation has been found to be effective in healing localized gingival recessions.[24]

A study completed by Ricci and colleagues found guided tissue regeneration to be preferable to connective tissue graft method when severe mucogingival defects are present and gaining a certain level of clinical attachment is mandatory.[25] However, Chambrone and colleagues concluded in a 2009 study that "Subepithelial connective tissue grafts, coronally advanced flap alone or associated with other biomaterial and guided tissue regeneration may be used as root coverage procedures for the treatment of localised recession-type defects." They further noted that"[i]n cases where both root coverage and gain in the keratinized tissue are expected, the use of subepithelial connective tissue grafts seems to be more adequate."[26]

Barrier Membranes

Barrier membranes used in guided tissue regeneration can be derived from natural or synthetic sources. Based on the ability to be resorbed by the body, the barrier membranes are of two types: non-resorbable and resorbable.

Non-Resorbable Membranes

As the name suggests, non-resorbable membranes are not resorbed by the body and need to be removed after a specific period of time through a second surgical procedure. Millipore filter barriers were used as non-resorbable membranes but were found to be quite impractical.[27] Gottlow and others introduced the use of expanded polytetrafluoroethylene (ePTFE) membranes as barriers in 1984.[4,5] ePTFE membranes are non-resorbable but biocompatible synthetic polymer membranes of the Teflon trade name. Use of ePTFE as barrier membrane has yielded excellent outcomes; however, many clinicians still have recommended that the frequency of surgical intervention needs to be minimized to reduce the risks associated with its use.[28] ePTFE membranes need to be surgically removed after 4 to 6 weeks because they can interfere with the healing process and become contaminated by bacteria through premature exposure. Such complications can, in turn, adversely affect the regeneration of tissues.

Trombelli and others used an ePTFE membrane to treat deep and wide buccal gingival recessions and found that there was a significant increase in clinical attachment gain. The study indicated the effectiveness of guided tissue regeneration to improve soft tissue conditions of deep mucogingival defects.[29] Ito and Murai also reported soft tissue coverage of the root surfaces with guided tissue regeneration using ePTFE membrane. Such coverage was also found to be effective in reducing hypersensitivity and improving the esthetics.[30] In a later study, Ito, Oshio, Shiomi, and Murai compared guided tissue regeneration with expanded polytetrafluoroethylene membranes to free gingival graft for treatment of adjacent facial gingival recession. They concluded that "[b]oth procedures produced the same average amount of root coverage, reduction in gingival recession, and gain in clinical attachment." However, they also noted that [t]he guided tissue regeneration procedure provided a better esthetic appearance without any difference in gingival color or architecture in cases of adjacent facial gingival recession."[31]

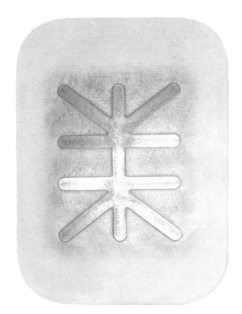

Figure 8-5 **Non-Resorbable Membrane (Titantium-reinforced ePTFE)**

Tinti and Vincenzi used titanium-reinforced membranes of expanded polytetrafluoroethylene (ePTFE, Fig. 8-5) to facilitate the creation and maintenance of secondary spaces in 12 patients with mucogingival recession defects, and reported that titanium-reinforced ePTFE membranes result in a simpler, faster, and more predictable surgical procedure.[17] Roccuzzo and Buser reported good outcomes in treatment of buccal recessions using ePTFE membranes and miniscrews.[32]

Resorbable Membranes

To avoid the limitations of ePTFE membranes, resorbable or bioabsorbable membranes were developed. These can be either animal-derived or synthetic polymers. As the name suggests, resorbable membranes are gradually hydrolyzed or degraded by the enzymes and do not require another surgical procedure for their removal.[33] An ideal resorbable barrier membrane should possess adequate mechanical strength to allow suturing of the membrane to the recipient tissue, be permeable to nutrients, and should not elicit antigenic response. In other words, it should be biocompatible. The various sources of resorbable membranes are rat collagen, bovine collagen, ox cecum cargile membrane, polylactic acid, polyacetic acid, polyglycolic acid, polyglactin 910 (Vicryl), synthetic skin, and freeze-dried dura mater. Recently developed membranes are combination of these materials.

Histological studies demonstrate the ability of a resorbable membrane to allow complete regeneration of the periodontal ligament in the coverage of gingival recessions.[34] Prato and others reported significant gains in probing attachment and root coverage with use of resorbable membranes for guided tissue regeneration.[35] Similar results were reported by Rachlin and colleagues.[36]

Jaspen and others reported favorable outcomes after using a new bioabsorbable barrier material for root coverage in recession type defects.[37] Vuddhakanok and others reported that a combination copolymer barrier of polylactide:polyglycolide did not prevent epithelial migration nor enhance connective tissue attachment to human roots with severe horizontal bone loss and active periodontal disease.[38] De Sanctis

and Zucchelli used a polyglycolactic membrane (Vicryl) for guided tissue regeneration to treat buccal recessions and found that root coverage was achieved in four out of six patients.[39] Waterman reported that use of a bioabsorbable membrane predictably and significantly increases root coverage and regenerates buccal bone when used to treat localized buccal recession defects.[40] A comparative study completed by Roccuzzo and colleagues showed no significant differences in the outcome in the two groups treated with bioresorbable and a non-resorbable membranes, except for the fact that the use of bioresorbable membrane was the choice of most patients, being a single step procedure.[41]

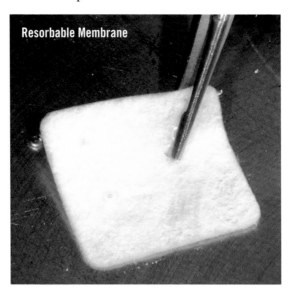

Resorbable Membrane

Collagen is basically a biocompatible material and has the property to promote wound healing. It is a natural protein and is broken down into amino acids by the body's own enzymes in about 4 to 38 weeks. This property makes it suitable as a barrier membrane in guided tissue regeneration. When used as barrier membranes, collagen membranes are absorbed by the recipient tissue and act as barriers for a specified period of time before being absorbed. It has been found that unmodified collagen membranes that are prepared in acidic pH cause acid leaching over the recipient area on application. Therefore, it is advisable to modify the collagen chemically and then reconstitute it at neutral pH.

Collagen is appropriate for use as barrier membrane due to its physical and biological properties.[42,43] The use of collagen reduces tissue-related problems and deficiencies associated with material type when compared to the nonresorbable membranes. Loe and Karring found that type 1 collagen is present in abundance in gingival connective tissue, hence qualifying for the ideal biomaterial to be used as barrier membrane in guided tissue regeneration.[44]

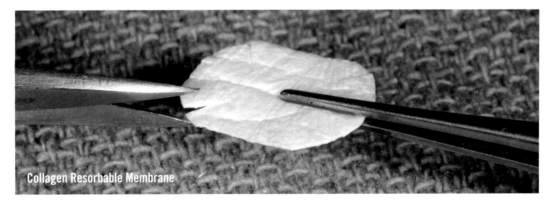

Collagen Resorbable Membrane

A collagen membrane is biocompatible, does not require a second surgery, interferes with migration of epithelial cells, and promotes development of new connective tissue attachment. It also promotes hemostasis by platelet aggregation, thereby forming blood clots and stabilizing the wound. It has been shown that collagen membranes facilitate primary wound closure via fibroblast chemotactic properties.[45] Blumenthal and others reported that placement of collagen does not enhance plaque accumulation or cause gingival inflammation.[46,47] Romagna reported significant reductions in probing depth in collagen treated groups when compared to sites without collagen.[48] To retard collagen membrane enzymatic degradation and to increase its mechanical strength, the diphenylphosphorylazide technique has been demonstrated to achieve natural cross-links between peptide chains of collagen without leaving any foreign product in the cross-linked molecule.[49]

Synthetic Resorbable Membranes

Synthetic membranes most widely used for guided tissue regeneration are polymers of lactic acid or glycolic acid. These contain ester bonds, which disintegrate over 30 to 60 days. However, their degradation produces free acids which are known to cause inflammation. Some brands of synthetic membranes used for guided tissue regeneration are Vicryl, Atrisorb, Atrisorb-FreeFlow, Arisorb-D, Resolut XT, EpiGide, and Gore Resolut Adapt.

Secondary Space

According to the principles proposed by Wang and Boyapati, creation and maintenance of space is important in guided tissue regeneration.[14] The space created between root surface and barrier membrane promotes the migration of periodontal progenitor cells toward and onto the detoxified root surface, which then differentiate into the desired tissue types. This space is difficult to maintain in gingival recessions because of the shape of the defect since the shape often causes the membrane to collapse over the recession defect. To prevent this collapse, clinicians have used many techniques, including reshaping the root surface to a concave shape, modifying the membrane by bending, using a thick film of fibrin/fibronectin between the surfaces, and using a titanium-reinforced membrane. Despite the efforts, none of the techniques achieved the aim of space maintenance. However, human histology studies have demonstrated that regeneration can occur following this procedure.[3,9] By contrast, Tinti and others, and Trombelli and colleagues have noted that no significant difference in probing depth reduction was detected between membrane-treated groups and non-membrane groups.[6,17,22,23,29]

Figure 8-6 **GBR During Iimplant Placement to Treat a Bony Dehiscence**

a

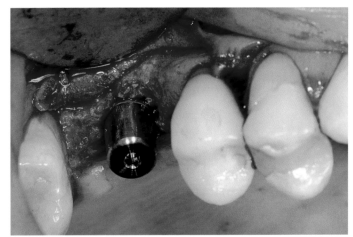

(a) Slight bony dehiscence with implant thread exposure and thin alveolar bone on the facial of the implant at the time of placement.

b

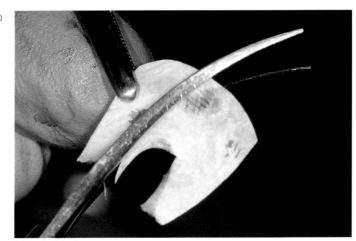

(b) Resorbable collagen membrane measured and trimmed to proper size and shape.

c

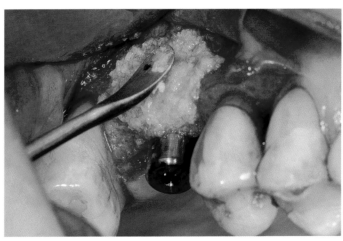

(c) Membrane inserted underneath the buccal flap and FDBA placed on the facial to cover the bony dehiscence and thin alveolar plate.

d

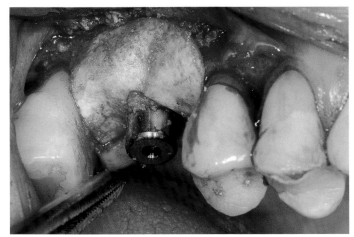

(d) Membrane placed over the grafted site.

e

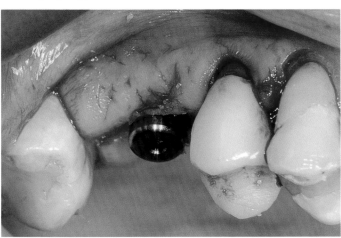

(e) Final position of the membrane with both ends tucked underneath the buccal and palatal flaps.

f

(f) Tension free closure of the flap around the implant with full coverage of the membrane and grafted site. ∎

Summary

Guided tissue regeneration has been widely used for regeneration of periodontal structures like cementum, periodontal ligaments, and alveolar bone. The procedure involves placing a barrier membrane for selective regeneration. The use of a membrane often requires the membrane to be permeable for nutrients but not for cells so that the membrane can serve as a cell barrier to guide the specific tissue regeneration. Exposure of the membrane occurs quite frequently, which adversely affects the surgical outcome. Although the procedure yields good clinical outcome in terms of root coverage, it is comparatively costly and technically demanding.

References

1. Hurley LA, Sticnhfield FE, Bassett AL, Lyon WH. The role of soft tissues in osteogenesis. An experimental study of canine spine fusions. J Bone Joint Surg Am. 1959 Oct;41-A:1243-54.

2. Melcher AH. On the repair potential of periodontal tissues. J Periodontol. 1976 May;47(5):256-60. Review.

3. Nyman S, Lindhe J, Karring T, Rylander H. New attachment following surgical treatment of human periodontal disease. J Clin Periodontol. 1982 Jul;9(4):290-6.

4. Gottlow J, Nyman S, Karring T, Lindhe J. New attachment formation as the result of controlled tissue regeneration. J Clin Periodontol. 1984 Sep;11(8):494-503.

5. Gottlow J, Nyman S, Lindhe J, Karring T, Wennström J. New attachment formation in the human periodontium by guided tissue regeneration. Case reports. J Clin Periodontol. 1986 Jul;13(6):604-16.

6. Tinti C, Vincenzi G, Cortellini P, Pini Prato G, Clauser C. Guided tissue regeneration in the treatment of human facial recession. A 12-case report. J Periodontol. 1992 Jun;63(6):554-60.

7. Tinti C, Vincenzi G, Cocchetto R. Guided tissue regeneration in mucogingival surgery. J Periodontol. 1993 Nov;64(11 Suppl):1184-91.

8. Pini Prato G, Tinti C, Vincenzi G, Magnani C, Cortellini P, Clauser C. Guided tissue regeneration versus mucogingival surgery in the treatment of human buccal gingival recession. J Periodontol. 1992 Nov; 63(11):919-28.

9. Cortellini P, Clauser C, Prato GP. Histologic assessment of new attachment following the treatment of a human buccal recession by means of a guided tissue regeneration procedure. J Periodontol. 1993 May; 64(5):387-91.

10. Rakhmatia YD, Ayukawa Y, Furuhashi A, Koyano K. Current barrier membranes: titanium mesh and other membranes for guided bone regeneration in dental applications. J Prosthodont Res. 2013 Jan;57(1):3-14.

11. Gentile P, Chiono V, Tonda-Turo C, Ferreira AM, Ciardelli G. Polymeric membranes for guided bone regeneration. Biotechnol J. 2011 Oct;6(10):1187-97.

12. Bottino MC, Thomas V, Schmidt G, Vohra YK, Chu TM, Kowolik MJ, Janowski GM. Recent advances in the development of GTR/GBR membranes for periodontal regeneration--a materials perspective. Dent Mater. 2012 Jul;28(7):703-21.

13. Dimitriou R, Mataliotakis GI, Calori GM, Giannoudis PV. The role of barrier membranes for guided bone regeneration and restoration of large bone defects: current experimental and clinical evidence. BMC Med. 2012 Jul 26;10:81. Review.

14. Wang HL, Boyapati L. "PASS" principles for predictable bone regeneration. Implant Dent. 2006 Mar;15(1):8-17. Review.

15. Aukhil I, Simpson DM, Suggs C, Pettersson E. In vivo differentiation of progenitor cells of the periodontal ligament. An experimental study using physical barriers. J Clin Periodontol. 1986 Oct;13(9):862-8.

16. Magnusson I, Nyman S, Karring T, Egelberg J. Connective tissue attachment formation following exclusion of gingival connective tissue and epithelium during healing. J Periodontal Res. 1985 Mar;20(2):201-8.

17. Tinti C, Vincenzi GP. Expanded polytetrafluoroethylene titanium-reinforced membranes for regeneration of mucogingival recession defects. A 12-case report. J Periodontol. 1994 Nov;65(11):1088-94.

18. Boltchi FE, Allen EP, Hallmon WW. The use of a bioabsorbable barrier for regenerative management of marginal tissue recession. I. Report of 100 consecutively treated teeth. J Periodontol. 2000 Oct; 71(10):1641-53.

19. Ling LJ, Hung SL, Lee CF, Chen YT, Wu KM. The influence of membrane exposure on the outcomes of guided tissue regeneration: clinical and microbiological aspects. J Periodontal Res. 2003 Feb;38(1):57-63.

20. Trombelli L, Scabbia A. Healing response of gingival recession defects following guided tissue regeneration procedures in smokers and non-smokers. J Clin Periodontol. 1997 Aug;24(8):529-33.

21. Villar CC, Cochran DL. Regeneration of periodontal tissues: guided tissue regeneration. Dent Clin North Am. 2010 Jan;54(1):73-92.

22. Trombelli L, Schincaglia G, Checchi L, Calura G. Combined guided tissue regeneration, root conditioning, and fibrin-fibronectin system application in the treatment of gingival recession. A 15-case report. J Periodontol. 1994 Aug;65(8):796-803.

23. Trombelli L, Schincaglia GP, Zangari F, Griselli A, Scabbia A, Calura G. Effects of tetracycline HCl conditioning and fibrin-fibronectin system application in the treatment of buccal gingival recession with guided tissue regeneration. J Periodontol. 1995 May;66(5):313-20.

24. Ozcan G, Kurtiş B, Baloş K. Combined use of root conditioning, fibrin-fibronectin system and a collagen membrane to treat a localized gingival recession: a 10-case report. J Marmara Univ Dent Fac. 1997 Sep;2(4):588-98.

25. Ricci G, Silvestri M, Tinti C, Rasperini G. A clinical/statistical comparison between the subpedicle connective tissue graft method and the guided tissue regeneration technique in root coverage. Int J Periodontics Restorative Dent. 1996 Dec;16(6):538-45.

26. Chambrone L, Sukekava F, Araújo MG, Pustiglioni FE, Chambrone LA, Lima LA. Root coverage procedures for the treatment of localised recession-type defects. Cochrane Database Syst Rev. 2009 Apr 15;(2). Review.

27. Miller N, Penaud J, Foliguet B, Membre H, Ambrosini P, Plombas M. Resorption rates of 2 commercially available bioresorbable membranes. A histomorphometric study in a rabbit model. J Clin Periodontol. 1996 Dec;23(12):1051-9.

28. Juodzbalys G, Raustia AM, Kubilius R. A 5-year follow-up study on one-stage implants inserted concomitantly with localized alveolar ridge augmentation. J Oral Rehabil. 2007 Oct;34(10):781-9.

29. Trombelli L, Schincaglia GP, Scapoli C, Calura G. Healing response of human buccal gingival recessions treated with expanded polytetrafluoroethylene membranes. A retrospective report. J Periodontol. 1995 Jan;66(1):14-22.

30. Ito K, Murai S. Adjacent gingival recession treated with expanded polytetrafluoroethylene membranes: a report of 2 cases. J Periodontol. 1996 Apr;67(4):443-50.

31. Ito K, Oshio K, Shiomi N, Murai S. A preliminary comparative study of the guided tissue regeneration and free gingival graft procedures for adjacent facial root coverage. Quintessence Int. 2000 May;31(5):319-26.

32. Roccuzzo M, Buser D. Treatment of buccal gingival recessions with e-PTFE membranes and miniscrews: surgical procedure and results of 12 cases. Int J Periodontics Restorative Dent. 1996 Aug;16(4):356-65.

33. Duskova M, Leamerova E, Sosna B, Gojis O. Guided tissue regeneration, barrier membranes and reconstruction of the cleft maxillary alveolus. J Craniofac Surg. 2006 Nov;17(6):1153-60.

34. Vincenzi G, De Chiesa A, Trisi P. Guided tissue regeneration using a resorbable membrane in gingival recession-type defects: a histologic case report in humans. Int J Periodontics Restorative Dent. 1998 Feb;18(1):24-33.

35. Prato GP, Clauser C, Magnani C, Cortellini P. Resorbable membrane in the treatment of human buccal recession: a nine-case report. Int J Periodontics Restorative Dent. 1995 Jun;15(3):258-67.

36. Rachlin G, Koubi G, Dejou J, Franquin JC. The use of a resorbable membrane in mucogingival surgery. Case series. J Periodontol. 1996 Jun;67(6):621-6.

37. Jepsen S, Heinz B, Kermanie MA, Jepsen K. Evaluation of a new bioabsorbable barrier for recession therapy: a feasibility study. J Periodontol. 2000 Sep;71(9):1433-40.

38. Vuddhakanok S, Solt CW, Mitchell JC, Foreman DW, Alger FA. Histologic evaluation of periodontal attachment apparatus following the insertion of a biodegradable copolymer barrier in humans. J Periodontol. 1993 Mar;64(3):202-10.

39. De Sanctis M, Zucchelli G. Guided tissue regeneration with a resorbable barrier membrane (Vicryl) for the management of buccal recession: a case report. Int J Periodontics Restorative Dent. 1996 Oct;16(5):435-41.

40. Waterman CA. Guided tissue regeneration using a bioabsorbable membrane in the treatment of human buccal recession. A re-entry study. J Periodontol. 1997 Oct;68(10):982-9.

41. Roccuzzo M, Lungo M, Corrente G, Gandolfo S. Comparative study of a bioresorbable and a non-resorbable membrane in the treatment of human buccal gingival recessions. J Periodontol. 1996 Jan;67(1):7-14.

42. Mundell RD, Mooney MP, Siegel MI, Losken A. Osseous guided tissue regeneration using a collagen barrier membrane. J Oral Maxillofac Surg. 1993 Sep;51(9):1004-12.

43. Cosci F, Cosci R. Guided bone regeneration for implant placement using absorbable collagen membranes: case presentations. Pract Periodontics Aesthet Dent. 1994 Mar;6(2):35-41; quiz 43.

44. Karring T, Löe H. A computerized method for quantitative estimation of the epithelium-connective tissue interface applied to the gingiva of various age groups. Acta Odontol Scand. 1973 Oct;31(4):241-8.

45. Kim DM, De Angelis N, Camelo M, Nevins ML, Schupbach P, Nevins M. Ridge preservation with and without primary wound closure: a case series. Int J Periodontics Restorative Dent. 2013 Jan-Feb;33(1):71-8.

46. Blumenthal NM. A clinical comparison of collagen membranes with e-PTFE membranes in the treatment of human mandibular buccal class II furcation defects. J Periodontol. 1993 Oct;64(10):925-33.

47. Van Swol RL, Ellinger R, Pfeifer J, Barton NE, Blumenthal N. Collagen membrane barrier therapy to guide regeneration in Class II furcations in humans. J Periodontol. 1993 Jul;64(7):622-9.

48. Romagna-Genon C. Comparative clinical study of guided tissue regeneration with a bioabsorbable bilayer collagen membrane and subepithelial connective tissue graft. J Periodontol. 2001 Sep;72(9):1258-64.

49. Zahedi S, Bozon C, Brunel G. A 2-year clinical evaluation of a diphenylphosphorylazide-cross-linked collagen membrane for the treatment of buccal gingival recession. J Periodontol. 1998 Sep;69(9):975-81.

Notes

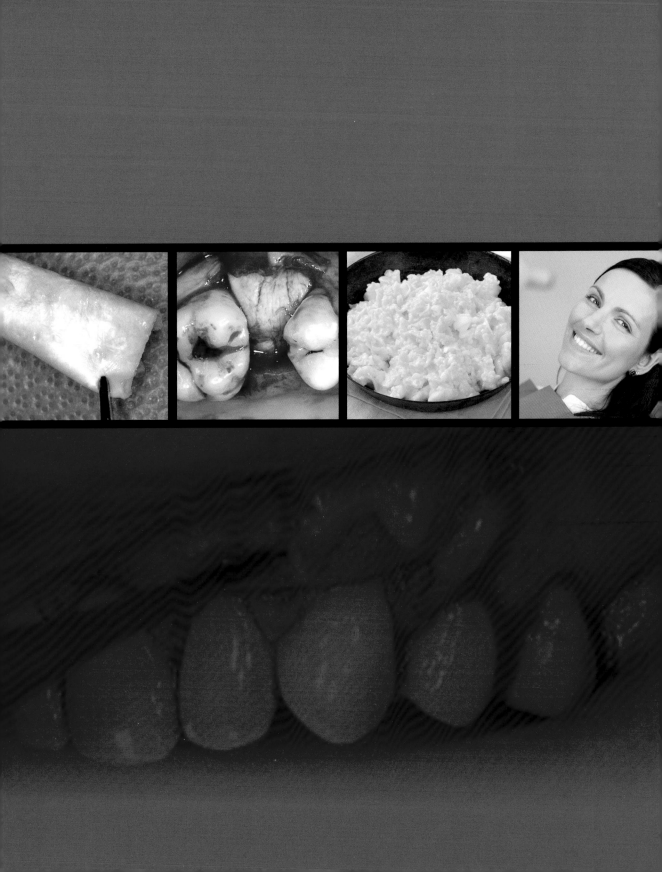

Acellular Dermal Matrix Graft

Harvested from human cadavers and used in medical procedures to promote soft tissue regeneration, the acellular dermal matrix graft is a non-immunogenic allograft because its cell components have been removed while the ultrastructural integrity of its extracellular matrix has been retained. This matrix has regenerative properties rich in collagen and elastin. These components help the body to regrow desired tissues, promote faster healing, and yield good esthetic results. The absence of cellular components reduces the likelihood of inflammatory response in the host tissue, and the graft is recognized by the recipient as "friendly" (biocompatible and safe) tissue. Studies suggest that the acellular dermal matrix graft does not produce scar tissue since the healing occurs not by granulation but by repopulation and revascularization.[1,2] An acellular dermal matrix graft can augment deficient gingival tissues without the discomfort and morbidity associated with the second surgical donor site. It is useful for patients who do not have sufficient donor tissue or who refuse to undergo a palatal harvest.

AlloDerm® is a commercially available acellular dermal matrix developed by LifeCell Corporation.[3] In this chapter, the term AlloDerm® is used synonymously with acellular dermal matrix graft. LifeCell Corporation accepts tissue only from organizations that meet the standards of the American Association of Tissue Banks (AATB) after the tissue passes FDA-approved guidelines. The donor tissue must go through strict screenings for the presence of diseases such as HIV and hepatitis, similar to any other tissues or organs being implanted. AlloDerm® was originally developed to treat burn patients; however, its use is widespread in other areas, such as general, orthopedic, urogenital, and dental surgery. In periodontology, the acellular dermal matrix graft has been used to increase the keratinized mucosa, to obtain root coverage in gingival recessions, and to increase gingival thickness in edentulous area.

History

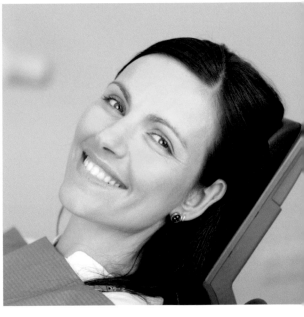

The drawbacks inherent with autografts have instigated a search for alternate approaches. In search for a substitute donor material for masticatory mucosa, clinicians speculated on the use of freeze-dried skin, and studies followed. Skin allografts are obtained from living donors or disease-free cadavers. The viability of human skin declines progressively after its removal from the living body; the rate of decline in viability depends in large part on the storage temperature. Generally, the higher the temperature, the more rapid the decline in viability. Freeze-drying, or lyophilization, is a process by which water is removed from the frozen biological material by sublimation under vacuum.[4] This freeze-dried tissue can be stored long term at room temperature in evacuated containers or waterproof envelopes at 17° C. Additionally, these tissues can be sterilized by either irradiation or by exposure to ethylene oxide gas. The freeze-dried skin is non-viable, non-immunogenic, and does not stimulate host response. Gher and others observed no evidence of hypersensitivity in the freeze-dried skin as determined by anti-HLA antibody and lymphocyte lysis assay.[5]

Freeze-dried skin allografts were developed for use as biologic bandages in treatment of burns. Carroll and colleagues demonstrated that freeze-dried skin allografts are biologically acceptable in the oral cavities of primates.[6] In 1977, Yukna and others demonstrated that allogenic freeze-dried skin graft is beneficial in treatment of mucogingival defects.[7] This study used freeze-dried allografts as a substitute for gingival autografts and found that allogenic freeze-dried skin and autogenous gingival tissue harvested at the time of the procedure yielded essentially similar clinical results when used as donor tissues.

Acellular dermal allograft tissue is used to treat full-thickness burns, depressed scars and nasal reconstruction, septal perforation, and facial defects; it is also used for lip augmentation and in a variety of procedures in neurosurgery, ophthalmology, and otolaryngology.[8-18] In dentistry, acellular dermal matrix allografts are used as substitutes for palatal donor tissue in mucogingival surgeries around natural teeth and implants to increase the zone of keratinized tissue, for tissue augmentation, ridge preservation, endosseous implant surgical applications, and for root coverage.[19-29] The technique is also used for soft tissue flap extension over bone grafts and correction of an amalgam tattoo. Studies have also reported that the replacement of subepithelial connective tissue grafts with the acellular dermal matrix allografts is effective for root coverage procedures.[22,30,31]

Advantages and Disadvantages of Acellular Dermal Matrix Allograft

Use of any skin allograft raises the risk of transmission of infection and the potential of eliciting an inflammatory host response. Replication of human pathogenic viruses

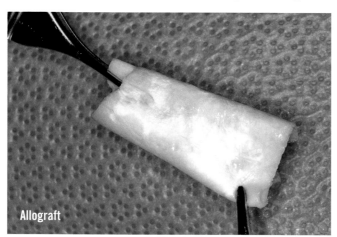

Allograft

has been found to occur only intracellularly. In addition, the host rejection response is stimulated by epidermal cells and the cells of endothelium and fibroblasts. An acellular dermal matrix graft overcomes all these drawbacks of skin allografts by virtue of its acellularity: the graft is incapable of transmitting diseases or eliciting rejection response. Therefore, acellular dermal matrix allograft is completely biocompatible and safe.

Studies report that an acellular dermal matrix allograft does not have undesirable dead cells with their associated class I and class II Human Leukocyte Antigen (HLA) antigens and potential transmission of cell-associated viruses.[32,33] A study of an acellular dermal matrix from frozen skin by Mizuno and Uchinuma concluded that the matrix "supported fibroblast infiltration and neovascularization....suggest[ing] that skin processed by...[this] simple method has the potential to be used as a dermal template together with the cultured epidermis in the closure of full-thickness wound."[34]

A study by Butler and Orgill attempted to show that "dermal and epidermal components can be supplied by grafting various substrates, concurrently or in stages" to reestablish "the normal function of skin." Their procedure "combine[d] disaggregated autologous keratinocytes and a highly porous, acellular collagen-glycosaminoglycan matrix...in a porcine model to regenerate a dermis and epidermis in vivo." They concluded, "The seeding process itself and the cell culture, when used, markedly expand the donor epithelial surface area, allowing large skin defects to be repaired using grafts created from very little donor tissue."[35]

When used for periodontal indications, an acellular dermal graft helps to treat larger recession areas containing multiple defects. The procedure does not require a second surgical site, it consumes less time, and results in good esthetic outcome. Since the acellular dermal matrix is commercially available, it offers unlimited availability and can be stored for more than a year. It is also easy to handle and suture. The allograft integrates consistently with the host tissue and can be used for different kinds of procedures. However, the acellular dermal matrix graft is expensive, and associated with longer healing time.

A 2006 review of the literature on acellular dermal matrix grafting by Zigdon and Horwitz commented on the widespread use of the graft in periodontal care, including "processing and mode of use, indications and contraindications, surgical techniques and clinical results for the treatment of localized and generalized gingival recessions... and comparisons with other methods of treatment for root recessions."[36] A 2008 review by Cairo, Pagliaro, and Nieri concluded that connective tissue grafting or enamel matrix derivative along with a coronally advanced flap "enhances the probability of obtaining" complete root coverage "in Miller Class I and II single gingival recessions." The results of their review showed that a "coronally advanced flap was associated with mean recession reduction and complete root coverage. The addition of connective tissue graft (CTG) or enamel matrix derivative enhanced the clinical outcomes of coronally advanced flap in terms of complete root coverage, while barrier membranes did not."

Interestingly, the study also showed "controversial" results concerning "the adjunctive use of acellular dermal matrix."[37] A 2012 review by Fu, Su, and Wang concluded that "[a]lthough these new materials [such as acellular dermal matrix, collagen matrix, guided tissue regeneration based root coverage, and biologic agent] do not surpass the gold standard (subepithelial connective graft), they do provide improved patient satisfaction and esthetics, are available in abundance, and lead to reduced postoperative discomfort and surgical time."[38]

Processing of the Acellular Dermal Graft Material

The donor skin is collected via a dermatome, and it is treated so that all cellular and immunogenic elements are removed without disrupting the architecture of the dermis or crosslinking of the collagen fibers. This aseptic process involves removal of the epidermis by incubation of the skin in sodium chloride, followed by removal of dermal fibroblasts and epithelial cells by treatment with detergents. This decellularization reduces major histocompatibility complex class I and class II molecules to undetectable levels. The matrix is cryoprotected and freeze dried without damage to the extracellular matrix proteins. The result is an acellular, non-immunogenic connective tissue matrix along with a base, or basement membrane complex and vascular channels. The acellular dermal matrix allograft has two distinct surfaces: a basement membrane side, which is smooth and does not absorb blood; and a connective tissue side, which is rougher and absorbs blood. Dodge, Henderson, and Greenwell found that the orientation of the material did not affect the treatment outcome.[21]

Techniques of Grafting with an Acellular Dermal Matrix Graft

The surgical procedure consists of a coronally positioned flap and placement of the acellular dermal graft material.[13] First, the teeth associated with the defect to be treated are scaled to remove any debris. The root is then conditioned with tetracycline, citric acid, or ethylenediaminetetraacetic acid. Bleeding points equivalent to the amount of buccal recession are marked in the interproximal papillae with a probe at the location of the intended new papillae tip. Scalloped sulcular incisions are accomplished and extended to the nearest line angle of the adjacent non-defective tooth. Oblique coronoapical incisions are made to release the full thickness flaps, which are reflected

Figure 9-1 Root Coverage Using Alloderm and Coronally Advanced Flap Technique

a

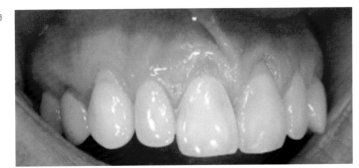

(a) Multiple gingival recessions of Miller Class I and II classification from right maxillary 2nd premolar to left maxillary 2nd premolar.

b

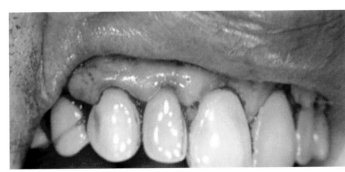

(b) Scalloped incision of the interdental papilla at the level of the CEJ in combination with intrasulcular incision around the cervical areas of the involved teeth.

c

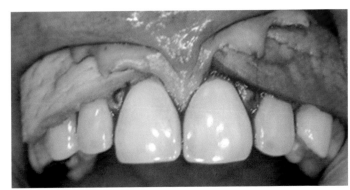

(c) Alloderm inserted underneath the flap after sufficient release of the periosteum to coronally advance the flap.

d

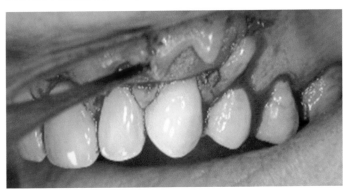

(d) Verification that the overlying flap is tension free.

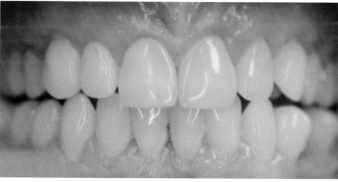

e

(e) Position of the coronally advanced flap and the Alloderm prior to suturing.

f

(f) Complete root coverage achieved after 12 weeks of healing. ■

to approximately 3 mm apical to the alveolar bone crest. To ensure sufficient mobility for coronal positioning, a split thickness flap is dissected from the coronal aspect. The papillae must be deepithelialized, which assures that the host tissue has good vascular supply and connective tissue.

The acellular dermal matrix allograft should be rehydrated in sterile saline or tetracycline solution. The graft is sized to cover the root defect and is positioned at the cementoenamel junction. The coronal border of the acellular dermal matrix allograft is approximated at the interproximal papillae to promote adequate blood flow between the papillae and the flap. The basement membrane side of the graft is placed against the host root defect. Sling sutures are performed to secure the graft to the host tissue. The ideal suture material for an acellular dermal matrix allograft is a resorbable monofilament suture that resorbs in about 10 weeks. A double sling suture technique is used to suture the coronally repositioned flap. Interrupted sutures are used to close the releasing incisions. The factors that affect the outcome in acellular dermal matrix grafting include a flap or pouch design that minimizes loss of vascular supply, coronal repositioning of the flap or pouch to cover the graft in such a way that it is tension free, and thorough root conditioning.

Acellular Dermal Matrix Allograft Used for Root Coverage

The acellular dermal matrix graft is useful for treating gingival recessions (Fig. 9-1). Various techniques have been described with mixed results.[21,22,32,39-45] Most often, a coronally positioned flap has been used to completely cover the acellular dermal matrix, but a tunnel procedure also has been reported. Many studies have reported root coverage using an acellular dermal matrix allograft greater than 90% while others have reported root coverage from 66% to 89%.[21,22,32,39,40,42-46]

Giannelli and Patore reported the efficacy of using an acellular dermal matrix allograft in the surgical treatment of even very wide gingival recessions.[47] AlloDerm® has demonstrated clinical and esthetic results equivalent to those with palatal tissue.[42,45,46,48] Multiple, randomized clinical trials have shown root coverage results with AlloDerm® to be equivalent to autogenous connective tissue, and they further concluded that the procedure was predictable and practical, including improved color and contour match, elimination of multiple surgeries, and unlimited availability.[49,50] Santos reported that AlloDerm® can be used as an alternative for root coverage to palatal donor tissue and that the product's application also overcomes the problems associated with guided tissue regeneration.[51] Multiple studies also have reported superior clinical efficacy of AlloDerm® over free gingival grafts. Wei conducted a study to investigate the clinical efficacy in acellular dermal matrix allograft for achieving increased keratinized tissue and found the acellular dermal matrix allograft superior to the free gingival graft.[52] Harris compared three surgical procedures and found that there was a greater increase in the width of gingival tissue with the free gingival graft and acellular dermal matrix allograft when compared to connective tissue grafting.[53] Harris reported similar results with a connective tissue of a partial thickness double pedicle graft and an acellular dermal matrix allograft used for complete root coverage, both clinically and histologically.[54] In another study by the same author, the acellular dermal matrix allograft yielded similar results as a coronally positioned pedicle graft combined with a connective tissue graft.[39]   Another study that compared short-term and long-term root coverage using AlloDerm® and subepithelial connective tissue grafting reported that breakdown occurs over a period of 2 months in root coverage obtained with an acellular dermal matrix allograft.[54]

Tal found that an acellular dermal matrix allograft can be a possible substitute for free autogenous connective tissue grafts and/or bioabsorbable barrier membranes.[32] In a comparative study, the same author found comparable results with an acellular dermal matrix allograft and a connective tissue graft in the treatment of gingival recession more than or equal to 4 mm.[55]

Similar results were reported by Aichelman and others, as well as by Arthur and colleagues, and Rahmani and others.[40,42,56]   Palatino compared the clinical results of two bilaminar techniques by autogenous connective tissue graft or acellular dermal matrix allograft and found that the connective tissue and acellular dermal matrix allograft can be used for treatment of recessions.[45]   Woodyard reported that treatment with a coronally positioned flap plus an acellular dermal matrix allograft significantly increased gingival thickness when compared with a coronally positioned flap alone.[43] Cortes and colleagues evaluated treatment of gingival recessions with the coronally positioned flap with or without an acellular dermal matrix allograft after a period of 24 months.[57]   When using the acellular dermal matrix allograft, clinicians produced a greater gingival thickness.   Papageorgakopoulos and others compared the coronally positioned flap plus the acellular dermal matrix allograft with a tunnel technique with an acellular dermal matrix allograft and found that the coronally positioned flap with the acellular dermal matrix allograft produced a defect coverage of 95% whereas the tunnel technique combined with the acellular dermal matrix produced only 78% coverage.[58] Pontes reported that an acellular dermal matrix allograft could be successfully used in the treatment of gingival recession in pediatric patients.[59]   Buduneli reported that an acellular dermal matrix allograft can be used in the treatment of epidermolysis bullosa cases to increase the width of attached gingiva and to facilitate maintenance of their dentition.[60]   The acellular dermal matrix allograft can also be used to treat gingival pigmentation caused by deposit of melanin.[61]

A number of more recent studies in the literature have shown the varied efficacy of using an acellular dermal matrix in dental care, particularly in the treatment of gingival recession.

Mahn's 2010 study, "Use of the tunnel technique and an acellular dermal matrix in the treatment of multiple adjacent teeth with gingival recession in the esthetic zone," notes that "[t]he proper management of gingival recession is critical to the establishment of a natural appearing soft tissue architecture," and that "[s]ubepithelial connective tissue grafts have been considered the 'gold standard' but are limited by the availability of palatal donor tissue." The study further notes that "[t]unnel techniques have improved the esthetic results of connective tissue grafting" and that "[a]cellular dermal matrices have been successful in the treatment of gingival recession and are not limited by the palatal anatomy."[62] Santos, Goumenos, Pascual, and Nart explain in their 2011 study, "Acellular dermal matrix grafts have become a good alternative to autogenous soft tissue grafts in root coverage," and that "[u]ntil now, the literature has reported short- or medium-term data regarding the stability of the gingival margin after the use of acellular dermal matrix on root coverage." However, their study included

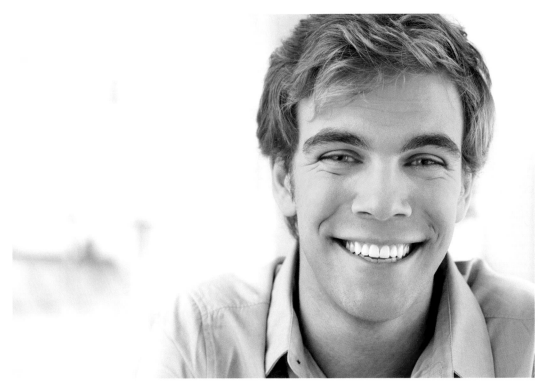

"a case report with 10 years of evaluation with creeping attachment that developed bucally on a moderate recession of a maxillary canine with an old composite restoration subsequent to an acellular dermal matrix" and that "[l]ong-term creeping attachment and complete root coverage on a restored tooth treated with acellular dermal matrix has not been previously reported in the dental literature."[63] Koudale, Charde, and Bhongade's 2012 comparative clinical evaluation of acellular dermal matrix allograft and subepithelial connective tissue graft for the treatment of multiple gingival recessions concluded that an acellular dermal matrix application "may be a useful substitute instead of subepithelial connective tissue graft for root coverage."[64] Shori, Kolte, Kher, Dharamthok, and Shrirao concisely note in their 2013 study that "[t]he most common problem encountered in [dental clinicians'] day to day practice is exposed root surface....[and that] [t]he main indication for root coverage procedures are esthetics and/or cosmetic demands followed by the management of root hypersensitivity, root caries or when [an exposed root] hampers proper plaque removal." Their comparative clinical study of the effectiveness of subpedicle acellular dermal matrix allograft with subepithelial connective tissue graft in the treatment of isolated marginal tissue recession concluded that "[b]oth...treatments produced a significant reduction in gingival recession and probing pocket depth and significant gain in clinical attachment level and width of keratinised gingiva."[65] Chavan, Bhongade, Tiwari, and Jaiswal, in their 2013 study entitled "Open flap debridement in combination with acellular dermal matrix allograft for the prevention of postsurgical gingival recession: a case series" concluded that the acellular dermal matrix "underneath the flap when combined with open flap debridement effectively minimizes postsurgical gingival recession."[66] Thombre, Koudale, and Bhongade's 2013 comparative evaluation of the effectiveness of coronally positioned flap with or without acellular dermal matrix allograft in the treatment of multiple marginal gingival recession defects concluded that the acellular dermal matrix allograft with a coronally positioned flap "is an effective procedure for the treatment of multiple gingival recessions."[67]

Subepithelial Allogenic Dermal Matrix Tissue Graft around Multiple Teeth: Histological Evidence

Clinical and in vitro studies suggest that the acellular dermal matrix allograft is a non-immunogenic scaffold that allows the host tissue to grow within it and that it heals by repopulation and revascularization rather than through a granulation process maturing to scar.[32] Due to its non-vital structure, the graft depends on cells and blood vessels from recipient sites to achieve reorganization.[68] A histological study that compared AlloDerm® and connective tissue found that both heal by forming dense collagenous tissue when placed under a coronally advanced flap. Further followup at six months reported similar overall histological outcomes for both connective tissue and AlloDerm® grafts.[22,69,70]

Silverstein and Callan demonstrated that AlloDerm® promotes fibroblast infiltration and neovascularization resulting in tissue regeneration.[23] This process does not cause infiltration of inflammatory cells, thus preventing cell-mediated immune responses. Wainright noted that AlloDerm® may undergo remodeling with time, being converted to the same histological configuration as the surrounding host tissues.[9] Haeri studied creeping attachments in autogenous and acellular dermal skin grafts in a patient with bilateral mucogingival defects in the canine and premolar areas and reported similar creeping attachments.[71] Lewis reported that after six months, AlloDerm® was well incorporated with new fibroblasts, vascular elements, and collagen while retaining the transplanted elastic fibers.[72] Similarly, Harris demonstrated that both the connective tissue graft and the AlloDerm® were incorporated into the surgical areas.[22] The matrix became a part of the tissue in that area.

A histological study by Wei and others compared the microstructure of AlloDerm® and free gingival sites treated earlier.[52] The connective tissue of AlloDerm® contained dense to extremely dense collagen fibers along with the scattered elastic fibers. A moderate to thin epithelial layer, with heterogeneous expression of keratinization and flat epithelium-connective tissue interface, covered the lamina propria. Both the thickness of epithelium and the degree of keratinization decreased in apical direction, being mostly para or othokeratinzed in the area close to the gingiva and non-keratinized adjacent to the alveolar mucosa.

Post-Operative Management and Patient Instructions

Post-operative medications include antibiotics (Clindamycin/Amoxicillin for 7–10 days), anti-inflammatory drugs (Ibuprofen for 7 days), and antiplaque mouthwash (an alcohol-free chlorhexidine digluconate rinse at least twice daily for one month). Post-operative swelling should be prevented because it can disturb the stability of the graft, causing the sutures to pull through the papillae. This result can displace the apical flap. The patient should be instructed to use mouth rinse twice daily for one month. Sutures are removed one month after surgery.

The patient should follow a soft diet, including scrambled eggs, cottage cheese, milkshakes, noodle casseroles, and liquid breakfasts. Care should be taken to avoid chewing on the treated areas. The patient should not brush the periodontal dressing. If the dressing becomes loose, it should be gently removed and discarded. A slight amount of bleeding may be seen for one to two days. However, if more bleeding occurs, the patient should place a gauze pad over the bleeding area and apply firm pressure for 30 minutes. Alternatively, a wet tea bag can also be used. The patient should avoid strenuous activity for a few days after surgery.

Summary

The acellular dermal matrix allograft has significant advantages. It is free of all cell components, which are the targets of the host immune system and, when present, can also contribute to disease transmission. The extracellular matrix consists of intact collagens, elastin and blood vessel channels. These components not only promote neoangiogenesis but also prevent inflammatory response. The matrix causes epithelial cells to migrate across its basement membrane through the development of creeping attachment. The host vascular supply infiltrates the acellular dermal matrix allograft, binding the two surfaces. Gradually, the allograft matrix is remodeled into the host tissue, filling the defect to be treated. The acellular dermal matrix allograft has been successfully used in various periodontal and soft tissue surgeries. Overall, the technique is acceptable, despite the high cost and expertise needed for handling the graft.

References

1. Rhee PH, Friedman CD, Ridge JA, Kusiak J. The use of processed allograft dermal matrix for intraoral resurfacing: an alternative to split-thickness skin grafts. Arch Otolaryngol Head Neck Surg. 1998 Nov;124(11):1201-4.

2. Girod DA, Sykes K, Jorgensen J, Tawfik O, Tsue T. Acellular dermis compared to skin grafts in oral cavity reconstruction. Laryngoscope. 2009 Nov;119(11):2141-9.

3. LifeCellTM [Internet]. Bridgewater (WI): LifeCell Corporation; 2013. AlloDerm®; 2013 [cited 2013 May 26]; [1 screen]. Available from: http://www.lifecell.com/health-care-professionals/lifecell-products/allodermr-regenerative-tissue-matrix/allodermr-tissue-matrix-defined/

4. Sailer, HF. Transplantation of lypophilized cartilage in maxillofacial surgery: Experimental foundations and clinical success. Karger, Basel, 1982. 3-7.

5. Gher ME Jr, Williams JE Jr, Vernino AR, Strong DM, Pelleu GB Jr. Evaluation of the immunogenicity of freeze-dried skin allografts in humans. J Periodontol. 1980 Oct; 51(10):571-7.

6. Carroll PB, Tow HD, Vernino AR. The use of allogeneic freeze-dried skin grafts in the oral environment. A clinical and histologic evaluation. Oral Surg Oral Med Oral Pathol. 1974 Feb;37(2):163-74.

7. Yukna RA, Tow HD, Carroll PB, Vernino AR, Bright RW. Evaluation of the use of freeze-dried skin allografts in the treatment of human mucogingival problems. J Periodontol. 1977 Apr;48(4):187-93.

8. Miller A, Brunelle J, Carlos J, Brown L, Loe H. Oral health of the United States adults. The National Survey of Oral Health in U.S. Employed Adults and Seniors: 1985-1986; NIH publication no. 87-2868.

9. Wainwright D, Madden M, Luterman A, Hunt J, Monafo W, Heimbach D, Kagan R, Sittig K, Dimick A, Herndon D. Clinical evaluation of an acellular allograft dermal matrix in full-thickness burns. J Burn Care Rehabil. 1996 Mar-Apr;17(2):124-36.

10. Lattari V, Jones LM, Varcelotti JR, Latenser BA, Sherman HF, Barrette RR. The use of a permanent dermal allograft in full-thickness burns of the hand and foot: a report of three cases. J Burn Care Rehabil. 1997 Mar-Apr;18(2):147-55.

11. Silverstein LH. Fundamentally changing soft tissue grafting. Dent Today. 1997 Mar; 16(3):56-9.

12. Kridel RW, Foda H, Lunde KC. Septal perforation repair with acellular human dermal allograft. Arch Otolaryngol Head Neck Surg. 1998 Jan;124(1):73-8.

13 chauer BM, VanderKam VM, Celikoz B, Jacobson DG. Augmentation of facial soft-tissue defects with Alloderm dermal graft. Ann Plast Surg. 1998 Nov;41(5):503-7.

14. Castor SA, To WC, Papay FA. Lip augmentation with AlloDerm acellular allogenic dermal graft and fat autograft: A comparison with autologous fat injection alone. Aesthetic Plast Surg. 1999 May-Jun;23(3):218-23.

15. Tobin HA, Karas ND. Lip augmentation using an alloderm graft. J Oral Maxillofac Surg. 1998 Jun;56(6):722-7.

16. Barret JP, Dziewulski P, McCauley RL, Herndon DN, Desai MH. Dural reconstruction of a class IV calvarial burn with decellularized human dermis. Burns. 1999 Aug;25(5):459-62.

17. Rubin PA, Fay AM, Remulla HD, Maus M. Ophthalmic plastic applications of acellular dermal allografts. Ophthalmology. 1999 Nov;106(11):2091-7.

18. McFeely WJ Jr, Bojrab DI, Kartush JM. Tympanic membrane perforation repair using AlloDerm. Otolaryngol Head Neck Surg. 2000 Jul;123(1 Pt 1):17-21.

19. Callan DP, Silverstein LH. Use of acellular dermal matrix for increasing keratinized tissue around teeth and implants. Pract Periodontics Aesthet Dent. 1998 Aug; 10(6):731-4.

20. Silverstein LH, Gornstein RA, Callan DP. The similarities between an acellular dermal allograft and a palatal graft for tissue augmentation: a clinical case. Dent Today. 1999 Mar;18(3):76-9.

21. Dodge JR, Henderson RD, Greenwell H. Root coverage without a palatal donor site using an acellular dermal graft. Periodontal Insights 1998;5(4):5-9.

22. Harris RJ. Root coverage with a connective tissue with partial thickness double pedicle graft and an acellular dermal matrix graft: a clinical and histological evaluation of a case report. J Periodontol. 1998 Nov;69(11):1305-11.

23. Silverstein LH, Callan DP. An acellular dermal matrix allograft substitute for palatal donor tissue. Post Grad Dentistry 1997;3(4):14-21.

24. Peacock ME, Cuenin MF, Hokett SD. Gingival augmentation with a dermal allograft. Gen Dent. 1999 Sep-Oct;47(5):526-8.

25. Fowler EB, Breault LG, Rebitski G. Ridge preservation utilizing an acellular dermal allograft and demineralized freeze-dried bone allograft: Part I. A report of 2 cases. J Periodontol. 2000 Aug;71(8):1353-9.

26. Callan DP. Use of acellular dermal matrix allograft material in dental implant treatment. Dental Surgery Products 1996;1:14-17.

27. Fowler EB, Breault LG, Rebitski G. Ridge preservation utilizing an acellular dermal allograft and demineralized freeze-dried bone allograft: Part II. Immediate endosseous implant placement. J Periodontol. 2000 Aug;71(8):1360-4. Erratum in: J Periodontol 2000 Oct;71(10):1670.

28. Harris RJ. A short-term and long-term comparison of root coverage with an acellular dermal matrix and a subepithelial graft. J Periodontol. 2004 May;75(5):734-43.

29. Andrade PF, Felipe ME, Novaes AB Jr, Souza SL, Taba M Jr, Palioto DB, Grisi MF. Comparison between two surgical techniques for root coverage with an acellular dermal matrix graft. J Clin Periodontol. 2008 Mar;35(3):263-9.

30. Henderson RD, Drisko CH, Greenwell H. Root coverage using Alloderm acellular dermal graft material. J Contemp Dent Pract. 1999 Nov 15;1(1):24-30.

31. Fowler EB, Breault LG. Root coverage with an acellular dermal allograft: a three-month case report. J Contemp Dent Pract. 2000 Aug 15;1(3):47-59.

32. Tal H. Subgingival acellular dermal matrix allograft for the treatment of gingival recession: a case report. J Periodontol. 1999 Sep;70(9):1118-24.

33. Livesey SA, Herndon DN, Hollyoak MA, Atkinson YH, Nag A. Transplanted acellular allograft dermal matrix. Potential as a template for the reconstruction of viable dermis. Transplantation. 1995 Jul 15;60(1):1-9.

34. Mizuno H, Takeda A, Uchinuma E. Creation of an acellular dermal matrix from frozen skin. Aesthetic Plast Surg. 1999 Sep-Oct;23(5):316-22.

35. Butler CE, Orgill DP. Simultaneous in vivo regeneration of neodermis, epidermis, and basement membrane. Adv Biochem Eng Biotechnol. 2005;94:23-41. Review.

36. Zigdon H, Horwitz J. [Using acellular dermal matrix (ADM) allograft in periodontal surgery--a literature review and case reports]. Refuat Hapeh Vehashinayim. 2006 Jul;24(3):19-29, 92. Review. Hebrew.

37. Cairo F, Pagliaro U, Nieri M. Treatment of gingival recession with coronally advanced flap procedures: a systematic review. J Clin Periodontol. 2008 Sep;35(8 Suppl):136-62.

38. Fu JH, Su CY, Wang HL. Esthetic soft tissue management for teeth and implants. J Evid Based Dent Pract. 2012 Sep;12(3 Suppl):129-42. Review.

39. Harris RJ. A comparative study of root coverage obtained with an acellular dermal matrix versus a connective tissue graft: results of 107 recession defects in 50 consecutively treated patients. Int J Periodontics Restorative Dent. 2000 Feb;20(1):51-9.

40. Novaes AB Jr, Grisi DC, Molina GO, Souza SL, Taba M Jr, Grisi MF. Comparative 6-month clinical study of a subepithelial connective tissue graft and acellular dermal matrix graft for the treatment of gingival recession. J Periodontol. 2001 Nov;72(11):1477-84.

41. Mahn DH. Treatment of gingival recession with a modified "tunnel" technique and an acellular dermal connective tissue allograft. Pract Proced Aesthet Dent. 2001 Jan-Feb;13(1):69-74; quiz 76.

42. Aichelmann-Reidy ME, Yukna RA, Evans GH, Nasr HF, Mayer ET. Clinical evaluation of acellular allograft dermis for the treatment of human gingival recession. J Periodontol. 2001 Aug;72(8):998-1005.

43. Woodyard JG, Greenwell H, Hill M, Drisko C, Iasella JM, Scheetz J. The clinical effect of acellular dermal matrix on gingival thickness and root coverage compared to coronally positioned flap alone. J Periodontol. 2004 Jan;75(1):44-56.

44. Harris RJ. Cellular dermal matrix used for root coverage: 18-month follow-up observation. Int J Periodontics Restorative Dent. 2002 Apr;22(2):156-63.

45. Paolantonio M, Dolci M, Esposito P, D'Archivio D, Lisanti L, Di Luccio A, Perinetti G. Subpedicle acellular dermal matrix graft and autogenous connective tissue graft in the treatment of gingival recessions: a comparative 1-year clinical study. J Periodontol. 2002 Nov;73(11):1299-307.

46. Henderson RD, Greenwell H, Drisko C, Regennitter FJ, Lamb JW, Mehlbauer MJ, Goldsmith LJ, Rebitski G. Predictable multiple site root coverage using an acellular dermal matrix allograft. J Periodontol. 2001 May;72(5):571-82.

47. Giannelli G, Pastore A. Root coverage with an acellular dermal matrix graft. J Clin Periodontol 2003. Supplement 4:98.

48. Santos A, Goumenos G, Pascual A. Management of gingival recession by the use of an acellular dermal graft material: a 12-case series. J Periodontol. 2005 Nov;76(11):1982-90.

49. Gapski R, Parks CA, Wang HL. Acellular dermal matrix for mucogingival surgery: a meta-analysis. J Periodontol. 2005 Nov;76(11):1814-22.

50. Shulman J. Clinical evaluation of an acellular dermal allograft for increasing the zone of attached gingiva. Pract Periodontics Aesthet Dent. 1996 Mar;8(2):201-8.

51. Santos A, Goumenos G. AlloDerm®: Alternative to root coverage. J Clin Periodontol 2003. Supplement 4:356:90.

52. Wei PC, Laurell L, Geivelis M, Lingen MW, Maddalozzo D. Acellular dermal matrix allografts to achieve increased attached gingiva. Part 1. A clinical study. J Periodontol. 2000 Aug;71(8):1297-305.

53. Harris RJ. Gingival augmentation with an acellular dermal matrix: human histologic evaluation of a case--placement of the graft on bone. Int J Periodontics Restorative Dent. 2001 Feb;21(1):69-75.

54. Harris RJ. A comparison of 2 root coverage techniques: guided tissue regeneration with a bioabsorbable matrix style membrane versus a connective tissue graft combined with a coronally positioned pedicle graft without vertical incisions. Results of a series of consecutive cases. J Periodontol. 1998 Dec;69(12):1426-34.

55. Tal H, Moses O, Zohar R, Meir H, Nemcovsky C. Root coverage of advanced gingival recession: a comparative study between acellular dermal matrix allograft and subepithelial connective tissue grafts. J Periodontol. 2002 Dec;73(12):1405-11.

56. Rahmani ME, Lades MA. Comparative clinical evaluation of acellular dermal matrix allograft and connective tissue graft for the treatment of gingival recession. J Contemp Dent Pract. 2006 May 1;7(2):63-70.

57. de Queiroz Côrtes A, Sallum AW, Casati MZ, Nociti FH Jr, Sallum EA. A two-year prospective study of coronally positioned flap with or without acellular dermal matrix graft. J Clin Periodontol. 2006 Sep;33(9):683-9.

58. Papageorgakopoulos G, Greenwell H, Hill M, Vidal R, Scheetz JP. Root coverage using acellular dermal matrix and comparing a coronally positioned tunnel to a coronally positioned flap approach. J Periodontol. 2008 Jun;79(6):1022-30.

59. Pontes AE, Novaes AB Jr, Grisi MF, Souza SL, Taba Júnior M. Use of acellular dermal matrix graft in the treatment of gingival recessions: a case report. J Clin Pediatr Dent. 2003 Winter;27(2):107-10.

60. Buduneli E, Ilgenli T, Buduneli N, Ozdemir F. Acellular dermal matrix allograft used to gain attached gingiva in a case of epidermolysis bullosa. J Clin Periodontol. 2003 Nov;30(11):1011-5.

61. Novaes AB Jr, Pontes CC, Souza SL, Grisi MF, Taba M Jr. The use of acellular dermal matrix allograft for the elimination of gingival melanin pigmentation: case presentation with 2 years of follow-up. Pract Proced Aesthet Dent. 2002 Oct;14(8):619-23; quiz 624.

62. Mahn DH. Use of the tunnel technique and an acellular dermal matrix in the treatment of multiple adjacent teeth with gingival recession in the esthetic zone. Int J Periodontics Restorative Dent. 2010 Dec;30(6):593-9.

63. Santos A, Goumenos G, Pascual A, Nart J. Creeping attachment after 10 years of treatment of a gingival recession with acellular dermal matrix: a case report. Quintessence Int. 2011 Feb;42(2):121-6.

64. Koudale SB, Charde PA, Bhongade ML. A comparative clinical evaluation of acellular dermal matrix allograft and sub-epithelial connective tissue graft for the treatment of multiple gingival recessions. J Indian Soc Periodontol. 2012 Jul;16(3):411-6.

65. Shori T, Kolte A, Kher V, Dharamthok S, Shrirao T. A comparative evaluation of the effectiveness of subpedicle acellular dermal matrix allograft with subepithelial connective tissue graft in the treatment of isolated marginal tissue recession: A clinical study. J Indian Soc Periodontol. 2013 Jan;17(1):78-81.

66. Chavan RS, Bhongade ML, Tiwari IR, Jaiswal P. Open flap debridement in combination with acellular dermal matrix allograft for the prevention of postsurgical gingival recession: a case series. Int J Periodontics Restorative Dent. 2013 Mar-Apr;33(2):217-21.

67. Thombre V, Koudale SB, Bhongade ML. Comparative evaluation of the effectiveness of coronally positioned flap with or without acellular dermal matrix allograft in the treatment of multiple marginal gingival recession defects. Int J Periodontics Restorative Dent. 2013 May-Jun;33(3):e88-94.

68. Batista EL Jr, Batista FC, Novaes AB Jr. Management of soft tissue ridge deformities with acellular dermal matrix. Clinical approach and outcome after 6 months of treatment. J Periodontol. 2001 Feb; 72(2):265-73.

69. Cummings LC, Kaldahl WB, Allen EP. Histologic evaluation of autogenous connective tissue and acellular dermal matrix grafts in humans. J Periodontol. 2005 Feb;76(2):178-86.

70. Richardson CR, Maynard JG. Acellular dermal graft: a human histologic case report. Int J Periodontics Restorative Dent. 2002 Feb;22(1):21-9.

71. Haeri A, Clay J, Finely JM. The use of an acellular dermal skin graft to gain keratinized tissue. Compend Contin Educ Dent. 1999 Mar;20(3):233-4, 239-42; quiz 244.

72. Cummings L, Kaldahl W, Bhattacharya I, Baritz BJ. Histologic evaluation of two techniques for root coverage in humans. J Periodontol 2003;74(10):1566.

Notes

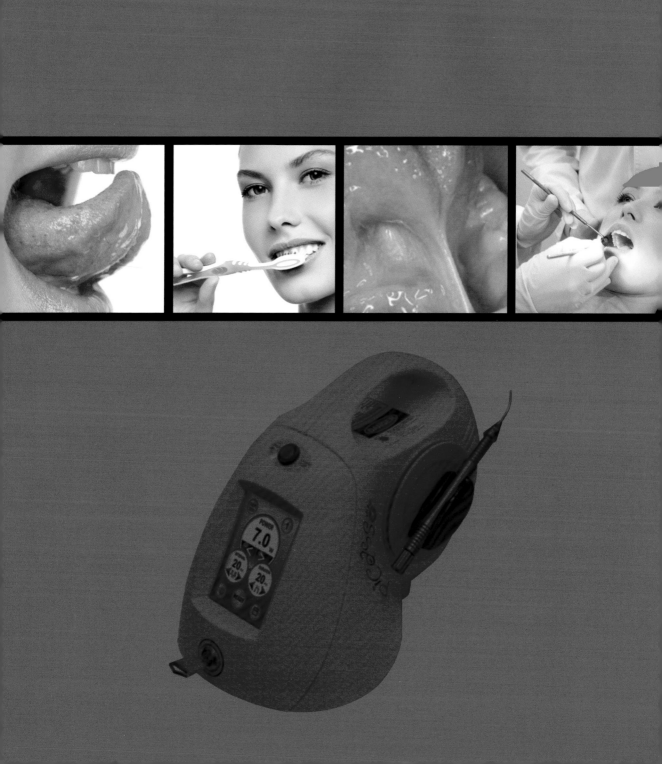

Frenectomy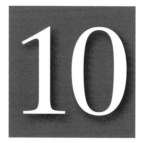

Afrenum is a tag of tissue connecting two body parts. A labial frenum is a fold of mucus membrane between the midline of the facial gingiva and the inner surface of the lip. A lingual frenum is found below the tongue. There are also several labial frena, or frenums, consisting of thin bands of fibrous tissue covered with mucosa extending from the lip and cheek to the alveolar mucosa. A frenum which extends inordinately along the tongue or the gingiva—or a frenum which is especially thick, short, or tight—could interfere with tooth alignment or hamper tongue or lip movement. Removal or alteration of the frenum, called a frenectomy, may be needed to correct such conditions.

The maxillary anterior frenum or *frenulum labii superioris* (superior labial frenum) and the inferior or mandibular labial frenum are thought to guide tooth growth. Specifically, the positioning and thickness of the frenum affect the growth of the teeth. Studies suggest that the prevalence of midline diastema is higher in the maxilla than in the mandible, and that the maxilla also has more papillary penetrating frenum attachments than the mandible. These discoveries were part of a 1998 study by Kaimenyi, whose aim "was to determine the prevalence of midline diastema, tongue tie and frenum attachments amongst school children in Nairobi." Over 1,800 children ranging in age from four to sixteen participated in the study, governed by multistage and proportionate sampling techniques to help ensure that the participants were randomly selected. Oral examinations determined the "[p]resence or absence of midline interdental spaces unusually bigger than other interdental spaces." A "morphological-functional classification of the labial frenum attachments" established by Placek and others was performed to determine precise frenum location. The study concluded that "the maxilla had a higher prevalence of midline diastema than the mandible, and that papillary penetrating frenum attachments amongst these patients were higher in the maxilla than the mandible."[1] A study in 2006 by Díaz-Pizán, Lagravère, and Villena attempted "to determine the prevalence of different types and insertions of labial frenums as well as midline diastema in Peruvian children between 0 and 6 years of age." In this study, over 1,300 children were examined clinically "to classify the labial frenum, measure gingival insertion levels, and quantify midline diastema." The simple frenum (nearly 60%) and the persistent tectolabial frenum (25%) comprised the majority of frenums catalogued. Other results found "[a] significant inverse correlation between the gingival insertion level and the midline diastema."[2] In 2011, a study by Boutsi and Tatakis focused on the "distribution of the attachment of the maxillary labial frenum in the children of different ethnic backgrounds." The study concluded that, "in children, ethnic background and gender are not associated with maxillary labial frenum attachment type, whereas age is strongly associated."[3]

Histology of the Frenum

There have been many attempts to describe the histology of frenum. A study by Edwards in 1977 arrived at the following conclusions:

1. **THE PRETREATMENT RELATIONSHIP** between a clinically "abnormal"-appearing maxillary midline frenum and a midline diastema showed a strong, but not absolute, correlation.

2. **DIASTEMA CASES** in which there were "abnormal" pretreatment frenums demonstrated a decidedly stronger potential for relapse after orthodontic closure.

3. **A THREE-STAGE SURGICAL PROCEDURE** was shown to be very effective in alleviating the relapse phenomenon following orthodontic treatment of diastemas. The surgical procedures were successful in avoiding many of the hazards to the periodontium associated with previous techniques.[4]

Henry, Levin, and Tsaknis performed biopsies on specimens in a 1977 study and found that there were no muscles in the frenum. The pull exerted by the frenum was, therefore, concluded to be due to elastic and connective tissues in the frenum itself.[5] However, in another study (1990), Ross, Brown, and Houston evaluated 40 frenal specimens from various intraoral sites and found that approximately 37.5% contained skeletal or striated muscle.[6] In a similar study, Gartner and Schein (1991) performed histological examinations of superior labial frena of cadavers or from frenectomies; they concluded that

[t]he frena were covered by stratified squamous nonkeratotic, orthokeratotic, or parakeratotic epithelia, depending upon the gingival extent of the frenum. In addition to the normal components of dense, irregular, collagenous connective tissue, almost all frena contained myelinated nerve fiber bundles and small vascular channels. Additionally, 35% of the frena examined contained a few small skeletal muscle fibers.[7]

Consequences of Abnormal Frenal Attachment

The labial frenum could potentially be a problem in patients of all age groups, from toddlers to adults. The height of frenal attachment varies in each individual. A normally attached frenum usually ends at the mucogingival junction. An abnormal frenum or high frenum has inadequate attached gingiva in the insertion area. The abnormal labial frenum can cause diastema (enlarged space between the central incisors), retraction of the gingival margin, and restricted lip movement. An abnormal labial frenum can also adversely affect esthetics by causing a high smile line.

Frenal attachments seldom cause a problem in dentate individuals; however, they can raise concern to restorative dentists, periodontists, and orthodontists. Abnormal frenal attachments can hamper proper fit and stability of prosthetic constructions.

In edentulous individuals wearing such a prosthesis, abnormal attachments can produce discomfort, prevent proper seating of the of prosthesis, and eventually lead to dislodgement. Additionally, frenal attachment abnormally located on the gingival margin may cause recession of gingival tissue or aggravate existing gingival recession. If the labial frenum attaches too low between the two upper front teeth, it can create a large gap between the teeth and cause recession of gingival tissue by pulling it off the bone. This condition (a large gap between the teeth) is called diastema, and is a concern mainly in children. Moreover, the presence of a thick fibrous frenal attachment can also make orthodontic closure of diastemas difficult.

Several studies have been conducted to find a correlation between frenal attachment and diastemas; however, none have yielded convincing results. In a comparative study of attached frena with and without diastemas, Ceremello found no correlation between the height of the frenum attachment and diastema present.[8] Mazzocchi and Clini found "no correlations between teeth diastema and frenum."[9] On the other hand, Angle found that the presence of abnormal frenum resulted in midline diastema.[10] Tait proposed that the frenum is an effect of, and not a cause for, the incidence of diastema, and reported other causes, such as ankylosed central incisor, flared or rotated central incisors, anodontia, macroglossia, dentoalveolar disproportion, localized spacing, closed bite, facial type, ethnic and familial characteristics, inter-premaxillary suture, and midline pathology.[11] Popovich, Thompson, and Main concluded that the frenum may be more a result of a diastema than a cause of it.[12]

Abnormal frenal attachment can also occur in labial aspect of the mandibular ridge, mostly in the central incisor area. The condition most commonly seen in individuals with a shallow vestibule can cause the frenum to pull on its attachment at the free marginal gingiva. In addition to causing recession, it can also lead to accumulation of food and plaque. If not treated, this condition may cause inflammation of the gingival tissue, formation of pockets, and subsequent loss of alveolar bone.

Classification of Maxillary Frenums

As cited by Lawrence A. Kotlow, frenums can be classified as follows:

CLASS I: Normal frenum that does not exhibit any abnormal attachments.

CLASS II: Frenum that is attached to the gingiva above the teeth. In children, this attachment does not cause any significant problem, but in adults who experience gingival recession due to aging, this attachment might need revision.

CLASS III: Frenum that attaches in the area between the teeth.

CLASS IV: Frenum that attaches onto the anterior papilla or palate behind the teeth.[13]

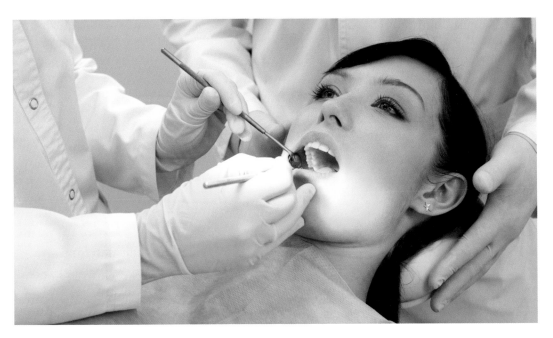

Indications for Frenectomy

Frenectomy (removal/alteration of the frenum) is indicated in cases of:

- Persistent gingival inflammation
- Progressive gingival recession
- Midline diastema

In an edentulous patient who wears dentures, lip movement may cause the frenum to pull, loosening the dentures. In these individuals, a frenectomy may help the dentures to fit well. One school of thought believes that a frenectomy may not help to close a diastema and that in certain cases the diastema may close on its own during normal development.[14] Many clinicians suggest closing the diastema orthodontically before performing a frenectomy. This closing would avoid the possibility of the development of surgical scar tissue, which may again maintain the diastema.[4,15,16] Surgical frenectomy in diastemas is not indicated unless the frenum is still attached to the incisive papilla by strong fibers which prevent physiological closure of the space between the incisors, and then not usually before the permanent cuspids have erupted between nine and ten years of age.

A very important factor when considering frenectomy is the best time to perform the procedure. Most researchers vary in their opinion of when to perform a frenectomy. Edwards suggested four factors that may guide a clinician in the decision.[4] The first one is that the frenal attachment inserts at the interdental margin or palatal/lingual to the incisors. The second factor is the unusually wider frenal attachment at the point of insertion. The third factor governing the decision to perform a frenectomy is the movement of the interdental and palatal tissue and subsequent blanching when the frenum is stretched. The fourth factor is the radiographic presence of an invagination of the interseptal bone between the teeth. In older children who have abnormal frenum attachment, a frenectomy should be performed when the permanent central incisors have just begun to erupt since it is likely that normal eruption pressures of the lateral incisors may push the central incisors together.[9,17]

Frenectomy Techniques

There are many techniques used to remove abnormal frenal attachments. Narrow frenal attachments can be treated with simple excision and Z-plasty techniques. However, wide frenal attachments may require a vestibuloplasty for removal. A simple excision can be performed under local anesthesia. The clinician administers 2% lidocaine at the surgical site to numb it. However, it should not be infiltrated into the frenum because infiltration may distort the shape of the frenum and misguide the surgeon.

Another way of identifying the frenum is by everting the lip. A pair of hemostats is used to grasp the frenum and clamp it. An elliptic incision is performed in a supraperiosteal fashion. A scissor is used to cut away and remove the frenum from both sides of the hemostats. Care is taken not to overextend the incision towards the lip. The wound margins are then approximated and closed by the clinician using resorbable sutures in an interrupted fashion. Sutures should be approximated close to the periosteum. Approximation helps in maintaining the height of the alveolar ridge and reducing hematoma formation. If the wound is left without suturing, it may take its previous form. The mucosal tissue is thus secured in place without loose wound margins. The sutures can be removed approximately one week after the frenectomy.

Another technique, called Z-plasty, involves excision of the connective tissue of the frenum in a similar fashion, except for the transpositioning of the flaps. Two releasing incisions are made in a Z-shape before undermining the flaps. These flaps are then rotated to close the initial vertical incision horizontally. The Z-technique is helpful in increasing the vestibular depth and in cases where there are chances of compromising the alveolar height.[18]

Puig, Lefebvre, and Landat used Z-plasty in the surgical treatment of hypertrophy of the superior labial frenum and recommended the technique for cases where there is hypertrophy of the frenum with a low insertion associated with an inter-incisor diastema and when the lateral incisors have appeared without causing the diastema to disappear.[19] A localized vestibuloplasty is an appropriate technique for treating frenal attachments of wide base. A supraperiosteal dissection is performed to the level of underlying periosteum. The mucosa is positioned superiorly, and, similar to the above technique, the incision is sutured just above the underlying periosteum. In this case, healing occurs by secondary intention.

Kahnberg compared frenum excision with vestibular extension of Z-plasty techniques for frenum removal and found that the differences between the preoperative and postoperative status were most marked where Z-plasty had been carried out and least marked after frenum excision. Postsurgical symptoms were most frequent after vestibular sulcus extension and least frequent after frenum excision.[20]

Edwards also described a technique for frenectomy. The frenum is apically positioned and the alveolar bone is denuded. The transseptal fibers are excised, followed by gingivoplasty or recontouring. Thereafter, the frenal attachment is sutured at a higher level. Edwards concluded that this technique greatly increases the long-term stability of an orthodontically closed maxillary midline diastema.[4]

Bagga, Bhat, Bhat, and Thomas described a novel frenectomy that results in good esthetics, excellent color match, gain in attached gingiva, and healing by primary intention at the site of the thick, extensive abnormal frenum.[21] Fowler and Breault have reported development of creeping attachment of 1.0 mm after a frenectomy procedure, which helped the patient avoid secondary graft surgery.[22] Frenectomy procedures are also performed in conjunction with free gingival grafting when there is extensive frenum attachment to create an area of attached gingiva and enhance healing, and laterally positioned pedicle graft for good esthetics.[23-25]

Laser-Assisted Frenectomy

Recently, laser-assisted frenectomies have also been reported. Frenectomy with laser does not require local anesthesia or suturing, and the wound heals with minimal postoperative complications. There is minimal patient discomfort and bleeding because the laser used in surgery seals the nerve endings and blood capillaries. One more advantage for the clinician is that the laser procedure provides a blood-free surgical area and allows for easy visualization for dissection. During the procedure, the frenum is grasped and pulled slightly. The laser tip is slowly touched upon the frenum and moved back and forth across it. The laser causes the frenum tissue to vaporize while simultaneously providing the benefit of hemostasis and coagulation. A low power setting is recommended to cause minimal thermal damage to the tissues.

A study that compared the degree of postoperative pain, discomfort, and functional complications in patients who underwent CO_2 laser-assisted frenectomy and conventional scalpel frenectomy found that CO_2 laser treatment used for frenectomy operations provides better patient perception in terms of postoperative pain and function than that obtained by the scalpel technique. These results are also applicable in pediatric patients undergoing frenectomy.[26,27]

Figure 10-1 **Laser-Assisted Lingual Frenectomy**

a

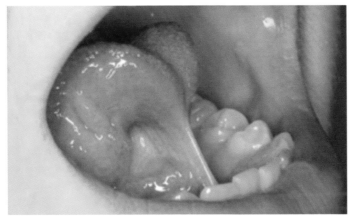

(a) Abnormal lingual frenum attachment.

b

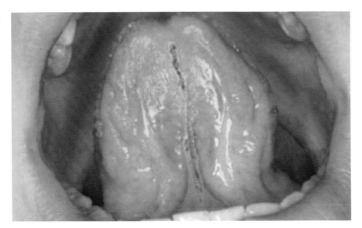

(c) Appearance of ventral surface of tongue after laser-assisted frenectomy.

c

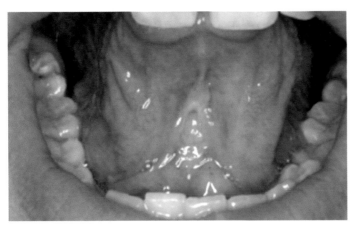

(c) Healing of the site after one week. ■

In a 2010 study, Olivi, Chaumanet, Genovese, Beneduce, and Andreana note that "[t]he labial frenum may impede oral hygiene and result in diastema between anterior teeth and traction of the attached gingiva. Surgical removal of the frenum during puberty has been recommended for these patients." Their study "evaluates the efficacy of an Er,Cr:YSGG laser in removing the labial frenum in an adolescent and pre-pubescent population." Part of the study evaluated patient acceptance of the procedure via the Wong-Baker FACES pain rating scale. The study concluded, "Patient acceptance was very high, and no postoperative adverse events were reported."[28]

A 2012 study by Pié-Sánchez, España-Tost, Arnabat-Domínguez, and Gay-Escoda attempted "[t]o compare upper lip frenulum reinsertion, bleeding, surgical time and surgical wound healing in frenectomies performed with the CO_2 laser versus the Er, Cr:YSGG laser." The study concluded,

> Upper lip laser frenectomy is a simple technique that results in minimum or no postoperative swelling or pain, and which involves upper lip frenulum reinsertion at the mucogingival junction. The CO_2 laser offers a bloodless field and shorter surgical times compared with the Er,Cr:YSGG laser. On the other hand, the Er,Cr:YSGG laser achieved faster wound healing.[29]

Home Care after Frenectomy

The patient should be instructed to follow certain procedures after the frenectomy to avoid interference with healing. The patient should brush the front teeth gently to prevent plaque accumulation since plaque buildup can complicate the healing process. In cases of maxillary frenectomy, the upper lip should be pulled upwards twice a day, and in cases of mandibular frenectomy, the lower lip should be pulled downward twice a day to prevent the operative area from healing together. A small amount of Vaseline can be put on the surgical site after pulling the lips apart. The patient should rinse the mouth with warm water after eating to promote healing. Pain medications as prescribed can be taken.

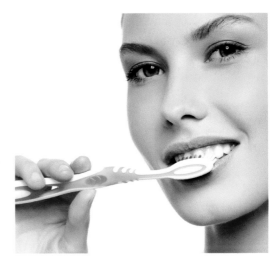

Summary

Abnormal frenal attachment is quite common; however, treatment may not be required in all cases. A frenectomy is necessary only when the frenal pull causes a diastema or gingival recession. Treatment of the abnormal frenum is usually delayed until the permanent incisors and cuspids have erupted, thus allowing the diastema to close naturally, if possible. Frenectomy is a simple procedure and can be performed in an office setting under local anesthesia. The procedure is associated with minimal postoperative complications, and it yields good results. The type of technique used for frenectomy depends on the degree of frenal attachment and associated functional or esthetic limitations. Laser-assisted surgeries, although expensive, should be considered as an alternative to conventional techniques whenever possible.

References

1. Kaimenyi JT. Occurrence of midline diastema and frenum attachments amongst school children in Nairobi, Kenya. Indian J Dent Res. 1998 Apr-Jun;9(2):67-71.

2. Díaz-Pizán ME, Lagravère MO, Villena R. Midline diastema and frenum morphology in the primary dentition. J Dent Child (Chic). 2006 Jan-Apr;73(1):11-4.

3. Boutsi EA, Tatakis DN. Maxillary labial frenum attachment in children. Int J Paediatr Dent. 2011 Jul;21(4):284-8.

4. Edwards JG. The diastema, the frenum, the frenectomy: a clinical study. Am J Orthod. 1977 May;71(5):489-508.

5. Henry SW, Levin MP, Tsaknis PJ. Histologic features of the superior labial frenum. J Periodontol. 1976 Jan;47(1):25-8.

6. Ross RO, Brown FH, Houston GD. Histologic survey of the frena of the oral cavity. Quintessence Int. 1990 Mar;21(3):233-7.

7. Gartner LP, Schein D. The superior labial frenum: a histologic observation. Quintessence Int. 1991 Jun;22(6):443-5.

8. Ceremello P. The superior labial frenum and midline diastema and their relation to growth and development of the oral structures. Am J Orthod Dentofacial Orthop 1993; 39(2):120-39.

9. Mazzocchi A, Clini F. [Indications for therapy of labial frenum]. Pediatr Med Chir. 1992 Nov-Dec;14(6):637-40. Italian.

10. Angle EH. Treatment of malocclusion of the teeth. 7th ed. S.S. White Dental Manufacturing Co: Philadelphia; 1907. pp. 103-4.

11. Tait CH. The median frenum of the upper lip and its influence on the spacing of the upper central incisor teeth. Dent Cosmos 1934;76:991-2.

12. Popovich F, Thompson GW, Main PA. The maxillary interincisal diastema and its relationship to the superior labial frenum and intermaxillary suture. Angle Orthod. 1977 Oct;47(4):265-71.

13. Kotlow LA. Lawrence A. Kotlow, D.D.S., P.C. [Internet]. Albany (NY): c2009. Preventive pediatric dental care; 2006 [cited 2013 June 2]; [about 28 screens]. Available from: http://www.kiddsteeth.com/articles/Maxillary%20Frenectomy2006adobenews.pdf

14. Koora K, Muthu MS, Rathna PV. Spontaneous closure of midline diastema following frenectomy. J Indian Soc Pedod Prev Dent. 2007 Mar;25(1):23-6.

15. Wilson HE. The labial fraenum. Trans Eur Orthod Soc 1960; 36:34.

16. Ben-Bassat Y, Brin I. Stability of upper incisors after surgical exposure and orthodontics. J Clin Orthod. 1985 Nov;19(11):815-8.

17. Belic D, Obrez-Oblak K. [Diastema verum and persistent labial frenum]. Zobozdrav Vestn. 1990 Summer;45(4-5):107-9. Croatian.

18. Sossi G, Casseler F, Radovich F, Ubiglia GP, Guidetti F. [Our experience in the correction of a short frenulum labialis by Z-plasty]. Minerva Stomatol. 1991 Jul-Aug;40(7-8):539-40. Italian.

19. Puig JR, Lefebvre E, Landat F. [Z-plasty technic, applied to hypertrophy of the upper labial frenum]. Rev Stomatol Chir Maxillofac. 1977;78(5):351-6. French.

20. Kahnberg KE. Frenum surgery. I. A comparison of three surgical methods. Int J Oral Surg. 1977 Dec;6(6):328-33.

21. Bagga S, Bhat KM, Bhat GS, Thomas BS. Esthetic management of the upper labial frenum: a novel frenectomy technique. Quintessence Int. 2006 Nov-Dec;37(10):819-23.

22. Fowler EB, Breault LG. Early creeping attachment after frenectomy: a case report. Gen Dent. 2000 Sep-Oct;48(5):591-3.

23. Breault LG, Fowler EB, Moore EA, Murray DJ. The free gingival graft combined with the frenectomy: a clinical review. Gen Dent. 1999 Sep-Oct;47(5):514-8.

24. Borghetti A, Guy JP, Cesano B. [Frenectomy associated with a triangular gingival graft]. J Parodontol. 1991 Nov;10(4):373-8. French.

25. Miller PD Jr. The frenectomy combined with a laterally positioned pedicle graft. Functional and esthetic considerations. J Periodontol. 1985 Feb;56(2):102-6.

26. Haytac MC, Ozcelik O. Evaluation of patient perceptions after frenectomy operations: a comparison of carbon dioxide laser and scalpel techniques. J Periodontol. 2006 Nov; 77(11):1815-9.

27. Shetty K, Trajtenberg C, Patel C, Streckfus C. Maxillary frenectomy using a carbon dioxide laser in a pediatric patient: a case report. Gen Dent. 2008 Jan-Feb;56(1):60-3.

28. Olivi G, Chaumanet G, Genovese MD, Beneduce C, Andreana S. Er,Cr:YSGG laser labial frenectomy: a clinical retrospective evaluation of 156 consecutive cases. Gen Dent. 2010 May-Jun;58(3):e126-33.

29. Pié-Sánchez J, España-Tost AJ, Arnabat-Domínguez J, Gay-Escoda C. Comparative study of upper lip frenectomy with the CO_2 laser versus the Er, Cr:YSGG laser. Med Oral Patol Oral Cir Bucal. 2012 Mar 1;17(2):e228-32.

Notes

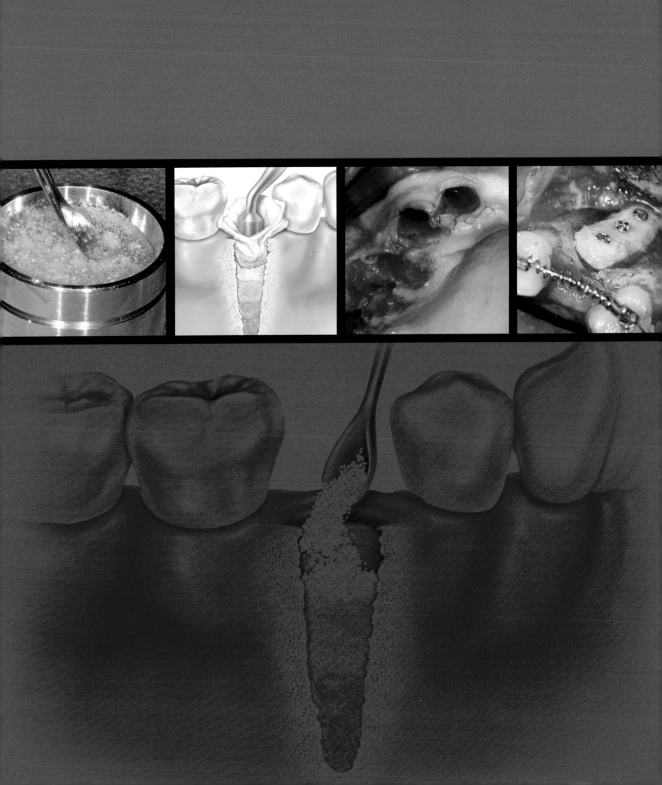

Preprosthetic Ridge Augmentation: Hard and Soft Tissue

Dental implants play an important role in enhancing the esthetics and functions of the oral cavity in individuals who have lost teeth and their supporting structures. Dental implants have become very common; however, the clinician must keep certain factors in mind before placement of implants. The most important factor is the presence of adequate alveolar bone height and width as well as the quality of bone itself. Availability of sufficient alveolar bone is important to support and retain the implant; the absence of sufficient alveolar bone can adversely affect the stability of the implant and subsequently the outcome of the implant surgery. In cases where the alveolar ridge is not sufficient to support the placement of implants, a ridge augmentation procedure may be helpful.[1] The treatment is generally recommended in cases of moderate to severely resorbed edentulous ridges. In extremely resorbed cases, the use of implants and the type of reconstructive procedure is still debatable.

Among the many factors that may reduce the dimension of alveolar ridge are tooth extraction, infection, cystic lesions, tooth/alveolar trauma, or congenital tooth agenesis. A deficient alveolar ridge may result in reduced volume and strength of residual alveolar bone, which can in turn affect the facial vertical dimensions. The patient may face difficulty in speech and masticatory function. There is also a likelihood of pathologic fractures.

Patients with a severely resorbed edentulous mandible often suffer from problems with the lower denture. These problems include insufficient retention of the lower denture, intolerance to loading by the mucosa, pain, difficulties with eating and

Figure 11-1 **Ridge Augmentation After Extraction of Maxillary 1st Premolar**

a

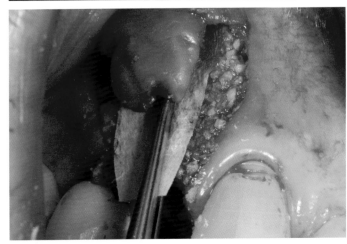

(a) Partial absence of buccal plate noted after extraction of maxillary 1st premolar.

b

(b) Area grafted with freeze-dried bone allograft (FDBA) and a resorbable membrane.

c

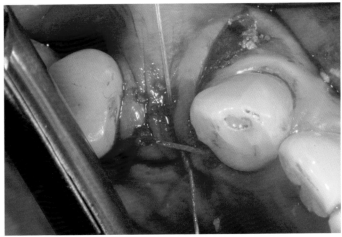

(c) Tension-free primary closure of the surgical site achieved after sufficient release of the periosteum. ■

speech, loss of soft tissue support, and altered facial appearance. These problems are a challenge for the prosthodontist and surgeon. Dental implants have been shown to provide a reliable solution for fixed and removable prostheses. This reliability has resulted in a drastic change in the treatment concepts for management of the severely resorbed edentulous mandible.

Alveolar ridge augmentation includes soft and hard tissue augmentations. The most common materials used are resorbable and nonresorbable membranes, graft biomaterials, xenografts, and bone morphogenetic proteins. Prosthetic rehabilitation of edentulous patients has always been a challenge. There are a number of pre-prosthetic surgeries used in order to improve the clinical outcome.[2] The early techniques included vestibuloplasties and grafting procedures.[3-9]

These techniques helped provide a wide denture-bearing area; however, they did not improve retention of implants or their stability. Moreover, these techniques were associated with a high morbidity rate.[10]

Need for Dental Ridge Augmentation

Alveolar ridge defects, which can lead to functional and/or esthetic compromise, can occur due to advanced periodontitis, formation of abscess, trauma, or tooth extractions. Once teeth are lost, the resorptive process is spontaneous. Studies report that after anterior tooth extraction without any type of ridge preservation, alveolar ridge resorption occurs at a rate of 40% to 60% during the first two to three years. Thereafter, the recession continues by the rate of 0.5-25% per year to the end of the patient's life.[11,12] Bone resorption will reduce retention and stability of complete dentures, which can progress to a stage that makes the denture useless.

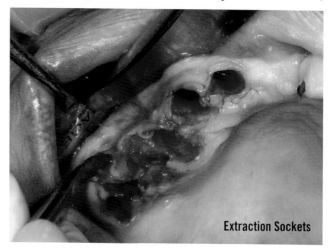

Extraction Sockets

Tissue loss caused by any of the reasons mentioned reduces the buccolingual and/or the apicocoronal ridge dimension, thus altering the alveolar ridge. These altered ridges pose a challenge for implants because the ridge alterations may not support prosthetic devices. Therefore, periodontal surgeries are necessary to establish a strong base for implant placement. Due to the complexity of the condition, the surgical approach requires coordination between the dental technician, periodontist, prosthodontist, and patients themselves. The patient-related factors include plaque control and cessation of smoking. These two factors have a very important role to play in the surgical outcomes.[13,14] Implants placed in a deformed ridge may pose many problems. Studies suggest that critical esthetic problems may arise when an anterior fixed prosthesis is fabricated over a deformed, collapsed edentulous ridge.[15]

Classification of Ridge Alterations

Many researchers have attempted to classify ridge defects to facilitate appropriate treatment selection. The classifications suggested by Siebert, Allen, and colleagues are widely accepted. Seibert's qualitative classification of ridge defects was based on the location of the deformity.[16-18]

- **CLASS I RIDGE DEFECTS** – Loss in the buccolingual width only.

- **CLASS II RIDGE DEFECTS** – Loss in the apicocoronal height only.

- **CLASS III RIDGE DEFECTS** – Combined loss of both buccolingual and apicocoronal loss resulting in both width and height loss

Allen and coworkers modified Seibert's classification and developed a quantitative classification of Type A, B, and C defects.[19]

- **TYPE A DEFICIENCY** – Apicocoronal loss of ridge contour.

- **TYPE B DEFICIENCY** – Buccolingual loss.

- **TYPE C DEFICIENCY** – Combination of buccolingual and apicocoronal loss.

The defects were further classified on the basis of the depth relative to the adjacent ridge.

- **MILD DEFICIENCIES** – Less than 3 mm.

- **MODERATE DEFICIENCIES** – From 3 to 6 mm.

- **SEVERE DEFICIENCIES** – Greater than 6 mm.

Procedures for Preprosthetic Ridge Augmentation

All the surgical techniques of alveolar ridge augmentation aim to restore the function of the alveolar ridge in anterior, posterior, vertical, and lateral directions; to augment the bone tissue in mandibular atrophy; to create adequate supportive structures for dentures and implants; and to provide biologic acceptance of implants. Various techniques are used to augment the hard and soft tissue before placement of prostheses. Soft tissue augmentation is accomplished using the roll technique or the inverted pouch technique, free gingival onlay grafts, connective tissue onlay grafts, wedge sandwich grafts, and acellular dermal matrix allografts.[20]

Free gingival onlay grafts and acellular dermal matrix allografts are used to treat Class I, Class II, and Class III defects. Connective tissue onlay grafts, the roll technique, and wedge sandwich grafts are used for the small to moderate Class I defects. Hard tissues are augmented using guided bone regeneration with autogenous bone grafts, bone allografts, xenografts, synthetic bone substitute, and block grafts.

Gingival Onlay Grafts

Gingival onlay grafts are thick, free gingival grafts derived from partial or total thickness palatal grafts. They can be used to increase ridge height. Gingival onlay grafts treat only apicocoronal ridge defects. The technique is associated with many disadvantages, the most important of which is the pale color of the healed tissue, which is not appealing esthetically. There are also risks of the graft undergoing shrinkage after the surgery.[21] Gingival onlay grafts need a rich supply of blood and rapid revascularization for graft survival.[16] As a result, this technique should not be used on areas with previous surgical trauma having compromised vascular supply.

Connective Tissue Onlay Grafts

The shortcomings associated with gingival onlay grafts can be overcome by the use of connective tissue grafts. When used for ridge augmentation, these grafts preserve the coloration and characteristics of overlying mucosa, resulting in a better esthetic outcome.[22] Connective tissue onlay grafts reduce the need for secondary surgery to fix the poor esthetic outcome. Mesimeris and Davis reported stability ranging from 7 to 12 years for the ridges augmented with connective tissue onlay grafts.[21]

Connective tissue onlay grafts are suitable for treating Class I defects but cannot be used alone in cases of severe apicocoronal ridge defects. The need for a second surgical site is the major disadvantage of connective tissue grafts although the donor area generally heals by primary intention. Along with soft tissue augmentation, severe ridge defects also require hard tissue augmentation to provide adequate support for the implant.

Autogenous Bone Grafts

Of all the procedures used for bone augmentation, autogenous bone grafting is the most predictable and is considered the gold standard. Autogenous bone grafts have osteogenic (bone producing), osteoinductive (bone inducing), and osteoconductive (bone supporting) properties. Thus, they are ideal for increasing hard tissue volume. Block bone grafts have reduced osteogenic activity and slower revascularization than particulate bone marrow grafts.

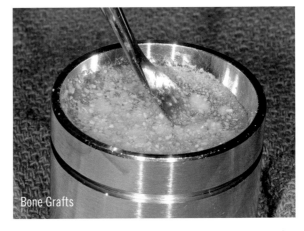
Bone Grafts

Autogenous bone grafts can be harvested either from intraoral or extraoral sites. Intraoral donor sites include the mandibular symphysis, mandibular ramus, and maxillary tuberosity. The iliac crest, tibia, scapula, clavicle, and calvarium are some extraoral sites for harvesting bone graft. There are no definite criteria for choosing a site for harvesting a graft; however, certain factors should be considered before a clinician chooses a graft harvesting site. These factors include anatomic limitation, access convenience, and proximity to the implant site. An intraoral harvested intramembraneous bone graft is optimal since it undergoes minimal resorption, enhances revascularization, and better incorporates at the donor site. Studies have reported higher stability of grafts harvested from calvaria when compared to iliac bone grafts.[23,24]

Vies, Tsirlis, and Parisis as well as Misch recommended the mandible for bone graft harvesting as it is associated with minimal resorption and early revascularization.[25,26] These qualities of mandibular bone may be due to its membranous origin while other long bones have an endochondral origin. Mandibular bone also incorporates easily with the maxillofacial region and has biochemical similarity. All these factors contribute to a better gain in bone tissue. In addition, mandibular bone can be harvested and placed as a corticocancellous bone block, which is much more capable of withstanding the forces of mastication after prosthetic reconstruction than any other bone. There is a high success rate and good long-term results with mandibular bone grafts.

It has been reported that there are more complications and morbidity related to donor area in patients treated with mandibular ramus graft than in those treated with mandibular symphysis graft. The most common complications are temporary sensory deficit in the lower lip and mental area.[27] Hwang, Shim, Yang, and Park described a noninvasive partial cortical ramal bone harvesting technique that is reproducible and predictable for preventing nerve damage while providing a sufficient block of bone needed for a dental implant.[28]

A 2005 study demonstrated that an intraoral bone block graft is a predictable procedure with high success rates that provides faciolingual and vertical bone addition. Onlay bone grafting has a low rate of complications and failures. Intraoral bone graft is not recommended for diabetic patients and smokers.[29] Pelo, Boniello, Gasparini, Longobardi, and Amoroso suggested a surgical technique to augment the alveolar ridge for vertical and horizontal defects through a localized alveolar osteotomy and interpositional bone graft. The onlay bone graft augments the palatobuccal dimension, and the interposed graft guarantees vertical augmentation.[30]

Figure 11-2 **Combined Orthodontic, Ridge Augmentation and Implant Therapy to Restore a Congenitally Missing Maxillary Lateral Incisor**

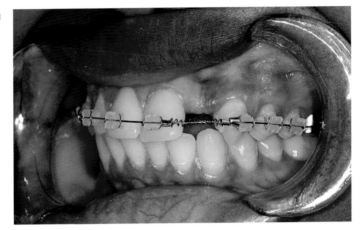

(a) Orthodontic treatment to create enough space(mesiodistally) in preparation for implant therapy.

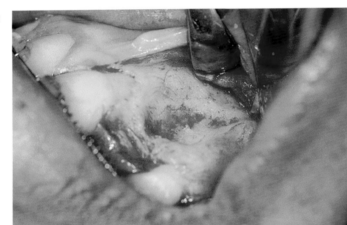

(b) Severe buccolingual ridge deficiency noted at the time of surgery.

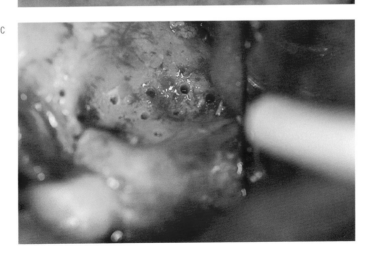

(c) Deficient ridge perforated with a #4 round bur to create the Rapid Accelatory Phenomenon(RAP).

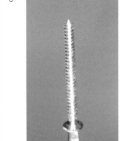

(d) Block graft shaped
and fitted into place.

(e) Titanium
retention screw.

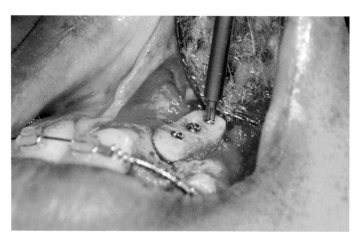

(f) Titanium screws being
placed with a driver. ▼

g

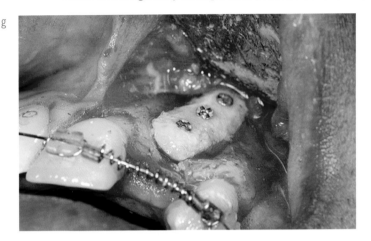

(g) Block graft stabilized in place with 3 retention screws.

h

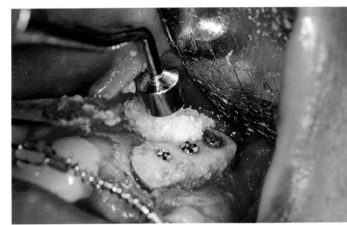

(h) Allograft particulate bone placed around the grafted site.

i

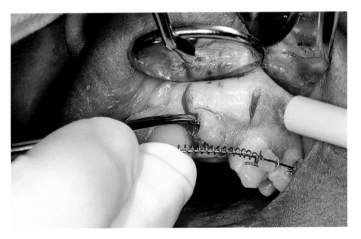

(i) Tension free passive positioning of the overlying flap.

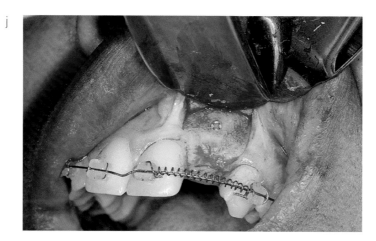

(j) Surgical exposure of the grafted site after 6 months of healing.

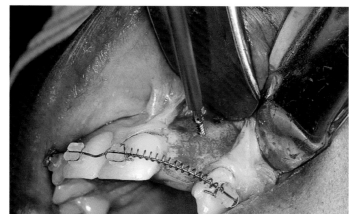

(k) Removal of titanium retension screw.

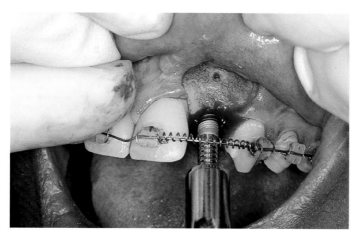

(l) Sufficient buccolingual ridge width achieved for implant placement. ∎

There are many drawbacks of using autogenous bone grafts. Such grafts require a second surgery for harvesting the grafts; this donor site may be associated with increased morbidity. There could be unpredictable bone resorption depending on the donor site selected for the graft. The techniques do not aid in augmenting the soft tissue structures. Such grafts take longer to heal, and treatment time is increased.

The surgery can be accomplished in either one stage or two stages depending on the clinical conditions. In one-stage surgery, the implants are placed at the same time as the ridge augmentation procedure. In two-stage procedures, endosseous implants are placed after the graft has been incorporated for three to four months. The advantage of a one-stage procedure is that the graft and the implant can be placed at the same time, thereby eliminating a second procedure.

An important disadvantage is that the positioning and angulation of the implants are more complicated, making this one-stage procedure undesirable from a prosthetic point of view. Another drawback of the one-step reconstruction with onlay bone grafts and endosseous implants is the unpredictable resorption of the grafted bone around the implants.[31-33] Resorption of the graft is less extensive than in the onlay technique, when one interposes a bone graft in the interforaminal area, in combination with the placement of endosseous implants in a one-stage or a two-stage procedure.[34-37] In particular, when the two-stage procedure is used, the bone-to-implant interface can, for the most part, be preserved. Although most studies report the use of an intraoral grafting approach for the edentulous mandible, a submental extraoral approach to prevent oral contamination of the graft has also been used.

An autogenous onlay bone graft, protected by titanium mesh, shows relatively less bone absorption when compared to bone grafts used alone. However, short-term exposure of the mesh should be avoided.[38,39] Tissue-engineered bone derived from periosteum has also been used to increase the vertical and horizontal dimensions of the alveolar ridge.[40] Long-term efficacy of PepGen P-15, a tissue-engineered particulate bone replacement graft, has also been reported.[41]

Figure 11-3 **Schematic Presentation of Socket Preservation Procedure**

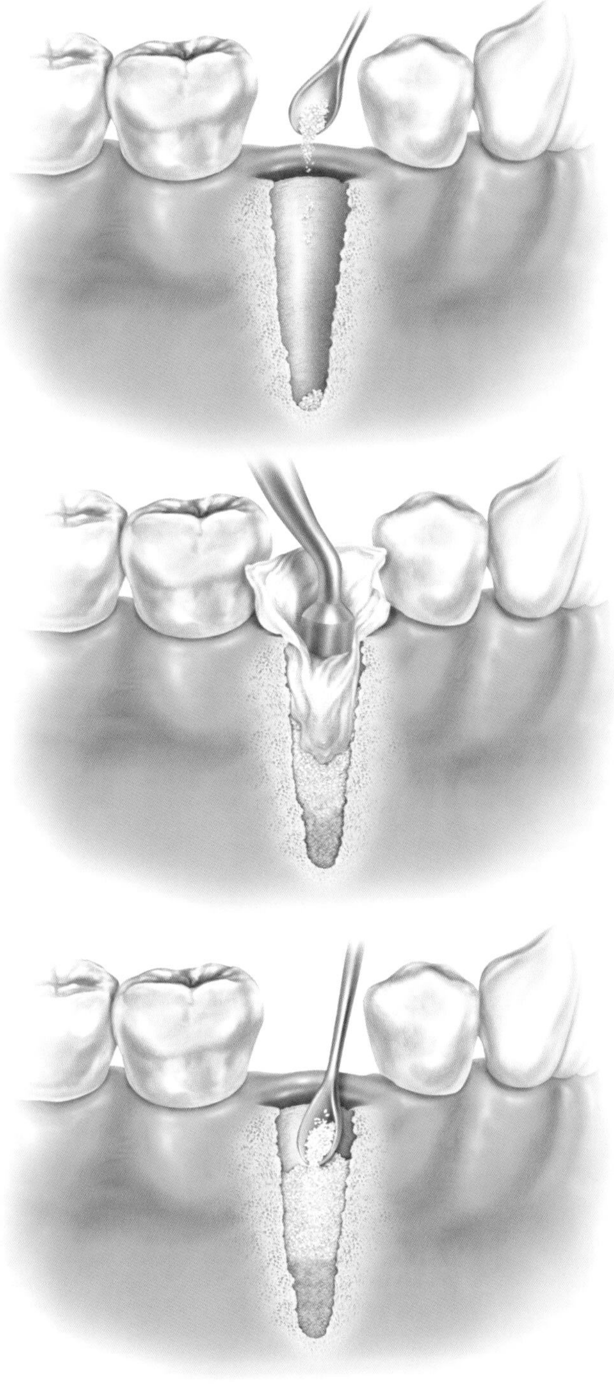

(a–g) Alternate, incremental placement of particulate FDBA and light condensing with lint-free gauze to fill the extraction socket. ■

d

e

f

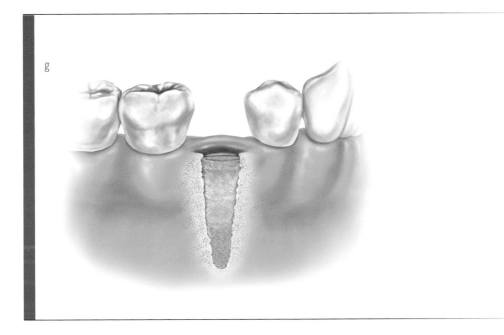

g

Allografts

Freeze-dried demineralized allogenic bone plays an important role in repairing osseous defects. Studies have shown that resorbable allogenic bone has osteogenic properties. It transforms fibroblasts into chondroblasts, resulting in bone formation even when implanted into non-skeletal tissue. In an eight-month autopsy study, Whittaker and colleagues conducted human subantral augmentation using freeze-dried demineralized bone in conjunction with resorbable hydroxyapatite and simultaneous placement of titanium fixtures.[42]   The results showed well-integrated fixtures in both the area of original bone and in the graft and also histological evidence of new bone, replacing 80% of the graft material in eight months.

Bone consists of organic and inorganic material; therefore, there are risks of a cellular reaction. This reaction depends on the methods that are followed to process the bone. Becker and colleagues demonstrated that mineralized bone obtained from a bone bank without removal of the organic matrix may not have an adverse antigenic response when implanted.[43] The various synthetic material used for bone augmentation include synthetic forms of calcium phosphate, materials including dense and porous hydroxyapatite, and other materials similar to it.[12] These materials retain alveolar bulk but are slow at resorption because of their chemical composition.

Hydroxyapatite

Hydroxyapatite is an appropriate synthetic bone material for ridge augmentation since it is osteoconductive and can adhere to the bones effectively.[44] Use of hydroxyapatite is also associated with fewer neural injuries during the procedure. Postoperative ridge resorption with hydroxyapatite is as low as 4% to 10% when compared to other methods. It is well tolerated by other tissues and does not cause local or systemic inflammation.

Hard Tissue Replacement (HTR)

Bioplant HTR (Hard Tissue Replacement) is another synthetic bone alloplast that has shown promising results in augmentation of altered ridge. It consists of a calcified co-polymer of polyhydroxyethylmethacrylate and polymethylmethacrylate and calcium hydroxide. It has shown good results at ridge augmentation as well as for ridge preservation after tooth extraction.[45-48] The material is extremely biocompatible, osteoconductive, and efficacious in periodontal defects.[48-50] In addition, in areas with a low potential for bone growth, use of HTR may stimulate dense collagen growth, thereby serving as a filler. This property can be used for expansion of connective tissue in areas where bone regeneration is not possible.

Bioglass

Bioglass, developed in 1971 by Hench and colleagues, has shown more osteoconduction activity when compared to hydroxyapatite.[51] It can prove a good material for ridge augmentation due to its inherent properties to adhere to the surrounding bone and remodel into normal bone over time.[51,52] It can also adhere to tissues other than bone, and it promotes hemostatic activity.[53] Tadjoedin and colleagues, as well as Cordioli and others, have reported use of bioactive glass for augmentation of maxillary sinus floor. They found that in particles close to the sinus floor, membrane bone tissue was formed.[54,55]

Figure 11-4 **Ridge Augmentation Using Allogenic Block Grafts**

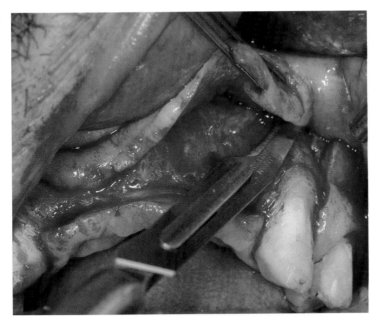

(a) Buccolingual and apicocoronal ridge deficiency in tha maxilla between the canines.

(b) Periosteal releasing incision accomplished to coronally advance the overlying flap without tension. ▼

Figure 11-4 **Ridge Augmentation Using Allogenic Block Grafts** (CONT.)

c

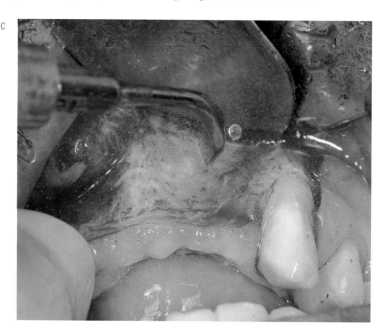

(c) Periosteum removed from the underlying bone of the recipient site with a Piezo instrument.

d

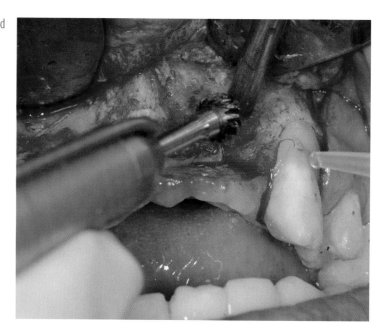

(d) Residual alveolar bone roughened with a #8 round carbide bur.

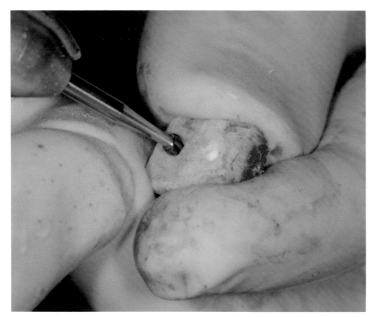

(e) Block graft shaped with a carbide bur to the required dimensions.

(f) Marks made on the block graft for proper positioning of the retention screws. ▾

Figure 11-4 **Ridge Augmentation Using Allogenic Block Grafts** (CONT.)

g

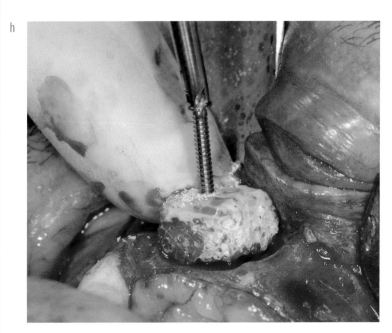

(g) Block graft prior to rounding off of the corners and placement.

h

(h) Stabilization of the block graft onto the recipient site with retention screws.

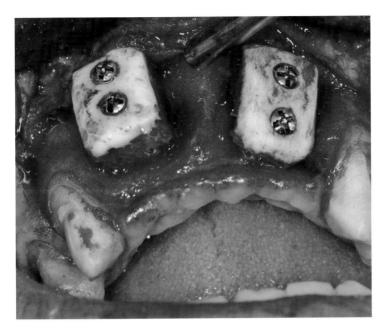

(i) Block grafts in position.

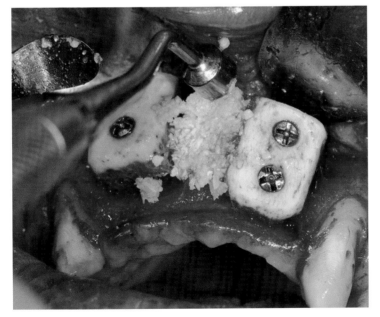

(j) Particulate bone allograft placed in between the block grafts. ▾

Figure 11-4 **Ridge Augmentation Using Allogenic Block Grafts** (CONT.)

k

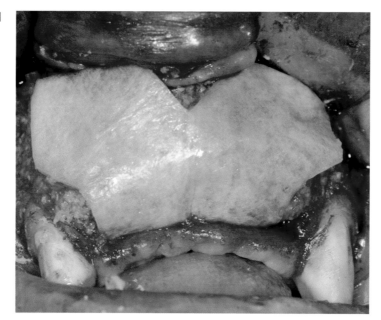

(k) Particulate bone allograft placed around and over the block grafts.

l

(l) A resorbable barrier membrane placed over the grafted site.

m

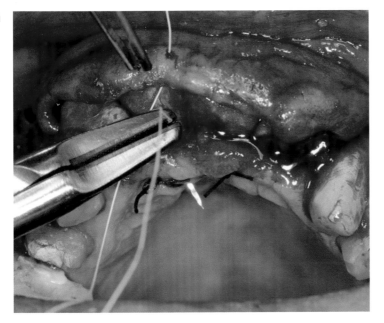

(m) Augmented ridge prior to closure.

n

(n) Area sutured with resorbable polyglycolic acid (PGA) suture. ▼

Figure 11-4 **Ridge Augmentation Using Allogenic Block Grafts** (CONT.)

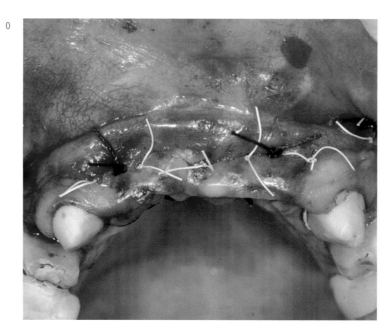

0

(o) Tension free primary closure of the grafted site. ∎

Xenografts: Deproteinized Bovine Bone

Xenografts are grafts harvested from nonhuman species and processed using various chemical and physical techniques to remove their antigenicity. The most common source is bovine bone. This deproteinized bovine bone, or DBB, is anorganic, pathogen-free, and shows minimal or no adverse reaction to host tissues; DBB can be used as bone grafts.

DBB has a crystalline with carbonate-containing apatite. The calcium phosphate ratio is similar to that of natural human bone. It shows osteoblast adhesion property suitable for ridge augmentation and for supporting bone formation around teeth and endosseous implants. Studies involving use of DBB for treating bone defects or extraction sites have shown comparable results with autogenous bone grafts.[56-58] van Steenbergh, Callens, Geers, and Jacobs reported use of DBB in grafting small defects between the implant and the labial bone in conjunction with immediate placement of implants in extraction sites.[59]

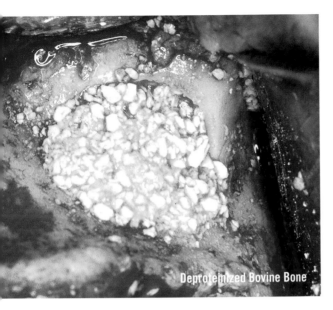

Deproteinized Bovine Bone

Deproteinized bovine graft in combination with recombinant human platelet-derived growth factor bovine bone has shown the potential to regenerate large three-dimensional alveolar defects in humans.[60] Deproteinized bovine bone mineral has also yielded good outcomes when used with expanded polytetrafluoroethylene titanium-reinforced membrane.[61,62] Hasson suggested the use of a subperiosteal tunneling technique combined with bovine bone graft and resorbable collagen membrane as an alternative surgical approach for augmenting the deficient alveolar lateral ridge.[63] The technique is a minimally invasive procedure that does not require a secondary site for bone harvesting and should be considered when performing augmentation of deficient lateral alveolar ridge.

Distraction Osteogenesis

In addition to the various grafting techniques, a method called distraction osteogenesis can also be used for augmenting the alveolar ridge dimensions. It is a technique for gradual bone lengthening wherein the natural healing process allows development of new bone tissue. In others it can also be called local guided bone regeneration.[64-66] The technique is used for ridges that have more than 5 mm vertical deficiency.

Typically, the procedure involves an osteotomy in the interforaminal area followed by placement of the distraction device. Five to seven days after surgery, osteogenesis by active distraction starts at the rate of 0.5 to 1 mm per day. Within four to six weeks, the newly formed bone gets mineralized enough to undergo implant placement. Although the consolidation period for optimum bone maturation of the distracted segment is unclear, it is recommended that the implant be left unloaded for at least three months to allow further mineralization and remodeling.

The technique results in development of vital bone to close the defect as well as the parallel gain of soft tissue. With distraction osteogenesis, there is no associated morbidity of the donor site. However, when used in edentulous, resorbed mandible, the procedure can cause fracture of the mandible, infection, and necrosis of the superior fragment. Another disadvantage of this approach is the long treatment period and the need for a suitable distractor.

The short-term clinical, radiographic and histomorphologic results of distraction osteogenesis are promising, as shown by several studies. The technique can also be used in combination with other procedures such as the split technique in the alveolar bone.[67-69]

There are not many studies that have reported success of implant therapy in distracted bone of an alveolar ridge since augmentation of the ridge improves the crown-implant ratio by increasing the implant dimension and decreasing the crown dimension, allowing the placement of a wider and longer implant for a better outcome. In one study, Wolvius and colleagues found distraction to be a suitable treatment for vertically deficient alveolar bone; however, a relatively high although manageable complication rate must be confronted, including considerable relapse.[70]

Guided Bone Regeneration

Guided bone regeneration is an effective method for increasing both width and height of a deformed ridge.[71-74] The technique helps to regenerate bone through selective exclusion of non-osteogenic tissues by a barrier membrane which could be resorbable or non-resorbable. The blood clot that fills the space between the membrane and the host tissue is gradually replaced with bone. Guided bone regeneration can be performed either with the implant placement as a one-stage procedure or as a separate surgery prior to placement of implants. The latter is chosen for ridges with large defects. Resorbable and non-resorbable membranes can be used as a barrier in the regeneration process.

Use of nonresorbable membranes requires a second surgery for its removal. Therefore, resorbable membranes are preferred as barriers. A resorbable membrane can be used alone or in combination with bone graft materials such as autogenous bone or mineralized freeze-dried bone allograft to prevent the collapse of the ridge following extraction.[22]

Combinations of Techniques and Comparative Analysis

Chiapasco, Zaniboni, and Rimondini reported similar outcomes with autogenous onlay bone grafts and alveolar distraction osteogenesis when used for ridge augmentation.[75] A comparative study of distraction osteogenesis and vertical guided bone regeneration demonstrated higher survival rates with distraction osteogenesis.[76] von Arx and Buser demonstrated successful horizontal ridge augmentation with high predictability by using a combination of autogenous block graft and guided bone regeneration technique with bovine bone mineral and collagen membranes.[77] von Arx and Buser note,

> In 42 patients with severe horizontal bone atrophy, a staged approach was chosen for implant placement following horizontal ridge augmentation. A block graft was harvested from the symphysis or retromolar area, and secured to the recipient site with fixation screws. The width of the ridge was measured before and after horizontal ridge augmentation. The block graft was subsequently covered with ABBM and a collagen membrane. Following a tension-free primary wound closure and a mean healing period of 5.8 months, the sites were re-entered, and the crest width was re-assessed prior to implant placement.

According to a 2008 study by Hämmerle, Jung, Yaman, and Lang, the combination of deproteinized bovine bone mineral and a collagen membrane is also reported to be an effective treatment option for horizontal bone augmentation before implant placement.[78] These researchers note,

> In all of the cases, but one, the bone volume following regeneration was adequate to place implants in a prosthetically ideal position and according to the standard protocol with complete bone coverage of the surface intended for osseointegration. Before the regenerative procedure, the average crestal bone width was 3.2 mm and to 6.9 mm at the time of implant placement. This difference was statistically significant ($P<0.05$, Wilcoxon's matched pairs signed-rank test).

Lyford and colleagues suggested that "a freeze-dried cancellous block allograft in conjunction with a resorbable membrane may be an acceptable alternative to the autogenous block graft in the treatment of compromised alveolar ridge deficiencies."[79] A combination of freeze-dried mineralized bone allograft mixed with recombinant human platelet derived-growth factor and a titanium-reinforced expanded polytetrafluoroethylene membrane showed promising results.[80]

A 2007 study demonstrated that vertical alveolar ridge augmentation using autogenous bone grafts and platelet-enriched fibrin glue with simultaneous implant placement may effectively increase vertical alveolar ridge height and allow for an acceptable level of osseointegration.[81] Results of the study showed that

> [i]mplant placement alone produced limited vertical alveolar height (0.6 +/- 0.4 mm). However, alveolar augmentation including a combination of autogenous bone grafts and platelet-enriched fibrin glue with simultaneous implant placement resulted in alveolar ridge augmentation amounting to 4.2 +/- 1.0 mm, comprising 63% of the defect height. New bone-implant contact was 40.5% in the defects treated with combined autogenous bone grafts and platelet-enriched fibrin glue, and was 48.4% in the resident bone; this difference was not statistically significant.

Another 2007 study that compared porous synthetic hydroxyapatite and bovine-derived hydroxyapatite showed that both can be used successfully as graft materials for maxillary sinus augmentation.[82]

Eratalay, Demiralp, Akincibay, and Tözüm reported the treatment of a localized edentulous ridge with an upside-down osteotomy technique at the symphysis region prior to implant placement. It was found that this technique may provide a successful result in partially edentulous ridges, in both maxilla and mandible.[83] The study reported that "[n]ine months after the augmentation procedure, the computed tomography (CT) examination of the area revealed that the width of the crest was 7 mm, and the height of the crest was in good relation with the cementoenamel junction of the adjacent teeth."

A 2008 study by Geurs and colleagues reported that a polyglycolic acid/trimethylene carbonate barrier membrane used in conjunction with an allograft provides lateral alveolar ridge augmentation comparable to that achieved with other materials without the necessity for bone graft harvesting or a second procedure to remove the barrier membrane.[84] A 2010 study by Binderman and colleagues describes a procedure called "periodontally accelerated osteogenic orthodontics," where particulate autogenous bone graft is used with corticotomy-assisted rapid orthodontic procedure to augment alveolar bone.[85] These researchers suggest that

> detachment of the bulk of dentogingival and interdental fibers from coronal part of root surfaces by itself should suffice to stimulate alveolar bone resorption mainly on its PDL surfaces, leading to widening of the periodontal ligament space which largely attributes to accelerated osteogenic orthodontics. Moreover this limited fiberotomy also disrupts transiently the positional physical memory of dentition (PPMD), allowing accelerated tooth movement. During retention period, a new biological and physical connectivity is generated that could be termed as new positional memory of the dental arch.

Rebaudi and colleagues suggested a new technique for ridge augmentation with autogenous cylindric bone grafts retrieved with trephine burs from intraoral donor sites. The clinical and histologic results suggested favorable outcomes.[86] Park reported good healing and increased keratinized tissue with a combination of acellular dermal matrix and deproteinized bovine bone.[87]

Alloderm has also been used in ridge preservation[88,89] and endosseous implant surgical applications.[90] In a 2010 study, Taylor and colleagues describe "a new surgical technique that addresses the unique and sensitive aspects of ADM [acellular dermal matrix] specifically to improve esthetic outcomes and gain increased clinical predictability when treating Miller Class I and II gingival recession defects."[91] In a 2011 study, Park proposes an "[i]mmediate implant placement combined with hard and soft tissue grafting has been suggested because it may preclude dramatic postextraction bone loss and may decrease overall discomfort with reduction in the number of surgeries and in treatment time."[92] Hsu, Shieh, and Wang's 2012 study describes using soft-tissue grafts as part of "a decision-making model to prevent midfacial mucosal recession following immediate implant placement," including the use of an acellular dermal matrix.[93]

Summary

Preprosthetic augmentation of deficient alveolar ridges is required for ridges that lack sufficient volume, contour, or height before implant placement. The deficient ridge often requires augmentation of both hard and soft tissues. Various techniques and their combinations are now available to suit different kinds of prosthetic needs. The selection of the surgical technique depends upon the type, size, and shape of the defect; the intended direction of the augmentation; and the surgical expertise or experience level of the clinician. Ridge augmentation can be carried out either vertically or horizontally. The clinician should have adequate knowledge of all the surgical techniques and their indications to choose the most appropriate technique for the patient.

References

1. Adell R, Lekholm U, Gröndahl K, Brånemark PI, Lindström J, Jacobsson M. Reconstruction of severely resorbed edentulous maxillae using osseointegrated fixtures in immediate autogenous bone grafts. Int J Oral Maxillofac Implants. 1990 Fall;5(3):233-46.

2. Jennings DE. Treatment of the mandibular compromised ridge: a literature review. J Prosthet Dent. 1989 May;61(5):575-9. Review.

3. Hillerup S. Preprosthetic vestibular sulcus extension by the operation of Edlan and Mejchar. A 2-year follow-up study-I. Int J Oral Surg. 1979 Oct;8(5):333-9.

4. Hillerup S. Preprosthetic surgery in the elderly. J Prosthet Dent. 1994 Nov;72(5):551-8. Review.

5. Härle F. Visor osteotomy to increase the absolute height of the atrophied mandible. A preliminary report. J Maxillofac Surg. 1975 Dec;3(4):257-60.

6. Curtis TA, Ware WH. Autogenous bone graft procedures for atrophic edentulous mandibles. J Prosthet Dent. 1977 Oct;38(4):366-79.

7. de Koomen HA, Stoelinga PJ, Tideman H, Huybers TJ. Interposed bone-graft augmentation of the atrophic mandible (a progress report). J Maxillofac Surg. 1979 May;7(2):129-35.

8. Lekkas K, Wes BJ. Absolute augmentation of the extremely atrophic mandible. (A modified technique). J Maxillofac Surg. 1981 May;9(2):103-7.

9. Peterson LJ. Augmentation of the mandibular residual ridge by a modified visor osteotomy. J Oral Maxillofac Surg. 1983 May;41(5):332-8.

10. Stoelinga PJ, Blijdorp PA, Ross RR, De Koomen HA, Huybers TJ. Augmentation of the atrophic mandible with interposed bone grafts and particulate hydroxylapatite. J Oral Maxillofac Surg. 1986 May;44(5):353-60.

11. Cawood JI, Howell RA. A classification of the edentulous jaws. Int J Oral Maxillofac Surg. 1988 Aug;17(4):232-6.

12. Ashman A. Postextraction ridge preservation using a synthetic alloplast. Implant Dent. 2000;9(2):168-76. Review.

13. Erley KJ, Swiec GD, Herold R, Bisch FC, Peacock ME. Gingival recession treatment with connective tissue grafts in smokers and non-smokers. J Periodontol. 2006 Jul;77(7):1148-55.

14. Trombelli L, Scabbia A. Healing response of gingival recession defects following guided tissue regeneration procedures in smokers and non-smokers. J Clin Periodontol. 1997 Aug;24(8):529-33.

15. Kaldahl WB, Tussing GJ, Wentz FM, Walker JA. Achieving an esthetic appearance with a fixed prosthesis by submucosal grafts. J Am Dent Assoc. 1982 Apr;104(4):449-52.

16. Seibert JS. Reconstruction of deformed, partially edentulous ridges, using full thickness onlay grafts. Part I. Technique and wound healing. Compend Contin Educ Dent. 1983 Sep-Oct;4(5):437-53.

17. Seibert JS. Reconstruction of deformed, partially edentulous ridges, using full thickness onlay grafts. Part II. Prosthetic/periodontal interrelationships. Compend Contin Educ Dent. 1983 Nov-Dec;4(6):549-62.

18. Seibert JS. Ridge augmentation to enhance esthetics in fixed prosthetic treatment. Compendium. 1991 Aug;12(8):548, 550, 552 passim.

19. Allen EP, Gainza CS, Farthing GG, Newbold DA. Improved technique for localized ridge augmentation. A report of 21 cases. J Periodontol. 1985 Apr;56(4):195-9.

20. Scharf DR, Tarnow DP. Modified roll technique for localized alveolar ridge augmentation. Int J Periodontics Restorative Dent. 1992;12(5):415-25.

21. Mesimeris V, Davis G. Use of subepithelial connective tissue grafts in combined periodontal prosthetic procedures. Periodontal Clin Investig. 1996 Spring;18(1):12-5.

22. Seibert JS. Treatment of moderate localized alveolar ridge defects. Preventive and reconstructive concepts in therapy. Dent Clin North Am. 1993 Apr;37(2):265-80. Review.

23. Carinci F, Farina A, Zanetti U, Vinci R, Negrini S, Calura G, Laino G, Piattelli A. Alveolar ridge augmentation: a comparative longitudinal study between calvaria and iliac crest bone grafts. J Oral Implantol. 2005;31(1):39-45.

24. Iizuka T, Smolka W, Hallermann W, Mericske-Stern R. Extensive augmentation of the alveolar ridge using autogenous calvarial split bone grafts for dental rehabilitation. Clin Oral Implants Res. 2004 Oct;15(5):607-15.

25. Veis AA, Tsirlis AT, Parisis NA. Effect of autogenous harvest site location on the outcome of ridge augmentation for implant dehiscences. Int J Periodontics Restorative Dent. 2004 Apr;24(2):155-63.

26. Misch CM. Comparison of intraoral donor sites for onlay grafting prior to implant placement. Int J Oral Maxillofac Implants. 1997 Nov-Dec;12(6):767-76.

27. Silva FM, Cortez AL, Moreira RW, Mazzonetto R. Complications of intraoral donor site for bone grafting prior to implant placement. Implant Dent. 2006 Dec;15(4):420-6.

28. Hwang KG, Shim KS, Yang SM, Park CJ. Partial-thickness cortical bone graft from the mandibular ramus: a non-invasive harvesting technique. J Periodontol. 2008 May; 79(5):941-4.

29. Schwartz-Arad D, Levin L, Sigal L. Surgical success of intraoral autogenous block onlay bone grafting for alveolar ridge augmentation. Implant Dent. 2005 Jun;14(2):131-8.

30. Pelo S, Boniello R, Gasparini G, Longobardi G, Amoroso PF. Horizontal and vertical ridge augmentation for implant placement in the aesthetic zone. Int J Oral Maxillofac Surg. 2007 Oct;36(10):944-8. Epub 2007 Jul 12.

31. Keller EE, Tolman DE. Mandibular ridge augmentation with simultaneous onlay iliac bone graft and endosseous implants: a preliminary report. Int J Oral Maxillofac Implants. 1992 Summer;7(2):176-84.

32. Vermeeren JI, Wismeijer D, van Waas MA. One-step reconstruction of the severely resorbed mandible with onlay bone grafts and endosteal implants. A 5-year follow-up. Int J Oral Maxillofac Surg. 1996 Apr;25(2):112-5.

33. Verhoeven JW, Cune MS, Terlou M, Zoon MA, de Putter C. The combined use of endosteal implants and iliac crest onlay grafts in the severely atrophic mandible: a longitudinal study. Int J Oral Maxillofac Surg. 1997 Oct;26(5):351-7.

34. Lew D, Hinkle RM, Unhold GP, Shroyer JV 3rd, Stutes RD. Reconstruction of the severely atrophic edentulous mandible by means of autogenous bone grafts and simultaneous placement of osseointegrated implants. J Oral Maxillofac Surg. 1991 Mar;49(3):228-33.

35. Satow S, Slagter AP, Stoelinga PJ, Habets LL. Interposed bone grafts to accommodate endosteal implants for retaining mandibular overdentures. A 1-7 year follow-up study. Int J Oral Maxillofac Surg. 1997 Oct;26(5):358-64.

36. Stellingsma C, Raghoebar GM, Meijer HJ, Batenburg RH. Reconstruction of the extremely resorbed mandible with interposed bone grafts and placement of endosseous implants. A preliminary report on outcome of treatment and patients' satisfaction. Br J Oral Maxillofac Surg. 1998 Aug;36(4):290-5.

37. Bell RB, Blakey GH, White RP, Hillebrand DG, Molina A. Staged reconstruction of the severely atrophic mandible with autogenous bone graft and endosteal implants. J Oral Maxillofac Surg. 2002 Oct;60(10):1135-41.

38. Roccuzzo M, Ramieri G, Bunino M, Berrone S. Autogenous bone graft alone or associated with titanium mesh for vertical alveolar ridge augmentation: a controlled clinical trial. Clin Oral Implants Res. 2007 Jun;18(3):286-94. Epub 2007 Feb 13.

39. Proussaefs P, Lozada J. Use of titanium mesh for staged localized alveolar ridge augmentation: clinical and histologic-histomorphometric evaluation. J Oral Implantol. 2006;32(5):237-47.

40. Strietzel FP. Tissue-engineered bone for lateral alveolar ridge augmentation: a case report. Int J Oral Maxillofac Implants. 2006 Jan-Feb;21(1):131-5.

41. Hahn J. 8-year onlay bone graft and ridge augmentation with PepGen P-15: a clinical and radiographic case study. Implant Dent. 2004 Sep;13(3):228-31.

42. Whittaker JM, James RA, Lozada J, Cordova C, GaRey DJ. Histological response and clinical evaluation of heterograft and allograft materials in the elevation of the maxillary sinus for the preparation of endosteal dental implant sites. Simultaneous sinus elevation and root form implantation: an eight-month autopsy report. J Oral Implantol. 1989;15(2):141-4.

43. Becker W, Urist M, Becker BE, Jackson W, Parry DA, Bartold M, Vincenzzi G, De Georges D, Niederwanger M. Clinical and histologic observations of sites implanted with intraoral autologous bone grafts or allografts. 15 human case reports. J Periodontol. 1996 Oct;67(10):1025-33.

44. Misch CE, Dietsh F. Bone-grafting materials in implant dentistry. Implant Dent. 1993 Fall;2(3):158-67. Review.

45. Szabó G, Suba Z, Barabás J. Use of Bioplant HTR synthetic bone to eliminate major jawbone defects: long-term human histological examinations. J Craniomaxillofac Surg. 1997 Apr;25(2):63-8.

46. Ashman A, Bruins P. Prevention of alveolar bone loss postextraction with HTR grafting material. Oral Surg Oral Med Oral Pathol. 1985 Aug;60(2):146-53.

47. Boyne PJ. Use of HTR in tooth extraction sockets to maintain alveolar ridge height and increase concentration of alveolar bone matrix. Gen Dent. 1995 Sep-Oct;43(5):470-3.

48. Ashman A, LoPinto J, Rosenlicht J. Ridge augmentation for immediate postextraction implants: eight year retrospective study. Pract Periodontics Aesthet Dent. 1995 Mar;7(2):85-94; quiz 95.

49. Kamen PR. Attachment of oral fibroblasts to HTR polymer. Compend Suppl. 1988;(10):S350-2.

50. Yukna RA, Yukna CN. Six-year clinical evaluation of HTR synthetic bone grafts in human grade II molar furcations. J Periodontal Res. 1997 Nov;32(8):627-33.

51. Hench LL, Paschall HA. Direct chemical bond of bioactive glass-ceramic materials to bone and muscle. J Biomed Mater Res. 1973; 7(3):25-42.

52. Furusawa T, Mizunuma K, Yamashita S, Takahashi T. Investigation of early bone formation using resorbable bioactive glass in the rat mandible. Int J Oral Maxillofac Implants. 1998 Sep-Oct;13(5):672-6.

53. Wheeler DL, Montfort MJ, McLoughlin SW. Differential healing response of bone adjacent to porous implants coated with hydroxyapatite and 45S5 bioactive glass. J Biomed Mater Res. 2001 Jun 15;55(4):603-12.

54. Tadjoedin ES, de Lange GL, Lyaruu DM, Kuiper L, Burger EH. High concentrations of bioactive glass material (BioGran) vs. autogenous bone for sinus floor elevation. Clin Oral Implants Res. 2002 Aug;13(4):428-36.

55. Cordioli G, Mazzocco C, Schepers E, Brugnolo E, Majzoub Z. Maxillary sinus floor augmentation using bioactive glass granules and autogenous bone with simultaneous implant placement. Clinical and histological findings. Clin Oral Implants Res. 2001 Jun;12(3):270-8.

56. Hallman M, Sennerby L, Zetterqvist L, Lundgren S. A 3-year prospective follow-up study of implant-supported fixed prostheses in patients subjected to maxillary sinus floor augmentation with a 80:20 mixture of deproteinized bovine bone and autogenous bone Clinical, radiographic and resonance frequency analysis. Int J Oral Maxillofac Surg. 2005 May;34(3):273-80.

57. Mordenfeld A, Hallman M, Johansson CB, Albrektsson T. Histological and histomorphometrical analyses of biopsies harvested 11 years after maxillary sinus floor augmentation with deproteinized bovine and autogenous bone. Clin Oral Implants Res. 2010 Sep;21(9):961-70.

58. Mordenfeld A, Albrektsson T, Hallman M. A 10-Year Clinical and Radiographic Study of Implants Placed after Maxillary Sinus Floor Augmentation with an 80:20 Mixture of Deproteinized Bovine Bone and Autogenous Bone. Clin Implant Dent Relat Res. 2012 Oct 15.

59. van Steenberghe D, Callens A, Geers L, Jacobs R. The clinical use of deproteinized bovine bone mineral on bone regeneration in conjunction with immediate implant installation. Clin Oral Implants Res. 2000 Jun;11(3):210-6.

60. Simion M, Rocchietta I, Dellavia C. Three-dimensional ridge augmentation with xenograft and recombinant human platelet-derived growth factor-BB in humans: report of two cases. Int J Periodontics Restorative Dent. 2007 Apr;27(2):109-15.

61. Simion M, Fontana F, Rasperini G, Maiorana C. Vertical ridge augmentation by expanded-polytetrafluoroethylene membrane and a combination of intraoral autogenous bone graft and deproteinized anorganic bovine bone (Bio Oss). Clin Oral Implants Res. 2007 Oct;18(5):620-9.

62. Canullo L, Malagnino VA. Vertical ridge augmentation around implants by e-PTFE titanium-reinforced membrane and bovine bone matrix: a 24- to 54-month study of 10 consecutive cases. Int J Oral Maxillofac Implants. 2008 Sep-Oct;23(5):858-66.

63. Hasson O. Augmentation of deficient lateral alveolar ridge using the subperiosteal tunneling dissection approach. Oral Surg Oral Med Oral Pathol Oral Radiol Endod. 2007 Mar;103(3):e14-9.

64. Urbani G. Alveolar distraction before implantation: a report of five cases and a review of the literature. Int J Periodontics Restorative Dent. 2001 Dec;21(6):569-79. Review.

65. Emtiaz S, Noroozi S, Caramês J, Fonseca L. Alveolar vertical distraction osteogenesis: historical and biologic review and case presentation. Int J Periodontics Restorative Dent. 2006 Dec;26(6):529-41.

66. Raghoebar GM, Vissink A. [Using distraction osteogenesis in pre-implant surgery]. Ned Tijdschr Tandheelkd. 2008 Jun;115(6):315-21. Review.

67. van Strijen PJ, Breuning KH, Becking AG, Perdijk FB, Tuinzing DB. Complications in bilateral mandibular distraction osteogenesis using internal devices. Oral Surg Oral Med Oral Pathol Oral Radiol Endod. 2003 Oct;96(4):392-7.

68. Gaggl A, Rainer H, Chiari FM. Horizontal distraction of the anterior maxilla in combination with bilateral sinus lift operation--preliminary report. Int J Oral Maxillofac Surg. 2005 Jan;34(1):37-44.

69. Matsushita K, Inoue N, Yamaguchi HO, Ooi K, Totsuka Y. Tooth-borne distraction of the lower anterior subapical segment for correction of class II malocclusion, subsequent to genioplasty. Oral Maxillofac Surg. 2011 Sep;15(3):183-8.

70. Wolvius EB, Scholtemeijer M, Weijland M, Hop WC, van der Wal KG. Complications and relapse in alveolar distraction osteogenesis in partially dentulous patients. Int J Oral Maxillofac Surg. 2007 Aug;36(8):700-5. Epub 2007 Jul 2.

71. Hermann JS, Buser D. Guided bone regeneration for dental implants. Curr Opin Periodontol. 1996;3:168-77. Review.

72. Chiapasco M, Zaniboni M. Clinical outcomes of GBR procedures to correct peri-implant dehiscences and fenestrations: a systematic review. Clin Oral Implants Res. 2009 Sep;20 Suppl 4:113-23.

73. Retzepi M, Donos N. Guided Bone Regeneration: biological principle and therapeutic applications. Clin Oral Implants Res. 2010 Jun;21(6):567-76.

74. Clementini M, Morlupi A, Canullo L, Agrestini C, Barlattani A. Success rate of dental implants inserted in horizontal and vertical guided bone regenerated areas: a systematic review. Int J Oral Maxillofac Surg. 2012 Jul;41(7):847-52.

75. Chiapasco M, Zaniboni M, Rimondini L. Autogenous onlay bone grafts vs. alveolar distraction osteogenesis for the correction of vertically deficient edentulous ridges: a 2-4-year prospective study on humans. Clin Oral Implants Res. 2007 Aug;18(4):432-40. Epub 2007 May 14.

76. Chiapasco M, Romeo E, Casentini P, Rimondini L. Alveolar distraction osteogenesis vs. vertical guided bone regeneration for the correction of vertically deficient edentulous ridges: a 1-3-year prospective study on humans. Clin Oral Implants Res. 2004 Feb;15(1):82-95.

77. von Arx T, Buser D. Horizontal ridge augmentation using autogenous block grafts and the guided bone regeneration technique with collagen membranes: a clinical study with 42 patients. Clin Oral Implants Res. 2006 Aug;17(4):359-66.

78. Hämmerle CH, Jung RE, Yaman D, Lang NP. Ridge augmentation by applying bioresorbable membranes and deproteinized bovine bone mineral: a report of twelve consecutive cases. Clin Oral Implants Res. 2008 Jan;19(1):19-25. Epub 2007 Oct 22.

79. Lyford RH, Mills MP, Knapp CI, Scheyer ET, Mellonig JT. Clinical evaluation of freeze-dried block allografts for alveolar ridge augmentation: a case series. Int J Periodontics Restorative Dent. 2003 Oct;23(5):417-25.

80. Fagan MC, Miller RE, Lynch SE, Kao RT. Simultaneous augmentation of hard and soft tissues for implant site preparation using recombinant human platelet-derived growth factor: a human case report. Int J Periodontics Restorative Dent. 2008 Feb;28(1):37-43.

81. Lee HJ, Choi BH, Jung JH, Zhu SJ, Lee SH, Huh JY, You TM, Li J. Vertical alveolar ridge augmentation using autogenous bone grafts and platelet-enriched fibrin glue with simultaneous implant placement. Oral Surg Oral Med Oral Pathol Oral Radiol Endod. 2008 Jan;105(1):27-31. Epub 2007 Sep 27.

82. Mangano C, Scarano A, Perrotti V, Iezzi G, Piattelli A. Maxillary sinus augmentation with a porous synthetic hydroxyapatite and bovine-derived hydroxyapatite: a comparative clinical and histologic study. Int J Oral Maxillofac Implants. 2007 Nov-Dec;22(6):980-6.

83. Eratalay K, Demiralp B, Akincibay H, Tözüm TF. Localized edentulous ridge augmentation with upside down osteotomy prior to implant placement. Dent Traumatol. 2004 Oct;20(5):300-4.

84. Geurs NC, Korostoff JM, Vassilopoulos PJ, Kang TH, Jeffcoat M, Kellar R, Reddy MS. Clinical and histologic assessment of lateral alveolar ridge augmentation using a synthetic long-term bioabsorbable membrane and an allograft. J Periodontol. 2008 Jul;79(7):1133-40.

85. Binderman I, Gadban N, Bahar H, Herman A, Yaffe A. Commentary on: periodontally accelerated osteogenic orthodontics (PAOO) - a clinical dilemma. Int Orthod. 2010 Sep;8(3):268-77. doi: 10.1016/j.ortho.2010.07.001. Epub 2010 Aug 23.

86. Rebaudi A, Massei G, Trisi P, Calvari F. A new technique for bone augmentation and papilla reconstruction with autogenous free gingival-bone grafts. Int J Periodontics Restorative Dent. 2007 Oct;27(5):429-39.

87. Park JB. Ridge expansion with acellular dermal matrix and deproteinized bovine bone: a case report. Implant Dent. 2007 Sep;16(3):246-51.

88. Luczyszyn SM, Papalexiou V, Novaes AB Jr, Grisi MF, Souza SL, Taba M Jr. Acellular dermal matrix and hydroxyapatite in prevention of ridge deformities after tooth extraction. Implant Dent. 2005 Jun; 14(2):176-84.

89. Novaes AB Jr, de Barros RR. Acellular dermal matrix allograft. The results of controlled randomized clinical studies. J Int Acad Periodontol. 2008 Oct;10(4):123-9.

90. El Helow K, El Askary Ael S. Regenerative barriers in immediate implant placement: a literature review. Implant Dent. 2008 Sep;17(3):360-71.

91. Taylor JB, Gerlach RC, Herold RW, Bisch FC, Dixon DR. A modified tensionless gingival grafting technique using acellular dermal matrix. Int J Periodontics Restorative Dent. 2010 Oct;30(5):513-21.

92. Park JB. Immediate implantation with ridge augmentation using acellular dermal matrix and deproteinized bovine bone: a case report. J Oral Implantol. 2011 Dec;37(6):717-21.

93. Hsu YT, Shieh CH, Wang HL. Using soft tissue graft to prevent mid-facial mucosal recession following immediate implant placement. J Int Acad Periodontol. 2012 Jul;14(3):76-82.

Notes

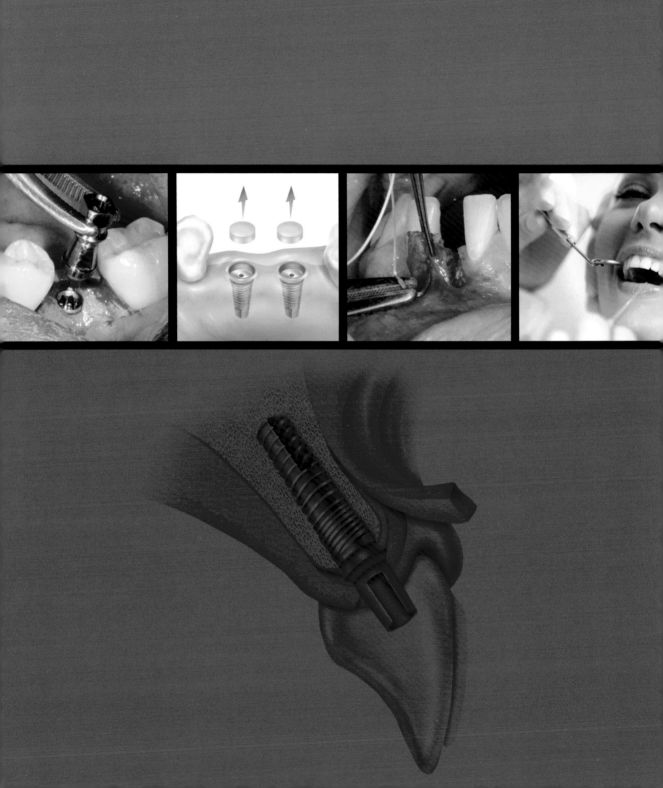

Soft Tissue Management and Dental Implants

D
ental implants are increasingly the treatment of choice for replacement of missing teeth and restoration of lost function and esthetics. Success of any dental implant depends not only on osseointegration of the implant with the underlying bone but also on the development of a healthy interface between the soft tissue and the implant. Soft tissue considerations are very important in implant dentistry. If the soft tissues are not included in the treatment planning, the outcome may be compromised by inadequate zone of keratinzed tissue, gingival recession, and compression of soft tissue by the prosthesis.

The soft tissue factors worth considering are the width of the existing gingiva, form of the interdental papillae, and space beneath the planned prosthesis or interocclusal space. The implant factors include the type and form of material surface, the type of implant component, and the time of implant placement. Too much space beneath the prosthesis can compromise the speech, function, and control of fluid. On the contrary, if the space is not adequate, there can be a rebound of compressed soft tissue, which can encroach upon the implant surface.[1]

Soft Tissue and Natural Teeth

Schroeder and colleagues reported that a healthy gingiva consists of 4% junctional epithelium, 27% oral epithelium, and 69% connective tissue that includes a small inflammatory cell infiltrate occupying about 3% to 6% of the gingival volume.[2] The oral epithelium consists of a keratinized, stratified squamous epithelium. The junctional epithelium forms a collar around the tooth and is about 2 mm high and 100 μm thick.

The inner cells of the junctional epithelium make a tight seal, called the epithelial attachment apparatus, against the tooth surface.[3] Salonen and others reported that the epithelial attachment consists of hemidesmosomes at the plasma membrane of the cells (directly attached to the tooth cells) and a basal lamina-like extracellular matrix.[4] The junctional epithelium has many protective functions. It acts as a barrier against infective agents, inhibiting colonization of the microorganisms by rapid cell division and exfoliation. It also provides a pathway for gingival crevicular fluid and transmigration of leucocytes.[5,6]

Schroeder and colleagues reported that the lamina propria of the gingival tissue consists of about 60% collagen fibers, 5% fibroblasts, and 35% vessels and nerves.[3] The collagen fiber bundles (Sharpey's fibers), composed of collagen type I and type III, are classified as circular, dentogingival, dentoperiostal, and transseptal fiber based upon their distinct direction of arrangement.[7,8] The function of these fibers is to attach the gingiva to the root cementum and to the alveolar bone, making the gingiva more rigid and resistant. Type I collagen is found in dense fibers whereas type III collagen is detected in subepithelial and perivascular compartments. Connective tissue is populated by fibroblasts and mast cells. The fibroblasts produce fibers and a matrix; the mast cells produce matrix components and vasoactive substances. A small number of inflammatory cells—such as macrophages, polymorphonuclear cells, lymphocytes, and plasma cells—are also present; however, their number may vary.[3] The lamina propria has a rich supply of blood vessels through the subepithelial plexus under the oral epithelium and the dentogingival plexus along the junctional epithelium.[9]

Implant Soft Tissue Interface

A normal wound healing process consists of four phases: hemostasis, inflammation, proliferation, and remodeling.[10-12] Junker, Caterson, and Eriksson report in a 2013 study that

> [t]he development of a sealed polyurethane wound chamber has allowed... studies evaluating the effects of growth factors, transplanted cells, and other bioactive substances on wound healing. Studies have compared wet, moist, and dry healing, with the conclusion that a wet, incubator-like microenvironment

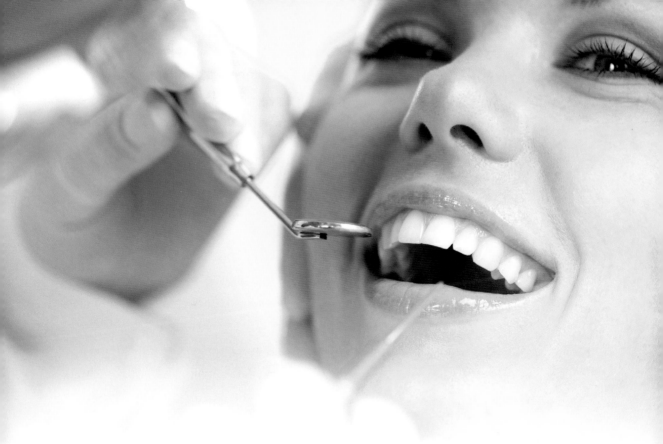

provides the fastest healing with fewest aberrations and least scar formation. The wet environment is also paramount for the survival and proliferation of transplanted cells or tissue, which has been shown in studies of porcine and human wounds....These findings have been used in clinical settings to treat wounds of different types. A titanium chamber has been developed to create an in vivo incubator, which will serve as a regenerative platform for in vivo tissue engineering.[13]

Each phase in the wound healing process is unique and gradually leads to the next phase, mediated by several cellular components.

In the first phase (hemostasis), platelets, endothelial cells, fibrin, and fibronectin are activated through growth factors and cytokines. In about two to five days, neutrophils, macrophages, and lymphocytes induce inflammation. The third stage of proliferation is mediated by fibroblasts and by epithelial and endothelial cells. This phase begins in two days to three weeks and is characterized by release of growth factors and collagen deposition. The remodeling phase is characterized by collagen cross-linking and collagen degradation, which increases scar strength. After dental implant surgery, the gingival tissue recovers by undergoing these same phases of healing.

The soft tissue around dental implants, called peri-implant mucosa, is very different from the gingival tissue found around the natural teeth. Implants are considered successful if they are osseointegrated well, which means that there is a direct structural connection at the light microscopic level between bone and the surface of a load-carrying implant.[14]   However, there is no soft tissue or periodontal ligament-like connection between the bone and implant. Electron microscopy reveals that the bone is found approximately 20 nm from the implant surface[15] or in contact with the implant surface.[16] A 2012 study by Sakka, Baroudi, and Nassani concludes that

> [o]sseointegration is a good indication of the clinical success of titanium implants referring to the direct anchorage of such implants to the surrounding host bone. Despite the high success rate of endosseous dental implants, they do fail. A lack of primary stability, surgical trauma, and infection seem to be the most important causes of early implant failure. Early signs of infection may be an indication of a much more critical result than if the same complications occur later, because of disturbance of the primary bone healing process. Occlusal overload and periimplantitis seem to be the most important factors associated with late failure. Suboptimal implant design and improper prosthetic constructions are among those risk factors responsible for implant complications and failure.[17]

Studies have shown no evidence of Sharpey's fibers between an implant or implant abutment and bone.

The soft tissue between the implant and the peri-implant mucosa is comprised of one epithelial component and one connective tissue component. The epithelial component, called the barrier epithelium, is similar to the junctional epithelium around natural teeth.[18-31] Studies conducted on an epoxy resin implant showed the development of a basal lamina and hemidesmosomes two weeks after implant placement.[32] In cases of vitallium implants, hemidesmosomes were found developing after 2-3 days of healing.[33]

However, many studies have shown structural dissimilarities between the junctional epithelium around teeth and the barrier epithelium around implants.[34-37] Some biopsy results showed the presence of inflammatory infiltrates, which indicated the presence of an immune response.[38-41]

Other studies reported functional similarities regarding antigen presentation and density of leukocytes in the gingiva and peri-implant mucosa.[42,43] Human biopsy studies have shown collagen type I as the main constituent in the connective tissue of the peri-implant mucosa.[44] Distribution of collagen III, IV, VII, and fibronectin are similar, whereas collagen type V is abundant in peri-implant tissues.[45] Unlike the gingival tissue, collagen fiber bundles in the peri-implant mucosa are aligned mostly in a parallel direction with the implant surface.[29,46-55] However, other studies report collagen fiber bundles to be functionally orientated and running in different directions.[23,24,30,56] Circular collagen fibers[26,51,53,57,58] and perpendicularly attached collagen fibers in the peri-implant mucosa[59-63] also have been reported. The peri-implant mucosa is found to be poorly vascularized.[53, 64,65]

Biological Dimension

Similar to the biological width around natural teeth, a minimum width of peri-implant mucosa is important for a stable epithelial-connective tissue attachment to form. This width includes a 2 mm long epithelial portion and a connective tissue portion about 1 mm-1.5 mm long.[47,64,66] In cases, where the thickness of the peri-implant mucosa was reduced, the alveolar bone resorbed and the mucosal dimensions were reestablished.[67] It was also reported that this dimension remained the same in loaded and unloaded conditions.[66,68]

Clinical Monitoring of the Soft Tissues around Dental Implants

Clinical monitoring of the soft tissue around dental implants is important to ensure a healthy gingiva and a stable implant. This monitoring is completed through traditional methods using periodontal probing. However, there are concerns regarding which type of periodontal probe should be used and whether a relationship exists between bone and attachment levels around a dental implant. Quirynen and others, and

Hermann and colleagues, found that in cases of dental implants with healthy soft tissues, a relationship between the bone and attachment level exists, and the clinical attachment level is a reliable indicator of bone level.[68,69] In another study, Etter and colleagues observed that healing of the epithelial attachment after probing around dental implants is complete after five days.[70] All these monitoring methods rely upon the

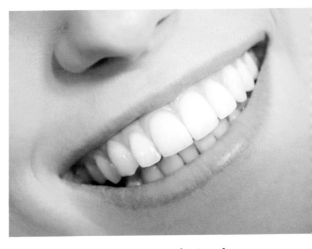

state of periodontal tissue to infer the state of the bone that is supporting the implant. These methods have been challenged by many clinicians who believe that periodontal indices are not reliable indicators of success of osseointegrated dental implants.[71,72]

One Stage Vs. Two Stage Surgery: Effect on Soft Tissue

In one-stage surgery, the implants are placed either with a transmucosal healing abutment (Figs. 12-1) or a temporary abutment and crown at the same time as the implant placement. Two-stage surgery involves placement of the implant with a cover screw and primary closure at the initial stage. After sufficient healing time, the patient then undergoes a second uncovering stage with placement of a transmucosal healing abutment(Figs.12-2 and 12-3)and /or temporarization (Fig. 12-4) and loading of final restoration (Fig. 12-5). Soft tissue recession is a major concern after implant surgery. Studies report similar amounts of tissue recession for both one-stage and two-stage surgery. The amount of soft tissue recession for single-stage dental implants is similar to that of two-stage approaches. Oates and others reported significant recession of 0.5 mm within the first three months, and a mean decrease in tissue levels of 1.6 mm after 24 months for a single-stage surgery.[73] Furthermore, a long-term study showed 1.75 mm tissue loss over nine years and 1.7 mm over three years after single-stage surgery.[38,74] Becker and Becker reported that a flap design included in the second-stage surgery can reduce tissue recessions after dental implant surgery.[75]

Figure 12-1 **One Stage Implant Surgery** (A case of a mandibular 2nd molar)

a

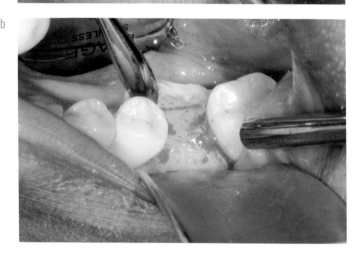

(a) Midcrestal incision from the distal of the 2nd premolar to the mesial of the 2nd molar.

b

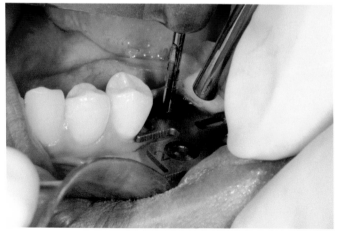

(b) Full thickness flap reflection.

c

(c) Pilot hole placed in the proper position with the aid of the ITT guide system. ▾

Figure 12-1 **One Stage Implant Surgery** (A case of a mandibular 2nd molar, CONT.)

d

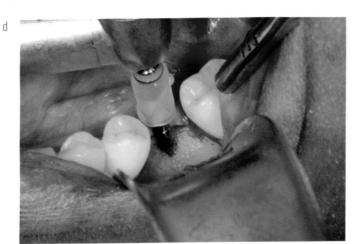

(d) Osteotomy site prepared with a drill stop for proper depth.

e

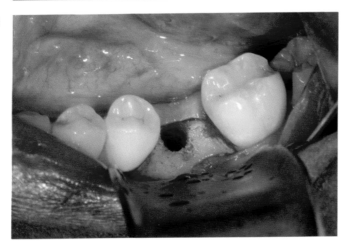

(e) Completed implant osteotomy.

f

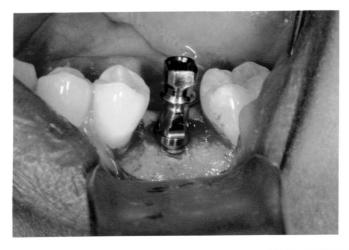

(f) Implant in place.

g

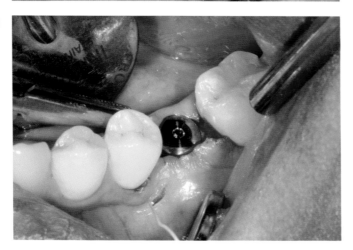

(g) Removal of implant carrier/abutment.

h

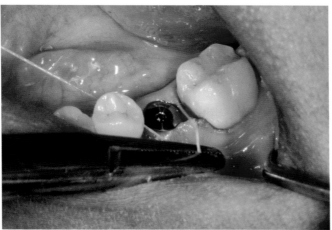

(h) A transmucosal healing abutment placed.

i

(i, j & k) Flap sutured around the transmucosal abutment with a polyglycolic acid suture and interrupted suturing technique. ▼

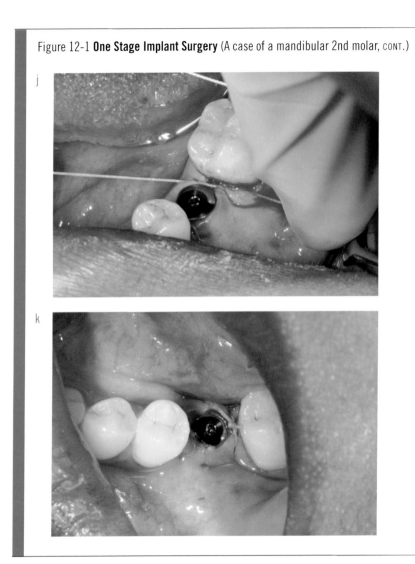

Figure 12-1 **One Stage Implant Surgery** (A case of a mandibular 2nd molar, CONT.)

j

k

Microgap

Dental implants can be a one-part system or two-part system. A one-part system has the osseous component in continuation with the transmucosal component whereas a two-part system has separate osseous and transmucosal components. The two-part system, due to separate components, has a microgap between the components. The position of the microgap relative to the crestal bone largely affects the bone loss around implants. An animal study on the traditional Brånemark implant showed the presence of an inflammatory cell infiltrate at the level of the interface between the

Figure 12-2 **Two-stage Implant Surgery** (X-incision Design)

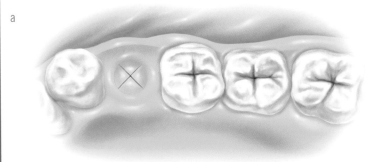

a

(a-d) Schematic drawing of uncovering and placemnet of transmucosal healing abutment using **x-incision design.** ∎

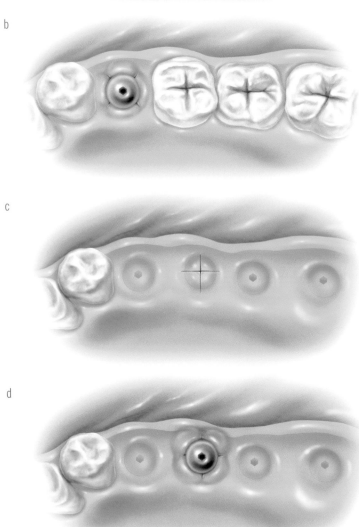

b

c

d

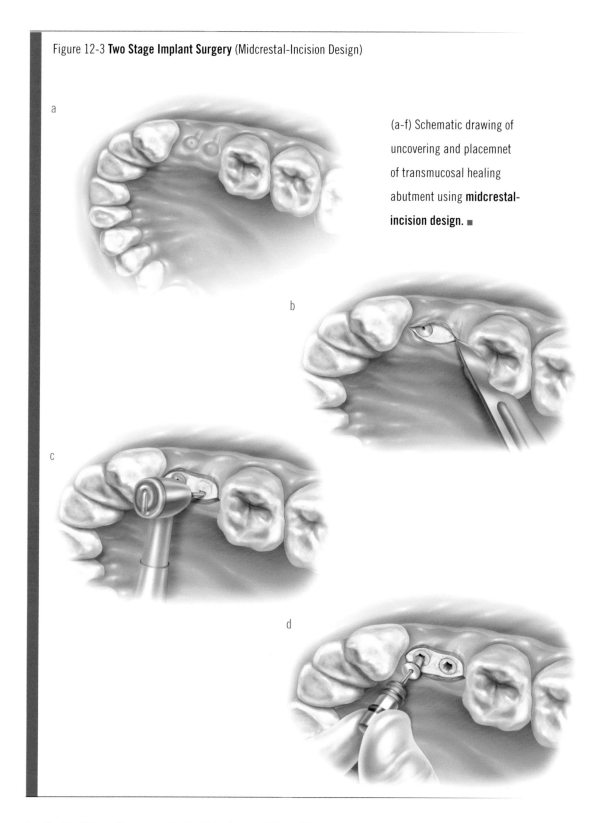

Figure 12-3 **Two Stage Implant Surgery** (Midcrestal-Incision Design)

(a-f) Schematic drawing of uncovering and placemnet of transmucosal healing abutment using **midcrestal-incision design.** ▪

a

b

c

d

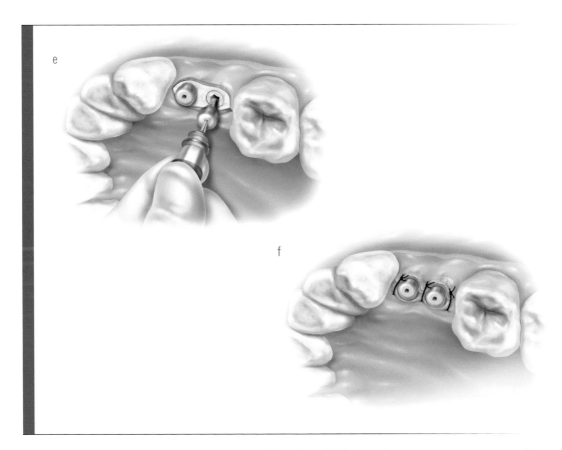

two components. The crestal bone was found to be located 1 mm to 1.5 mm apical to the microgap.[76] Animal studies comparing one-part implants and two-part implants have shown that the most coronal bone-to-implant contact of a two-part implant was consistently located approximately 2 mm below the junction level of the components.[77] Additionally, the position of microgap at different levels of crestal bone resulted in different amounts of bone loss.[78-82]

Hermann and others, and King and colleagues, reported that micromovements at the microgap between two components may influence the location of the marginal bone-to-implant contact.[83,84]

Animal studies were also completed to determine the inflammatory reaction to the microgap. Broggini and colleagues found clusters of inflammatory cells around the microgap in two-part implant systems whereas only scattered inflammatory cells were found in the tissue surrounding one-part implants.[85] In another study, Broggini

Figure 12-4 **Two Stage Implant Surgery** (Trapezoidal-Incision Design)

a

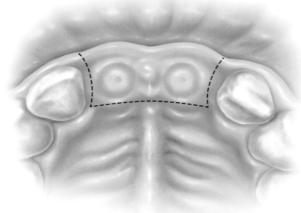

(a-g) Schematic drawing of uncovering and placemnet of transmucosal healing abutment using **trapezoidal-incision design** for maximum increase in facial and interproximal soft tissue dimensions. ▾

b

c

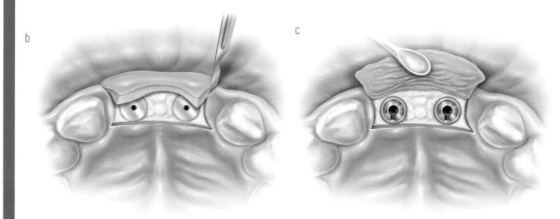

d

e

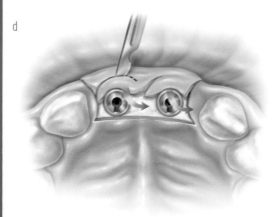
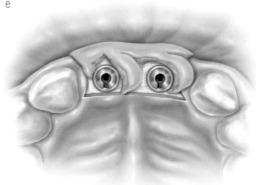

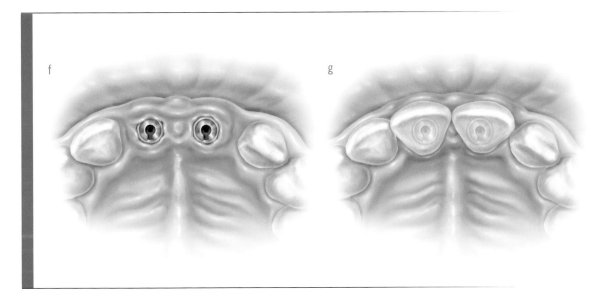

observed that the number of inflammatory cells increases with the depth of the implant-abutment interface.[86]

Effect of Implant Materials on Soft Tissues

The soft tissue reactions to implants vary based on the type of material used. For a long time, pure titanium had been used as abutment material because it was found to be biocompatible. The mechanical properties of titanium make it an ideal material for implants.[38]

However, other materials were also tried to improve esthetics and functions of the final implants. McKinney and others, for example, showed that soft tissues formed around alumina (Al_2O_3) and that single crystal sapphire had structures such as basal lamina, hemidesmosomes, and a connective tissue with collagen fibers that were mainly oriented parallel to the implant surface.[21,22 ,24,46] Microscopic biopsy studies, however, found no difference between single-crystal sapphire implants and titanium implants regarding the organization of the epithelium, the arrangement of collagen fibers, nerves, vessels, and different connective tissue cells.[87]

A comparative animal study on abutments made of titanium, gold alloy, dental porcelain, and Al_2O_3 ceramic indicated the absence of soft tissue attachments with gold alloy and dental porcelain implants.[88] On the other hand, soft tissue attachments

Figure 12-5 **Two Stage Implant Surgery**

A case of maxillary central incisors from the time of uncovering, immediate temporarization and final restoration.

a

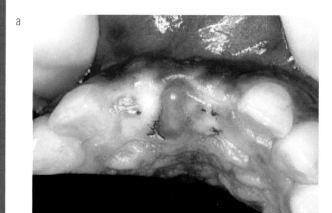

(a) Healed implant site at the time of second stage uncovering procedure.

b

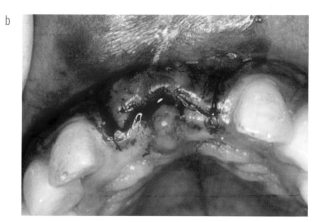

(b) Trapezoidal-incision design to increase the facial and interproxiaml dimensions of the soft tissues.

c

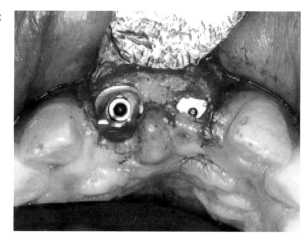

(c) Full thickness flap reflection.

d

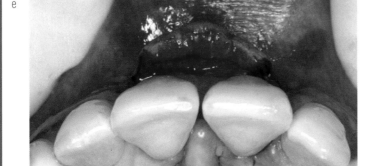

(d) Custom-made abutment secured in place.

e

(e) Temporary crowns cemented.

f

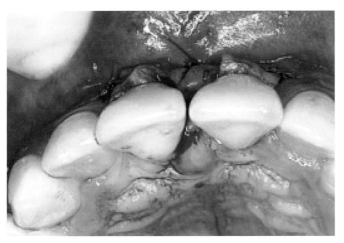

(f) Soft tissues sutured around the properly contoured temporary crowns to obtain an optimum soft tissue emergence profile. ▾

Figure 12-5 **Two Stage Implant Surgery** (CONT.)

g

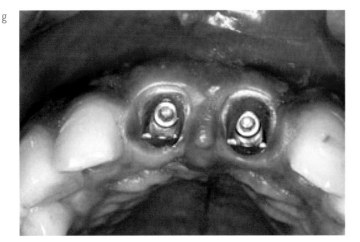

(g & h) Healed implant uncovered sites at 12 weeks. Note the presence of interproximal soft tissues in between the implants and the nice soft tissue emergence profile.

h

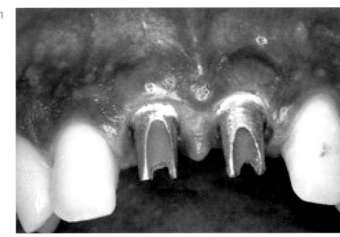

i

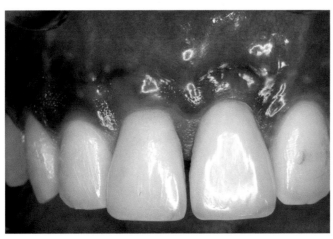

(i) Final implant prosthesis in place. ■

of similar dimensions and tissue structures were found with titanium and ceramic abutments. Vigolo and colleagues reported no difference in perimucosal response around abutments made of gold alloy and titanium.[89] Other researchers found no differences in soft tissue response with transmucosal collars and abutments of titanium and dental ceramics.[90-92]

A comparative study demonstrated less bacteria and plaque accumulation on zirconia abutments than on titanium discs.[93,94] Degidi and others reported lower inflammatory levels in the zirconia healing caps than in the titanium healing caps.[95] Similar soft tissue dimensions were found with both types of abutment materials.[96] Abutments made of zirconia and alumina zirconia demonstrated favorable hard tissue and soft tissue responses.[97,98]

Effect on Soft Tissues from Surface Treatments of Titanium Implants

Many methods have been tried to modify the surface of the titanium implant to increase the stability of implants and decrease the tissue reaction against it. The use of hydroxyapatite and other coatings on titanium implants was intended to promote soft tissue formation with structures resembling the soft tissue attachment to teeth. Some of these methods are polishing, particle blasting, etching, and anodization. These surface treatments were thought to enhance formation of gingival tissue and the structures resembling the soft tissue attachment to teeth. These surface-modified implants may result in a different tissue reaction.

In their 2002 study, Abrahamsson and colleagues found that soft tissue dimensions did not differ around implants with a polished smooth surface or a thermal dual acid etched surface.[99] Other studies have suggested that surface roughness of the implants does not affect plaque accumulation.[100-102] Animal studies on implants coated with calcium phosphate coatings demonstrated that epithelium and supra alveolar collagen fibers formed around dense calcium hydroxyapatite titanium implants.[102] The collagen fibers were parallel to the hydroxyapatite-coated implants placed.[50] A comparative study of the submerged and nonsubmerged hydroxyapatite implants indicated no difference in soft tissue dimensions.[103]

Piatelli and colleagues found parallel and perpendicular collagen fiber bundles around plasma-sprayed titanium implants on analysis of autopsy materials.[60] Another study that compared titanium implants with a solgel-derived nanoporous TiO2 film found hemidesmosomes of the cells in the junctional epithelium facing the surface. Surface-treated implants showed a shorter distance between the implant margin and the bone crest.[31]

Peri-Implant Mucositis and Peri-Implantitis

The peri-implant tissues may demonstrate pathological changes. These changes, when confined to the soft tissue, are termed peri-implant mucositis.[104-106] These implants are called "ailing implants."[107] In their 2012 study, Sakka, Idrees, Alissa, and Kujan note that

> [t]he distinction between ailing and failing implants is clinically important. Changes in the peri-implant soft or hard tissues will indicate whether the implant is ailing, failing, or has failed. This article discusses these clinical situations and provides an overview and description of peri-implant diseases and their treatment alternatives.[108]

Before loading an implant, the clinician should evaluate the overall design of the prosthesis and the state of the soft tissues. In order to prevent bacterial invasion, the clinician must be sure that there is an adequate amount of keratinized tissue to provide a peri-implant seal. Soft tissue grafting may be needed to augment the tissues if found to be insufficient.

When pathological changes involve the alveolar bone, causing bone loss, the changes are termed peri-implantitis.[106,109,110] The implant in this condition is called a failing implant. Peri-implantitis usually begins at the coronal portion of the implant; however, the implant may not be clinically mobile as the more apical portion of the implant maintains an osseointegrated status.[111,112] The implant may become mobile once the bone loss progresses to involve the whole implant surface.[111]

Appropriate therapy is needed to arrest the progression of these pathological changes to ensure the success of dental implants. Therapy depends on the severity of bone loss, the kind of bone defect, and the type of implants used. There are many factors that may lead to peri-implant problems. The two major factors are bacterial infection and biomechanical overload. There are other factors, such as inappropriate technique, surgical trauma, inadequate alveolar bone, and unfavorable host response. In cases of patients presenting with peri-implant problems, the clinician should try to identify the actual cause and treat it accordingly. Great care must be exercised to prevent plaque formation on the implant. Plaque accumulated on the implant can cause inflammation in the adjoining connective tissues, resulting in progressive tissue destruction.[104,106,109,110] These changes differ according to the type of implants used.

Biomechanical forces are a major cause of peri-implant problems. Excessive forces can put high stress on the bone-to-implant contact, leading to microfractures and loss of osseointegration.[113,114] Soft tissue grafting is performed in conjunction with dental implant surgery either at the first stage or at the second stage to augment the gingival tissue around the implant. These options include the free gingival graft, apically and coronally positioned grafts, subepithelial connective tissue grafts, inverted pouch procedure or roll technique, and combination techniques.

Connective tissue grafts have been used to reestablish normal tissue volume, contour, and architecture around dental implants.[115,116] A technique combining subepithelial connective tissue grafts and immediate implant placement and provisionalization has been devised to achieve a more stable peri-implant tissue in conditions that include thin biotype.[117] Acellular dermal matrix allografts can be used as a grafting material to increase the width of peri-implant keratinized mucosa. This procedure appears to have some benefits for oral hygiene.[118] One study reported that the width of keratinized tissues around implants was increased by using the acellular dermal matrix allograft but by a lesser amount than seen with the autogenous gingival graft.[119]

Guided Bone Regeneration for Dental Implants

Guided bone regeneration (GBR) procedures are helpful in augmenting the ridge dimensions before, during (Fig. 12-7) or after (Fig. 12-6) dental implant placement. Such procedures ensure adequate tissue height and width for stability of the implant.[120-123] Small bone defects can be treated with particulate bone graft materials. Resorbable

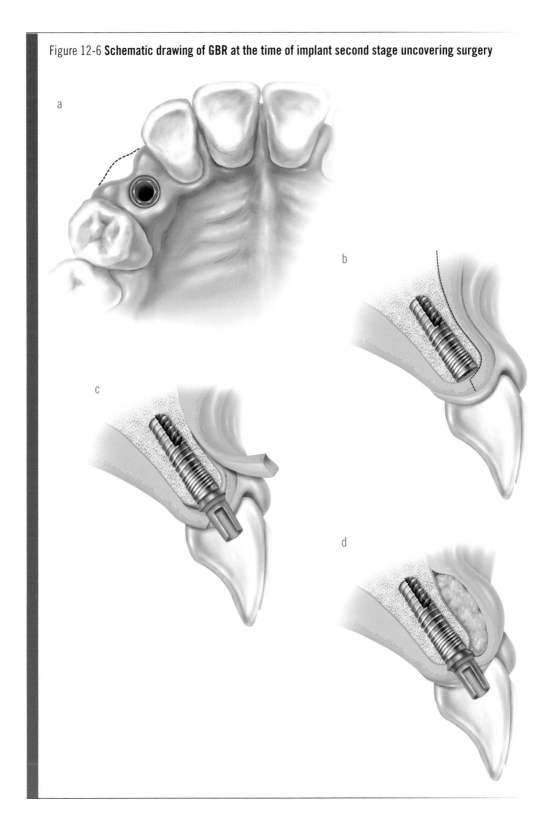

Figure 12-6 **Schematic drawing of GBR at the time of implant second stage uncovering surgery**

Figure 12-7 **GBR at the time of implant placement** (A case of mandibular central incisor)

a

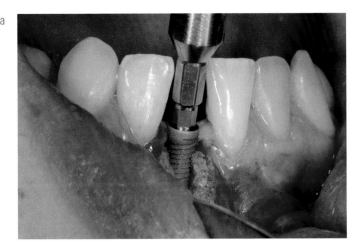

(a & b) Facial bony dehiscence exposing the coronal 1/3 of the implant threads at the time of placement

b

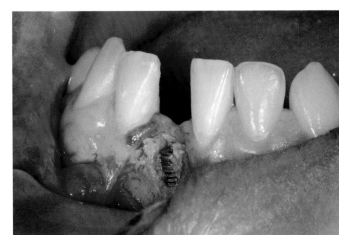

c

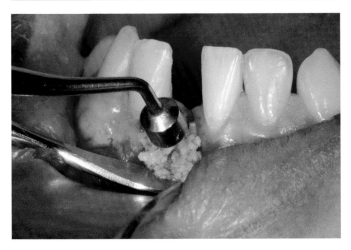

(c & d) Particulate allograft bone (FDBA) placed on facial dehiscence site. ▼

Figure 12-7 **GBR at the time of implant placement** (A case of mandibular central incisor, CONT.)

d

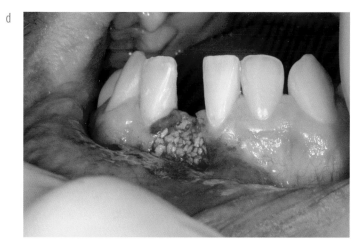

e

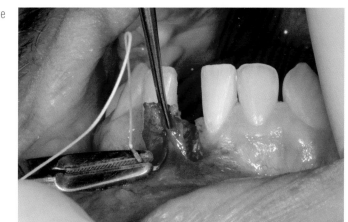

(e & f) Tension free closure of the area with a polyglycolic acid (PGA) suture and interrupted suturing technique. ■

f

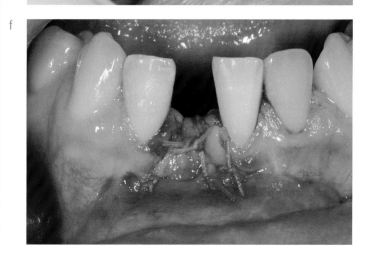

or nonresorbable membranes can also be used along with particulate bone grafting.[124] Bone blocks with a barrier membrane are used to treat large defects.[125] Bone blocks can effectively create alveolar bone height, which is quite difficult when compared to augmentation of bone width. Bischof and colleagues suggested that vertical alveolar bone length should be able to support at least a 10-mm implant with a crown-to-implant ratio of 1:1.[126] Guided bone regeneration should only be performed in patients who have adequate keratinized tissue to cover the wound.[127]

Summary

An implant is successful when it completely integrates with the soft and hard tissue of the oral cavity. Adequate bone tissue is necessary to provide firm support to the implant and restorations. In addition to hard tissues, soft tissues have an important role in the success of dental implants. Soft tissue acts as a barrier to prevent microbial entry to the implants and their components. Any compromise with soft tissues during implant surgery may jeopardize the esthetic and functional outcome of the implant. Inadequate soft tissue around the implant may lead to recession, plaque formation, and eventual inflammation of the peri-implant tissues. Therefore, an adequate amount of gingiva at the surgical site is crucial.

References

1. Taylor TD. Osteogenesis of the mandible associated with implant reconstruction: a patient report. Int J Oral Maxillofac Implants. 1989 Fall;4(3):227-31.

2. Schroeder HE, Münzel-Pedrazzoli S, Page R. Correlated morphometric and biochemical analysis of gingival tissue in early chronic gingivitis in man. Arch Oral Biol. 1973 Jul;18(7):899-923.

3. Schroeder HE, Listgarten MA. The gingival tissues: the architecture of periodontal protection. Periodontol 2000. 1997 Feb; 13:91-120.

4. Salonen JI, Kautsky MB, Dale BA. Changes in cell phenotype during regeneration of junctional epithelium of human gingiva in vitro. J Periodontal Res. 1989 Nov;24(6):370-7.

5. Löe H, Karring T. Mitotic activity and renewal time of the gingival epithelium of young and old rats. J Periodontal Res Suppl. 1969; (4):18-9.

6. Schiött CR, Löe H. The origin and variation in number of leukocytes in the human saliva. J Periodontal Res. 1970;5(1):36-41.

7. FENEIS H. [Anatomy and physiology of the normal gingiva]. Dtsch Zahnarztl Z. 1952 Apr 15;7(8):467-76. Undetermined Language.

8. Page RC, Ammons WF, Schectman LR, Dillingham LA. Collagen fibre bundles of the normal marginal g-ngiva in the marmoset. Arch Oral Biol. 1974 Nov;19(11):1039-43.

9. Egelberg J. The blood vessels of the dento-gingival junction. J Periodontal Res. 1966;1(3):163-79.

10. Kiwanuka E, Junker J, Eriksson E. Harnessing growth factors to influence wound healing. Clin Plast Surg. 2012 Jul;39(3):239-48. Epub 2012 May 23. Review.

11. Werner S, Grose R. Regulation of wound healing by growth factors and cytokines. Physiol Rev. 2003 Jul;83(3):835-70. Review.

12. Squier CA, Kremenak CR. Quantitation of the healing palatal mucoperiosteal wound in the beagle dog. Br J Exp Pathol. 1982 Oct;63(5):573-84.

13. Junker JP, Caterson EJ, Eriksson E. The microenvironment of wound healing. J Craniofac Surg. 2013 Jan;24(1):12-6.

14. Brånemark PI. Introduction to osseointegration. In: Brånemark PI, Zarb G, Albrektsson T, eds. Tissue integrated prostheses: Osseointegration in clinical dentistry. Chicago: Quintessence; 1995; 11-76.

15. Albrektsson T. Bone tissue response. In: Brånemark PI, Zarb G, Albrektsson T. eds. Tissue integrated prostheses: Osseointegration in Clinical Dentistry. Chicago: Quintessence; 1985;129-143.

16. Listgarten MA, Lang NP, Schroeder HE, Schroeder A. Periodontal tissues and their counterparts around endosseous implants [corrected and republished with original paging, article originally printed in Clin Oral Implants Res 1991 Jan-Mar;2(1):1-19]. Clin Oral Implants Res. 1991 Jul-Sep;2(3):1-19. Review.

17. Sakka S, Baroudi K, Nassani MZ. Factors associated with early and late failure of dental implants. J Investig Clin Dent. 2012 Nov;3(4):258-61. Epub 2012 Aug 27. Review.

18. James RA, Schultz RL. Hemidesmosomes and the adhesion of junctional epithelial cells to metal implants--a preliminary report. Oral Implantol. 1974 Winter;4(3):294-302.

19. Hansson HA, Albrektsson T, Brånemark PI. Structural aspects of the interface between tissue and titanium implants. J Prosthet Dent. 1983 Jul;50(1):108-13.

20. Gould TR, Westbury L, Brunette DM. Ultrastructural study of the attachment of human gingiva to titanium in vivo. J Prosthet Dent. 1984 Sep;52(3):418-20.

21. McKinney RV Jr, Steflik DE, Koth DL. Evidence for a junctional epithelial attachment to ceramic dental implants. A transmission electron microscopic study. J Periodontol. 1985 Oct;56(10):579-91.

22. Hashimoto M, Akagawa Y, Nikai H, Tsuru H. Ultrastructure of the peri-implant junctional epithelium on single-crystal sapphire endosseous dental implant loaded with functional stress. J Oral Rehabil. 1989 May;16(3):261-70.

23. Arvidson K, Bystedt H, Ericsson I. Histometric and ultrastructural studies of tissues surrounding Astra dental implants in dogs. Int J Oral Maxillofac Implants. 1990 Summer;5(2):127-34.

24. Fartash B, Arvidson K, Ericsson I. Histology of tissues surrounding single crystal sapphire endosseous dental implants: an experimental study in the beagle dog. Clin Oral Implants Res. 1990 Dec;1(1):13-21.

25. Mackenzie IC, Tonetti MS. Formation of normal gingival epithelial phenotypes around osseo-integrated oral implants in humans. J Periodontol. 1995 Nov;66(11):933-43.

26. Fujii N, Kusakari H, Maeda T. A histological study on tissue responses to titanium implantation in rat maxilla: the process of epithelial regeneration and bone reaction. J Periodontol. 1998 Apr;69(4):485-95.

27. Kawahara H, Kawahara D, Mimura Y, Takashima Y, Ong JL. Morphologic studies on the biologic seal of titanium dental implants. Report II. In vivo study on the defending mechanism of epithelial adhesions/attachment against invasive factors. Int J Oral Maxillofac Implants. 1998 Jul-Aug;13(4):465-73.

28. Marchetti C, Farina A, Cornaglia AI. Microscopic, immunocytochemical, and ultrastructural properties of peri-implant mucosa in humans. J Periodontol. 2002 May;73(5):555-63.

29. Glauser R, Schüpbach P, Gottlow J, Hämmerle CH. Periimplant soft tissue barrier at experimental one-piece mini-implants with different surface topography in humans: A light-microscopic overview and histometric analysis. Clin Implant Dent Relat Res. 2005;7 Suppl 1:S44-51.

30. Nevins M, Nevins ML, Camelo M, Boyesen JL, Kim DM. Human histologic evidence of a connective tissue attachment to a dental implant. Int J Periodontics Restorative Dent. 2008 Apr;28(2):111-21.

31. Rossi S, Tirri T, Paldan H, Kuntsi-Vaattovaara H, Tulamo R, Närhi T. Peri-implant tissue response to TiO2 surface modified implants. Clin Oral Implants Res. 2008 Apr;19(4):348-55. Epub 2008 Feb 5.

32. Listgarten MA, Lai CH. Ultrastructure of the intact interface between an endosseous epoxy resin dental implant and the host tissues. J Biol Buccale. 1975 Mar;3(1):13-28.

33. Swope EM, James RA. A longitudinal study on hemidesmosome formation at the dental implant-tissue overflow. J Oral Implantol. 1981;9(3):412-22.

34. Inoue T, Takeda T, Lee CY, Abiko Y, Ayukawa Y, Tanaka T, Yoshinari M, Shimono M. Immunolocalization of proliferating cell nuclear antigen in the peri-implant epithelium. Bull Tokyo Dent Coll. 1997 Aug;38(3):187-93.

35. Carmichael RP, McCulloch CA, Zarb GA. Quantitative immunohistochemical analysis of keratins and desmoplakins in human gingiva and peri-implant mucosa. J Dent Res. 1991 May;70(5):899-905.

36. Ikeda H, Yamaza T, Yoshinari M, Ohsaki Y, Ayukawa Y, Kido MA, Inoue T, Shimono M, Koyano K, Tanaka T. Ultrastructural and immunoelectron microscopic studies of the peri-implant epithelium-implant (Ti-6Al-4V) interface of rat maxilla. J Periodontol. 2000 Jun;71(6):961-73.

37. Fujiseki M, Matsuzaka K, Yoshinari M, Shimono M, Inoue T. An experimental study on the features of peri-implant epithelium: immunohistochemical and electron-microscopic observations. Bull Tokyo Dent Coll. 2003 Nov;44(4):185-99.

38. Adell R, Lekholm U, Rockler B, Brånemark PI, Lindhe J, Eriksson B, Sbordone L. Marginal tissue reactions at osseointegrated titanium fixtures (I). A 3-year longitudinal prospective study. Int J Oral Maxillofac Surg. 1986 Feb;15(1):39-52.

39. Lekholm U, Adell R, Lindhe J, Brånemark PI, Eriksson B, Rockler B, Lindvall AM, Yoneyama T. Marginal tissue reactions at osseointegrated titanium fixtures. (II) A cross-sectional retrospective study. Int J Oral Maxillofac Surg. 1986 Feb;15(1):53-61.

40. Liljenberg B, Gualini F, Berglundh T, Tonetti M, Lindhe J. Some characteristics of the ridge mucosa before and after implant installation. A prospective study in humans. J Clin Periodontol. 1996 Nov;23(11):1008-13.

41. Seymour GJ, Gemmell E, Lenz LJ, Henry P, Bower R, Yamazaki K. Immunohistologic analysis of the inflammatory infiltrates associated with osseointegrated implants. Int J Oral Maxillofac Implants. 1989 Fall;4(3):191-8.

42. Tonetti MS, Imboden M, Gerber L, Lang NP. Compartmentalization of inflammatory cell phenotypes in normal gingiva and peri-implant keratinized mucosa. J Clin Periodontol. 1995 Oct;22(10):735-42.

43. Tonetti MS, Schmid, J., Hämmerle, C.H., Lang, N.P. Intraepithelial antigen-presenting cells in the keratinized mucosa around teeth and osseointegrated implants. Clin Oral Impl Res 1993; 4:177-186.

44. Chavrier CA, Couble ML. Ultrastructural immunohistochemical study of interstitial collagenous components of the healthy human keratinized mucosa surrounding implants. Int J Oral Maxillofac Implants. 1999 Jan-Feb;14(1):108-12.

45. Romanos GE, Schröter-Kermani C, Weingart D, Strub JR. Health human periodontal versus peri-implant gingival tissues: an immunohistochemical differentiation of the extracellular matrix. Int J Oral Maxillofac Implants. 1995 Nov-Dec;10(6):750-8.

46. Hashimoto M, Akagawa Y, Nikai H, Tsuru H. Single-crystal sapphire endosseous dental implant loaded with functional stress--clinical and histological evaluation of peri-implant tissues. J Oral Rehabil. 1988 Jan;15(1):65-76.

47. Berglundh T, Lindhe J, Ericsson I, Marinello CP, Liljenberg B, Thomsen P. The soft tissue barrier at implants and teeth. Clin Oral Implants Res. 1991 Apr-Jun;2(2):81-90.

48. Listgarten MA, Buser D, Steinemann SG, Donath K, Lang NP, Weber HP. Light and transmission electron microscopy of the intact interfaces between non-submerged titanium-coated epoxy resin implants and bone or gingiva. J Dent Res. 1992 Feb;71(2):364-71. Erratum in: J Dent Res 1992 May;71(5):1267.

49. Chavrier C, Couble ML, Hartmann DJ. Qualitative study of collagenous and noncollagenous glycoproteins of the human healthy keratinized mucosa surrounding implants. Clin Oral Implants Res. 1994 Sep;5(3):117-24.

50. Comut AA, Weber HP, Shortkroff S, Cui FZ, Spector M. Connective tissue orientation around dental implants in a canine model. Clin Oral Implants Res. 2001 Oct;12(5):433-40.

51. Schierano G, Ramieri G, Cortese M, Aimetti M, Preti G. Organization of the connective tissue barrier around long-term loaded implant abutments in man. Clin Oral Implants Res. 2002 Oct;13(5):460-4.

52. Tenenbaum H, Schaaf JF, Cuisinier FJ. Histological analysis of the Ankylos peri-implant soft tissues in a dog model. Implant Dent. 2003;12(3):259-65.

53. Schupbach P, Glauser R. The defense architecture of the human periimplant mucosa: a histological study. J Prosthet Dent. 2007 Jun;97(6 Suppl):S15-25. Erratum in: J Prosthet Dent. 2008 Mar;99(3):167.

54. Subramani K, Jung RE, Molenberg A, Hammerle CH. Biofilm on dental implants: a review of the literature. Int J Oral Maxillofac Implants. 2009 Jul-Aug;24(4):616-26. Review.

55. Pivodova V, Frankova J, Ulrichova J. Osteoblast and gingival fibroblast markers in dental implant studies. Biomed Pap Med Fac Univ Palacky Olomouc Czech Repub. 2011 Jun;155(2):109-16. Review.

56. Schroeder A, van der Zypen E, Stich H, Sutter F. The reactions of bone, connective tissue, and epithelium to endosteal implants with titanium-sprayed surfaces. J Maxillofac Surg. 1981 Feb;9(1):15-25.

57. Akagawa Y, Takata T, Matsumoto T, Nikai H, Tsuru H. Correlation between clinical and histological evaluations of the peri-implant gingiva around the single-crystal sapphire endosseous implant. J Oral Rehabil. 1989 Nov;16(6):581-7.

58. Ruggeri A, Franchi M, Marini N, Trisi P, Piatelli A. Supracrestal circular collagen fiber network around osseointegrated nonsubmerged titanium implants. Clin Oral Implants Res. 1992 Dec;3(4):169-75.

59. Buser D, Stich, H., Krekeler, G. & Schroeder, A. Faserstrukturen der periim-plantären Mukosa bei Titanimplantaten. Zeitschrift für Zahnärztliche Implantologie 1989; V:15-23.

60. Piattelli A, Scarano A, Piattelli M, Bertolai R, Panzoni E. Histologic aspects of the bone and soft tissues surrounding three titanium non-submerged plasma-sprayed implants retrieved at autopsy: a case report. J Periodontol. 1997 Jul;68(7):694-700.

61. Choi BH. Periodontal ligament formation around titanium implants using cultured periodontal ligament cells: a pilot study. Int J Oral Maxillofac Implants. 2000 Mar-Apr;15(2):193-6.

62. Schwarz F, Herten M, Sager M, Wieland M, Dard M, Becker J. Histological and immunohistochemical analysis of initial and early osseous integration at chemically modified and conventional SLA titanium implants: preliminary results of a pilot study in dogs. Clin Oral Implants Res. 2007 Aug;18(4):481-8. Epub 2007 Apr 30.

63. Schwarz F, Ferrari D, Herten M, Mihatovic I, Wieland M, Sager M, Becker J. Effects of surface hydrophilicity and microtopography on early stages of soft and hard tissue integration at non-submerged titanium implants: an immunohistochemical study in dogs. J Periodontol. 2007 Nov;78(11):2171-84.

64. Buser D, Weber HP, Donath K, Fiorellini JP, Paquette DW, Williams RC. Soft tissue reactions to non-submerged unloaded titanium implants in beagle dogs. J Periodontol. 1992 Mar;63(3):225-35.

65. Berglundh T, Lindhe J, Jonsson K, Ericsson I. The topography of the vascular systems in the periodontal and peri-implant tissues in the dog. J Clin Periodontol. 1994 Mar;21(3):189-93.

66. Cochran DL, Hermann JS, Schenk RK, Higginbottom FL, Buser D. Biologic width around titanium implants. A histometric analysis of the implanto-gingival junction around unloaded and loaded nonsubmerged implants in the canine mandible. J Periodontol. 1997 Feb;68(2):186-98.

67. Berglundh T, Lindhe J. Dimension of the periimplant mucosa. Biological width revisited. J Clin Periodontol. 1996 Oct;23(10):971-3.

68. Hermann JS, Buser D, Schenk RK, Schoolfield JD, Cochran DL. Biologic Width around one- and two-piece titanium implants. Clin Oral Implants Res. 2001 Dec;12(6):559-71.

69. Quirynen M, van Steenberghe D, Jacobs R, Schotte A, Darius P. The reliability of pocket probing around screw-type implants. Clin Oral Implants Res. 1991 Oct-Dec;2(4):186-92.

70. Etter TH, Håkanson I, Lang NP, Trejo PM, Caffesse RG. Healing after standardized clinical probing of the periimplant soft tissue seal: a histomorphometric study in dogs. Clin Oral Implants Res. 2002 Dec;13(6):571-80.

71. Chaytor DV, Zarb GA, Schmitt A, Lewis DW. The longitudinal effectiveness of osseointegrated dental implants. The Toronto Study: bone level changes. Int J Periodontics Restorative Dent. 1991;11(2):112-25.

72. Kim BS, Kim YK, Yun PY, Yi YJ, Lee HJ, Kim SG, Son JS. Evaluation of peri-implant tissue response according to the presence of keratinized mucosa. Oral Surg Oral Med Oral Pathol Oral Radiol Endod. 2009 Mar;107(3):e24-8.

73. Oates TW, West J, Jones J, Kaiser D, Cochran DL. Long-term changes in soft tissue height on the facial surface of dental implants. Implant Dent. 2002;11(3):272-9.

74. Apse P, Zarb GA, Schmitt A, Lewis DW. The longitudinal effectiveness of osseointegrated dental implants. The Toronto Study: peri-implant mucosal response. Int J Periodontics Restorative Dent. 1991;11(2):94-111.

75. Becker W, Becker BE. Flap designs for minimization of recession adjacent to maxillary anterior implant sites: a clinical study. Int J Oral Maxillofac Implants. 1996 Jan-Feb;11(1):46-54.

76. Ericsson I, Persson LG, Berglundh T, Marinello CP, Lindhe J, Klinge B. Different types of inflammatory reactions in peri-implant soft tissues. J Clin Periodontol. 1995 Mar;22(3):255-61.

77. Hermann JS, Cochran DL, Nummikoski PV, Buser D. Crestal bone changes around titanium implants. A radiographic evaluation of unloaded nonsubmerged and submerged implants in the canine mandible. J Periodontol. 1997 Nov;68(11):1117-30.

78. Hermann JS, Buser D, Schenk RK, Cochran DL. Crestal bone changes around titanium implants. A histometric evaluation of unloaded non-submerged and submerged implants in the canine mandible. J Periodontol. 2000 Sep;71(9):1412-24.

79. Piattelli A, Vrespa G, Petrone G, Iezzi G, Annibali S, Scarano A. Role of the microgap between implant and abutment: a retrospective histologic evaluation in monkeys. J Periodontol. 2003 Mar; 74(3):346-52.

80. Alomrani AN, Hermann JS, Jones AA, Buser D, Schoolfield J, Cochran DL. The effect of a machined collar on coronal hard tissue around titanium implants: a radiographic study in the canine mandible. Int J Oral Maxillofac Implants. 2005 Sep-Oct;20(5):677-86.

81. Valderrama P, Jones AA, Wilson TG Jr, Higginbottom F, Schoolfield JD, Jung RE, Noujeim M, Cochran DL. Bone changes around early loaded chemically modified sandblasted and acid-etched surfaced implants with and without a machined collar: a radiographic and resonance frequency analysis in the canine mandible. Int J Oral Maxillofac Implants. 2010 May-Jun;25(3):548-57.

82. Hermann JS, Jones AA, Bakaeen LG, Buser D, Schoolfield JD, Cochran DL. Influence of a machined collar on crestal bone changes around titanium implants: a histometric study in the canine mandible. J Periodontol. 2011 Sep;82(9):1329-38.

83. Hermann JS, Schoolfield JD, Schenk RK, Buser D, Cochran DL. Influence of the size of the microgap on crestal bone changes around titanium implants. A histometric evaluation of unloaded non-submerged implants in the canine mandible. J Periodontol. 2001 Oct;72(10):1372-83.

84. King GN, Hermann JS, Schoolfield JD, Buser D, Cochran DL. Influence of the size of the microgap on crestal bone levels in non-submerged dental implants: a radiographic study in the canine mandible. J Periodontol. 2002 Oct;73(10):1111-7.

85. Broggini N, McManus LM, Hermann JS, Medina RU, Oates TW, Schenk RK, Buser D, Mellonig JT, Cochran DL. Persistent acute inflammation at the implant-abutment interface. J Dent Res. 2003 Mar;82(3):232-7.

86. Broggini N, McManus LM, Hermann JS, Medina R, Schenk RK, Buser D, Cochran DL. Peri-implant inflammation defined by the implant-abutment interface. J Dent Res. 2006 May;85(5):473-8.

87. Arvidson K, Fartash B, Hilliges M, Köndell PA. Histological characteristics of peri-implant mucosa around Brånemark and single-crystal sapphire implants. Clin Oral Implants Res. 1996 Mar;7(1):1-10.

88. Abrahamsson I, Berglundh T, Glantz PO, Lindhe J. The mucosal attachment at different abutments. An experimental study in dogs. J Clin Periodontol. 1998 Sep;25(9):721-7.

89. Vigolo P, Givani A, Majzoub Z, Cordioli G. A 4-year prospective study to assess peri-implant hard and soft tissues adjacent to titanium versus gold-alloy abutments in cemented single implant crowns. J Prosthodont. 2006 Jul-Aug;15(4):250-6.

90. Barclay CW, Last KS, Williams R. The clinical assessment of a ceramic-coated transmucosal dental implant collar. Int J Prosthodont. 1996 Sep-Oct;9(5):466-72.

91. Rasperini G, Maglione M, Cocconcelli P, Simion M. In vivo early plaque formation on pure titanium and ceramic abutments: a comparative microbiological and SEM analysis. Clin Oral Implants Res. 1998 Dec;9(6):357-64.

92. Andersson B, Glauser R, Maglione M, Taylor A. Ceramic implant abutments for short-span FPDs: a prospective 5-year multicenter study. Int J Prosthodont. 2003 Nov-Dec;16(6):640-6.

93. Rimondini L, Cerroni L, Carrassi A, Torricelli P. Bacterial colonization of zirconia ceramic surfaces: an in vitro and in vivo study. Int J Oral Maxillofac Implants. 2002 Nov-Dec;17(6):793-8.

94. Scarano A, Piattelli M, Caputi S, Favero GA, Piattelli A. Bacterial adhesion on commercially pure titanium and zirconium oxide disks: an in vivo human study. J Periodontol. 2004 Feb;75(2):292-6.

95. Degidi M, Artese L, Scarano A, Perrotti V, Gehrke P, Piattelli A. Inflammatory infiltrate, microvessel density, nitric oxide synthase expression, vascular endothelial growth factor expression, and proliferative activity in peri-implant soft tissues around titanium and zirconium oxide healing caps. J Periodontol. 2006 Jan;77(1):73-80.

96. Kohal RJ, Weng D, Bächle M, Strub JR. Loaded custom-made zirconia and titanium implants show similar osseointegration: an animal experiment. J Periodontol. 2004 Sep;75(9):1262-8.

97. Glauser R, Sailer I, Wohlwend A, Studer S, Schibli M, Schärer P. Experimental zirconia abutments for implant-supported single-tooth restorations in esthetically demanding regions: 4-year results of a prospective clinical study. Int J Prosthodont. 2004 May-Jun;17(3):285-90.

98. Bae KH, Han JS, Seol YJ, Butz F, Caton J, Rhyu IC. The biologic stability of alumina-zirconia implant abutments after 1 year of clinical service: a digital subtraction radiographic evaluation. Int J Periodontics Restorative Dent. 2008 Apr;28(2):137-43.

99. Abrahamsson I, Zitzmann NU, Berglundh T, Linder E, Wennerberg A, Lindhe J. The mucosal attachment to titanium implants with different surface characteristics: an experimental study in dogs. J Clin Periodontol. 2002 May;29(5):448-55.

100. Bollen CM, Papaioanno W, Van Eldere J, Schepers E, Quirynen M, van Steenberghe D. The influence of abutment surface roughness on plaque accumulation and peri-implant mucositis. Clin Oral Implants Res. 1996 Sep;7(3):201-11.

101. Zitzmann NU, Abrahamsson I, Berglundh T, Lindhe J. Soft tissue reactions to plaque formation at implant abutments with different surface topography. An experimental study in dogs. J Clin Periodontol. 2002 May; 29(5):456-61.

102. Wennerberg A, Sennerby L, Kultje C, Lekholm U. Some soft tissue characteristics at implant abutments with different surface topography. A study in humans. J Clin Periodontol. 2003 Jan;30(1):88-94.

103. Kohal RJ, De LaRosa M, Patrick D, Hürzeler MB, Caffesse RG. Clinical and histologic evaluation of submerged and nonsubmerged hydroxyapatite-coated implants: a preliminary study in dogs. Int J Oral Maxillofac Implants. 1999 Nov-Dec;14(6):824-34.

104. Ericsson I, Berglundh T, Marinello C, Liljenberg B, Lindhe J. Long-standing plaque and gingivitis at implants and teeth in the dog. Clin Oral Implants Res. 1992 Sep;3(3):99-103.

105. Pontoriero R, Tonelli MP, Carnevale G, Mombelli A, Nyman SR, Lang NP. Experimentally induced peri-implant mucositis. A clinical study in humans. Clin Oral Implants Res. 1994 Dec;5(4):254-9.

106. Jovanovic SA, Donath K, Shayesteh H, Carranza FA, Kenney EB. Plaque-induced peri-implant disease in the mongrel dog. Dent Res 1995;74(Spec Iss):21.

107. Krauser JT. Hydroxylapatite-coated dental implants. Biologic rationale and surgical technique. Dent Clin North Am. 1989 Oct;33(4):879-903. Review.

108. Sakka S, Idrees M, Alissa R, Kujan O. Ailing and failing oral implants: initial therapy and surgical management. J Investig Clin Dent. 2012 Nov 27.

109. Lindhe J, Berglundh T, Ericsson I, Liljenberg B, Marinello C. Experimental breakdown of peri-implant and periodontal tissues. A study in the beagle dog. Clin Oral Implants Res. 1992 Mar;3(1):9-16.

110. Marinello CP, Berglundh T, Ericsson I, Klinge B, Glantz PO, Lindhe J. Resolution of ligature-induced peri-implantitis lesions in the dog. J Clin Periodontol. 1995 Jun;22(6):475-9.

111. Jovanovic SA. The management of peri-implant breakdown around functioning osseointegrated dental implants. J Periodontol. 1993 Nov;64(11 Suppl):1176-83. Review.

112. Isidor F. Loss of osseointegration caused by occlusal load of oral implants. A clinical and radiographic study in monkeys. Clin Oral Implants Res. 1996 Jun;7(2):143-52.

113. Roberts WE, Garetto LP, DeCastro RA. Remodeling of devitalized bone threatens periosteal margin integrity of endosseous titanium implants with threaded or smooth surfaces: indications for provisional loading and axially directed occlusion. J Indiana Dent Assoc. 1989 Jul-Aug;68(4):19-24.

114. Quirynen M, Naert I, van Steenberghe D. Fixture design and overload influence marginal bone loss and fixture success in the Brånemark system. Clin Oral Implants Res. 1992 Sep;3(3):104-11.

115. El-Askary AS. Use of connective tissue grafts to enhance the esthetic outcome of implant treatment: a clinical report of 2 patients. J Prosthet Dent. 2002 Feb;87(2):129-32.

116. Silverstein LH, Lefkove MD. The use of the subepithelial connective tissue graft to enhance both the aesthetics and periodontal contours surrounding dental implants. J Oral Implantol. 1994;20(2):135-8.

117. Kan JY, Rungcharassaeng K, Lozada JL. Bilaminar subepithelial connective tissue grafts for immediate implant placement and provisionalization in the esthetic zone. J Calif Dent Assoc. 2005 Nov;33(11):865-71.

118. Yan JJ, Tsai AY, Wong MY, Hou LT. Comparison of acellular dermal graft and palatal autograft in the reconstruction of keratinized gingiva around dental implants: a case report. Int J Periodontics Restorative Dent. 2006 Jun;26(3):287-92.

119. Park JB. Increasing the width of keratinized mucosa around endosseous implant using acellular dermal matrix allograft. Implant Dent. 2006 Sep;15(3):275-81.

120. Fiorellini JP, Nevins ML. Localized ridge augmentation/preservation. A systematic review. Ann Periodontol. 2003 Dec;8(1):321-7. Review.

121. Horowitz R, Holtzclaw D, Rosen PS. A review on alveolar ridge preservation following tooth extraction. J Evid Based Dent Pract. 2012 Sep;12(3 Suppl):149-60. Review.

122. Esposito M, Maghaireh H, Grusovin MG, Ziounas I, Worthington HV. Soft tissue management for dental implants: what are the most effective techniques? A Cochrane systematic review. Eur J Oral Implantol. 2012 Autumn;5(3):221-38. Review.

123. Agarwal G, Thomas R, Mehta D. Postextraction maintenance of the alveolar ridge: rationale and review. Compend Contin Educ Dent. 2012 May;33(5):320-4, 326; quiz 327, 336. Review.

124. Rose LF, Rosenberg E. Bone grafts and growth and differentiation factors for regenerative therapy: a review. Pract Proced Aesthet Dent. 2001 Nov-Dec;13(9):725-34; quiz 736, 721-2. Review.

125. Bahat O. Interrelations of soft and hard tissues for osseointegrated implants. Compend Contin Educ Dent. 1996 Dec;17(12):1161-8, 1170; quiz 1172. Review.

126. Bischof M, Nedir R, Szmukler-Moncler S, Bernard JP, Samson J. Implant stability measurement of delayed and immediately loaded implants during healing. Clin Oral Implants Res. 2004 Oct;15(5):529-39.

127. Yildirim M, Hanisch O, Spiekermann H. Simultaneous hard and soft tissue augmentation for implant-supported single-tooth restorations. Pract Periodontics Aesthet Dent. 1997 Nov-Dec;9(9):1023-31; quiz 1032. Review.

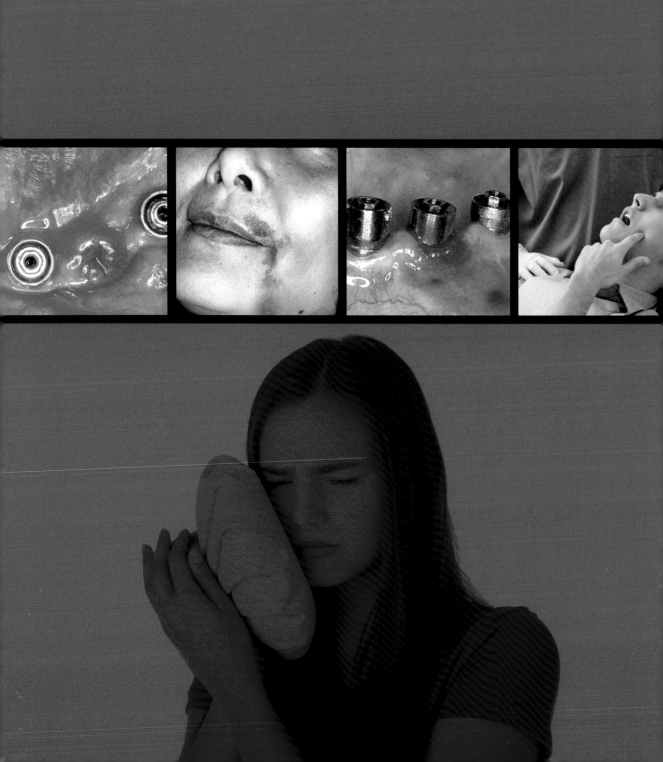

Soft Tissue Surgery Complications and Failures: Prevention and Treatment

13

Periodontal soft tissue surgeries may sometimes yield unintended results, leading to complications. Even minor complications during and after these surgeries can have significant adverse effects on the treatment outcome. The dental team should take all precautions to prevent complications and to manage them efficiently when they occur.[1,2]

Postoperative pain, swelling, and bleeding are the most common complications following soft tissue procedures. Most of the complications involve the local operative site. Systemic involvement is quite rare in postoperative periodontal complications. The clinician should exercise all precautions in preventing a complication. Factors like proper preoperative assessment and treatment planning (including a detailed diagnostic work up and appropriate patient selection) are very important in increasing the predictability of the procedure and preventing complications. For dental implants in particular, especially when a multidisciplinary approach is taken, "[s]uccessful implant treatment is the result of careful planning and integration of various areas of dentistry, not just those of prosthodontics and surgery."[3]

Preoperative Assessment

Proper patient selection is very important in prevention of complications both during and after the surgery. A detailed assessment of the patient, including a careful assessment of the patient's overall present condition, previous medical history, and personal history is necessary.

As Petranker, Nikoyan, and Ogle point out, "A thorough preoperative evaluation to identify correctable medical abnormalities and understand the residual risk is mandatory for all patients undergoing any surgical procedure, including oral surgery. Routine preoperative evaluation will vary among patients, depending on age and general health."[4] Such thorough assessment helps identify the patients who are at risk of developing surgical and medical complications. The medical history should also include details such as drug therapy, including anti-coagulants and steroids in the past and present, any procedures involving local and general anesthesia, and drug allergies. In addition, a detailed examination and diagnostics should be performed to decide the most suitable treatment for the presenting condition. The treatment of choice should also be based on the clinician's own expertise and skill.[5]

Soft Tissue Damage from Mechanical Trauma

Oral tissue needs to be handled gently during the surgery to avoid mechanical trauma. Most tissues eventually heal due to the rich blood supply; however, traumatized tissues are more prone to complications and delayed healing. Trauma to the soft tissue may also affect the final esthetic outcome of the procedure. Tension-free flap retraction and tension-free tissue closure are very important to ensure optimal results.

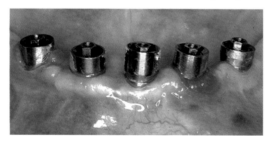 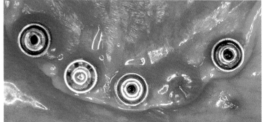

Complications and Management

The most common complications of periodontal surgery are bleeding, pain, and swelling. The incidences of these complications vary from one procedure to another. Gingival grafts are associated with higher incidences of postoperative pain and bleeding when compared to connective tissue grafts.[6,7] The acellular dermal matrix graft is associated with fewer incidences of swelling and bleeding. It is also observed that duration of surgical procedures highly correlates with post-surgical pain and swelling. As Fu, Su, and Wang conclude, "Although these new materials do not surpass the gold standard (subepithelial connective graft), they do provide improved patient satisfaction and esthetics, are available in abundance, and lead to reduced postoperative discomfort and surgical time."[2] In addition, smokers are more prone to develop procedure-related complications than nonsmokers.[8,9]

Bleeding and Hematoma Formation

Bleeding is the most common complication associated with soft tissue surgeries. Bleeding can occur during and after surgery. When bleeding occurs during surgery, the surgeon should localize the source of the bleeding. The bleeding should be controlled by using compressive sutures proximal to the bleeding point. A few drops of lidocaine with 1/100,000 epinephrine can also be infiltrated around the bleeding point to attain hemostasis. After the clinician completes the surgery, the site should be compressed with wet gauze for 5 to 10 minutes. If these methods do not work, the bleeding vessel should be cauterized. When bleeding occurs after surgery, the surgeon should instruct the patient to apply a wet tea bag to the site and compress the area for 10-15 minutes. The patient should come back to office if the bleeding does not stop.

In cases of bleeding from donor sites, in addition to the above-mentioned methods, hemostatic agents like oxidized regenerated cellulose and absorbable gelatin sponge can also be used.[10] Kim and colleagues concluded in their 2010 study that bismuth subgallate can be used as a topical hemostatic for palatal wounds as an option for soft tissue graft surgery.[11] Hematomas are collections of blood within soft tissues from hemorrhage leading to tissue enlargement. Mishandling of tissues may traumatize the capillary bed, leading to extravasation of the blood into surrounding connective tissue. Additionally, poor circulation in the operative site further contributes to the pooling of blood and the release of prostaglandins, resulting in inflammation. This result can be prevented by gentle handling of the soft tissues and timely management of intraoperative and postoperative bleeding.

The selection of flap design and method of closure are also important factors in preventing bleeding and hematoma formation. For example, Hunt reported that in procedures requiring flap reflection, intact elevation of the periosteum using a full thickness flap design, including the blood vessels within the flap, reduces the surgical trauma more commonly experienced with periosteal perforation.[12] Osbon found that postoperative application of direct pressure on the surgical site helps to ensure close adaptation of the mucoperiosteum to bone, thereby reducing the incidence of hematoma formation.[13]

Postoperative Pain

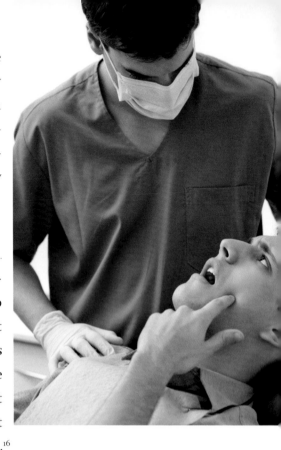

Pain is the most common postoperative complication. Soft tissue surgeries are more likely to cause pain than hard tissue surgeries. The most important factor affecting postoperative pain is the duration of the surgery. Lengthy surgeries are associated with more pain.[14,15] Studies show that the first 24 hours following surgery are the most painful, and thereafter the pain gradually subsides.[16]

To manage pain and associated inflammation, Jackson and colleagues have suggested administration of 800 mg Ibuprofen one hour prior to surgery, followed by 800 mg Ibuprofen twice daily.[17] Dionne and colleagues confirmed the analgesic and anti-inflammatory benefits of this treatment, recommending the safety range of 1600 mg per day to 3200 mg per day.[18] However, a more recent study showed that administration of ibuprofen before surgery can increase bleeding during and after surgery.[19]

Wessel and Tatakis reported greater incidence of donor site pain with gingival grafts when compared to connective tissue graft donor sites.[20] De Rossi notes that "[n]ew scientific evidence is constantly providing insight into the cause and pathophysiology of orofacial pain including temporomandibular disorders, cranial neuralgias, persistent idiopathic facial pains, headache, and dental pain."[21] In their 2007 study, Canakçi and Canakçi conclude, "Discomfort during periodontal treatments, postoperative pain and postoperative dentin hypersensitivity were associated significantly with age, type of therapy and higher scores on Corah's Dental Anxiety Scale." Regarding the clinical implications of pain management, they further note that "[p]eriodontal treatment is experienced as painful by substantial numbers of patients. Therefore, the [clinician] should count the pain responses during and after treatment and estimate the degree of pain according to sex, age and therapy type."[22] In their 2009 study concerning dentinal hypersensitivity, Porto, Andrade, and Montes noted that "[t]he availability of a wide variety of treatment could be an indicator that there is still no effective desensitizing agent to completely resolve the patient's discomfort, or that it is difficult to treat, irrespective of the available treatment options. Even with the large number of published studies, it has not been possible to reach a consensus about the product that represents the gold standard in the treatment of dentinal hypersensitivity."[23]

Swelling and Bruising

Swelling and bruising are common after surgery, and both gradually decrease over time. The patients should be instructed to use a cold compress over the operative area for the first 24 hours. Thereafter, the patient should apply warm pads. Anti-inflammatory drugs are also prescribed to decrease swelling. In their 2007 study entitled "Pain and swelling after periapical surgery related to oral hygiene and smoking," Garcia and colleagues attempted "[t]o evaluate pain and swelling during the first week after periapical surgery and its relation to patient age, gender, oral hygiene, and smoking," concluding that "[p]eriapical surgery caused little pain and moderate swelling during the first 2 days after the intervention; these findings were more distinct in patients with poor oral hygiene before surgery and in smokers."[24]

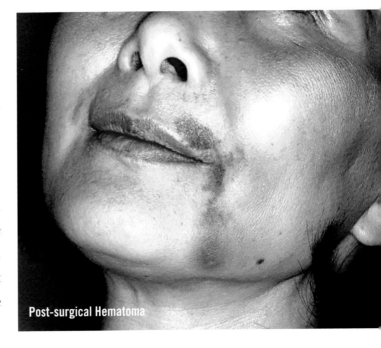

Post-surgical Hematoma

A follow up study by Garcia and others concluded,

> In the majority of published studies there was no statistically significant relationship between age and sex and the postoperative symptoms. However, greater pain and swelling is observed in patients with poor oral hygiene before surgery, and higher pain in patients who smoke, and in those with pain before surgery. Surgery of anterior teeth and molars is associated with greater pain.[25]

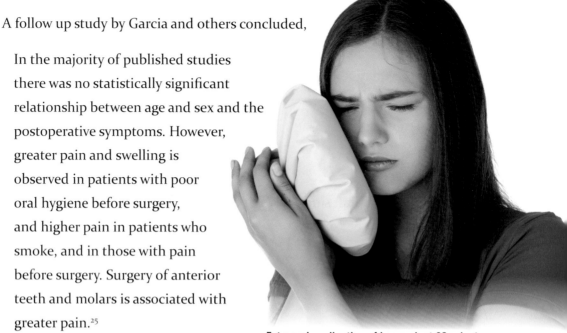

Extraoral application of ice pack at 20-minute intervals for the first 24 hours after surgery helps decrease post-operative hematoma and swelling.

Infection

Infection is the most serious complication after soft tissue/periodontal surgery because it directly affects the healing and outcome of the procedure. Generally, fever, body ache, and swollen lymph nodes indicate infection. Many clinicians recommend preoperative antibiotic prophylaxis and/or postoperative antibiotics to reduce risk of infection. Maestre and others have suggested that periodontal procedures induce bacteremia and may present risk of developing systemic complication; therefore, antibiotic prophylaxis is crucial for its prevention.[26] However, another school of thought advocates that unless there is a medical indication, there is no justification for using prophylactic antibiotic therapy to prevent infection following periodontal surgery.[27] Similarly, Tseng has suggested that the routine prescription of antibiotics is not necessary following periodontal surgery that follows aseptic surgical techniques.[28]

An acellular dermal matrix graft can also become infected, which would require its removal. Greenwell and colleagues have suggested antibiotic prophylaxis to prevent such an outcome.[29] In their 2009 study, Podgórska, Jakimiak, Röhm-Rodowald, and

Chojecka note, "There is still need for improvement in disinfection and sterilization in dental practice, especially including: monitoring and documentation of sterilization process, proper use of disinfectants according to manufactures [sic] instructions, [and] frequent disinfection of surfaces which come in contact with patients. Dental staff should take part in advanced training courses about disinfection and sterilization."[30]

Graft Mobility

Mobility of the graft in graft surgeries can occur if the graft was placed on the recipient site without adequate bed preparation. Pedicle grafts may also undergo necrosis or loosening due to poor patient selection or use of faulty techniques. Patients with thin biotype are not candidates for pedicle flap.

Recession at the Donor Site

Donor site recession is the most common complication in pedicle grafting procedures. This outcome occurs in patients with thin biotype who lack adequate gingiva and underlying bone for raising a pedicle graft. The procedure in these cases may compromise the esthetics of the adjacent area from which the flap was raised. Gingival recession can also occur after crown lengthening procedures.[31]

Membrane Exposure

In guided tissue regeneration procedures, exposure of the barrier membrane may affect the overall outcome of the surgery. Management of such cases differs based on the types of barrier membranes used and whether infection is present. Resorbable membranes without any signs of infection can be managed only by chlorhexidine gluconate mouth rinse since the membrane would disintegrate on its own. A patient treated with a non-resorbable membrane not having signs of infection should be started on antibiotics in addition to the chlorhexidine gluconate mouth rinse. The membrane should then be removed after six weeks. A non-resorbable membrane which is infected will need immediate removal.[32]

Conclusion

The dental clinician must view periodontal soft tissue surgeries with a keen eye for avoiding complications. Treatment outcomes for such surgeries should avoid even minor complications since such complications can have adverse functional and esthetic results. The most common complications after soft tissue procedures include postoperative pain, swelling, and bleeding involving the local operative site. Rarely are such complications systemic in nature. Proper preoperative assessment and treatment planning are essential elements for avoiding complications, especially for soft tissue surgeries involving dental implants.

References

1. Griffin TJ, Cheung WS, Zavras AI, Damoulis PD. Postoperative complications following gingival augmentation procedures. J Periodontol. 2006 Dec;77(12):2070-9.

2. Fu JH, Su CY, Wang HL. Esthetic soft tissue management for teeth and implants. J Evid Based Dent Pract. 2012 Sep;12(3 Suppl):129-42. Review.

3. Ng DY, Wong AY, Liston PN. Multidisciplinary approach to implants: a review. N Z Dent J. 2012 Dec;108(4):123-8. Review.

4. Petranker S, Nikoyan L, Ogle OE. Preoperative evaluation of the surgical patient. Dent Clin North Am. 2012 Jan;56(1):163-81, ix. Review.

5. Miloro M, DeLeeuw KA, Ruggiero SL. Patient assessment. J Oral Maxillofac Surg. 2012 Nov;70(11 Suppl 3):e12-30. Review.

6. de Castro LA, Vêncio EF, Mendonça EF. Epithelial inclusion cyst after free gingival graft: a case report. Int J Periodontics Restorative Dent. 2007 Oct;27(5):465-9.

7. Corsair AJ, Iacono VJ, Moss SS. Exostosis following a subepithelial connective tissue graft. J Int Acad Periodontol. 2001 Apr; 3(2):38-41.

8. Martins AG, Andia DC, Sallum AW, Sallum EA, Casati MZ, Nociti Júnior FH. Smoking may affect root coverage outcome: a prospective clinical study in humans. J Periodontol. 2004 Apr;75(4):586-91.

9. Andia DC, Martins AG, Casati MZ, Sallum EA, Nociti FH. Root coverage outcome may be affected by heavy smoking: a 2-year follow-up study. J Periodontol. 2008 Apr;79(4):647-53.

10. Rossmann JA, Rees TD. A comparative evaluation of hemostatic agents in the management of soft tissue graft donor site bleeding. J Periodontol. 1999 Nov; 70(11):1369-75.

11. Kim SH, Tramontina VA, Papalexiou V, Luczyszyn SM. Bismuth subgallate as a topical hemostatic agent at palatal donor sites. Quintessence Int. 2010 Sep;41(8):645-9.

12. Hunt PR. Safety aspects of mandibular lingual surgery. J Periodontol. 1976 Apr;47(4):224-9.

13. Osbon DB. Postoperative complications following dentoalveolar surgery. Dent Clin North Am. 1973 Jul;17(3):483-504.

14. Strahan JD, Glenwright HD. Pain experience in periodontal surgery. J Periodontal Res. 1967;2(2):163-6.

15. Glenwright HD, Strahan JD. Observations on pain following periodontal surgery. Dent Pract Dent Rec. 1968 May;18(9):323-4.

16. Seymour RA. Efficacy of paracetamol in reducing post-operative pain after periodontal surgery. J Clin Periodontol. 1983 May; 10(3):311-6.

17. Jackson DL, Moore PA, Hargreaves KM. Preoperative nonsteroidal anti-inflammatory medication for the prevention of postoperative dental pain. J Am Dent Assoc. 1989 Nov;119(5):641-7. Review.

18. Dionne RA, Campbell RA, Cooper SA, Hall DL, Buckingham B. Suppression of postoperative pain by preoperative administration of ibuprofen in comparison to placebo, acetaminophen, and acetaminophen plus codeine. J Clin Pharmacol. 1983 Jan;23(1):37-43.

19. Braganza A, Bissada N, Hatch C, Ficara A. The effect of non-steroidal anti-inflammatory drugs on bleeding during periodontal surgery. J Periodontol. 2005 Jul;76(7):1154-60.

20. Wessel JR, Tatakis DN. Patient outcomes following subepithelial connective tissue graft and free gingival graft procedures. J Periodontol. 2008 Mar;79(3):425-30.

21. De Rossi SS. Orofacial pain: a primer. Dent Clin North Am. 2013 Jul;57(3):383-92. Epub 2013 Jun 4.

22. Canakçi CF, Canakçi V. Pain experienced by patients undergoing different periodontal therapies. J Am Dent Assoc. 2007 Dec;138(12):1563-73.

23. Porto IC, Andrade AK, Montes MA. Diagnosis and treatment of dentinal hypersensitivity. J Oral Sci. 2009 Sep;51(3):323-32. Review.

24. García B, Penarrocha M, Martí E, Gay-Escodad C, von Arx T. Pain and swelling after periapical surgery related to oral hygiene and smoking. Oral Surg Oral Med Oral Pathol Oral Radiol Endod. 2007 Aug;104(2):271-6. Epub 2007 May 15.

25. García B, Larrazabal C, Peñarrocha M, Peñarrocha M. Pain and swelling in periapical surgery. A literature update. Med Oral Patol Oral Cir Bucal. 2008 Nov 1;13(11):E726-9. Review.

26. Maestre JR, Mateo M, Sánchez P. [Bacteremia after periodontal procedures]. Rev Esp Quimioter. 2008 Sep;21(3):153-6. Spanish.

27. Pack PD, Haber J. The incidence of clinical infection after periodontal surgery. A retrospective study. J Periodontol. 1983 Jul;54(7):441-3.

28. Tseng CC, Huang CC, Tseng WH. Incidence of clinical infection after periodontal surgery: a prospective study. J Formos Med Assoc. 1993 Feb;92(2):152-6.

29. Greenwell H, Vance G, Munninger B, Johnston H. Superficial-layer split-thickness flap for maximal flap release and coronal positioning: a surgical technique. Int J Periodontics Restorative Dent. 2004 Dec;24(6):521-7.

30. Podgórska M, Jakimiak B, Röhm-Rodowald E, Chojecka A. [Assessment of disinfection and sterilization processes in dental practice as an important factors in prevention of infections]. Przegl Epidemiol. 2009;63(4):545-50. Polish.

31. Brägger U, Lauchenauer D, Lang NP. Surgical lengthening of the clinical crown. J Clin Periodontol. 1992 Jan;19(1):58-63.

32. Nowzari H, Matian F, Slots J. Periodontal pathogens on polytetrafluoroethylene membrane for guided tissue regeneration inhibit healing. J Clin Periodontol. 1995 Jun;22(6):469-74.

About the Authors

ARUN K. GARG, D.M.D.

DR. ARUN K. GARG earned engineering and dental degrees from the University of Florida and then completed his residency training at the University of Miami/Jackson Memorial Hospital. For nearly twenty years, he served as a full-time Professor of Surgery in the Division of Oral and Maxillofacial Surgery and as Director of Residency Training at the University of Miami School of Medicine. He was frequently recognized as "faculty member of the year" by his residents. Dr. Garg is the founder of Implant Seminars, the nation's largest provider of dental implant continuing education. He is considered the world's preeminent authority on bone biology, bone harvesting, and bone grafting for dental implant surgery. He has written and published seven books (*Practical Implant Dentistry: A Thorough Understanding; Bone Biology, Harvesting & Grafting for Dental Implants: Rationale and Clinical Applications; Dental and Craniofacial Applications of Platelet-Rich Plasma; Dental Implantology Dictionary; Implant Dentistry: A Practical Approach; Practical Soft Tissue Management for Natural Teeth and Dental Implants;* and *Implant Excellence*), which have been translated into multiple languages and distributed worldwide.

Dr. Garg is the president of the International Dental Implant Association. He is a highly respected clinician and educator who has been a featured speaker at dozens of state, national and international dental association conventions and meetings, including the American Academy of Periodontology and the American College of Oral and Maxillofacial Surgeons. ▾

Dr. Garg has received numerous awards, including outstanding educator and an award for best article published by the *Implant Dentistry Journal.* In addition, Dr. Garg has developed and refined many surgical techniques and devices that simplify surgery while making it more predictable. He is a consultant and advisor to numerous companies. His private practices are located in Miami and Ft. Lauderdale, Florida.

LILIBETH AYANGCO, DMD, MS

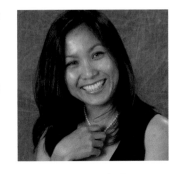

LILIBETH AYANGCO, DMD, MS received a DMD degree from the University of the East, Manila, Philippines in 1991 and maintained a private practice until she moved to Florida in 1995. She completed a two-year General Practice Residency at the University of Miami-Jackson Memorial Hospital in 1997 and went on to the University of Florida to receive a certificate from a two-year Foreign Trained Dental program in 1999. She has been a clinical instructor since 1996 on workshops teaching advanced bone and soft tissue grafting and implant surgeries both nationally and internationally.

Dr. Ayangco is a Diplomate of the American Board of Periodontology. She received a certificate in Periodontics from The Mayo Clinic in Rochester, Minnesota and a Masters in Science from The Mayo Medical School in 2002. While at Mayo, she published several articles in peer reviewed journals on the surgical management of implant complications, oral pathology and the oral and dermal complications of certain antibiotics. She authored a chapter on *Erythema Multiforme* in a multiple volume dermatology book in collaboration with consultants at The Mayo Clinic. In 2002, after completing her time at Mayo, Dr. Ayangco established a private practice limited to periodontics, oral pathology and implant surgery in Deerfield Beach, Florida. She strongly believes and advocates the Mayo philosophies of "the welfare of the patient always come first" and "evidence-based, data-driven care".